Essentials of Bayley™-4 Assessment

Essentials of Psychological Assessment Series

Series Editors, Alan S. Kaufman and Nadeen L. Kaufman

Essentials of 16PF® Assessment
by Heather E. P. Cattell and James M. Schuerger

Essentials of Adaptive Behavior Assessment of Neurodevelopmental Disorders
by Celine A. Saulnier and Cheryl Klaiman

Essentials of ADHD Assessment for Children and Adolescents
by Elizabeth P. Sparrow and Drew Erhardt

Essentials of Assessing, Preventing, and Overcoming Reading Difficulties
by David A. Kilpatrick

Essentials of Assessment Report Writing, Second Edition
by W. Joel Schneider, Elizabeth O. Lichtenberger, Nancy Mather, Nadeen L. Kaufman, and Alan S. Kaufman

Essentials of Assessment with Brief Intelligence Tests
by Susan R. Homack and Cecil R. Reynolds

Essentials of Autism Spectrum Disorders Evaluation and Assessment
by Celine A. Saulnier and Pamela E. Ventola

Essentials of Bayley Scales of Infant Development-II Assessment
by Maureen M. Black and Kathleen Matula

Essentials of Behavioral Assessment
by Michael C. Ramsay, Cecil R. Reynolds, and R. W. Kamphaus

Essentials of Career Interest Assessment
by Jeffrey P. Prince and Lisa J. Heiser

Essentials of CAS2 Assessment
by Jack A. Naglieri and Tulio M. Otero

Essentials of Child and Adolescent Psychopathology, Second Edition
by Linda Wilmshurst

Essentials of Cognitive Assessment with KAIT and Other Kaufman Measures
by Elizabeth O. Lichtenberger, Debra Y. Broadbooks, and Alan S. Kaufman

Essentials of Conners Behavior Assessments™
by Elizabeth P. Sparrow

Essentials of Creativity Assessment
by James C. Kaufman, Jonathan A. Plucker, and John Baer

Essentials of Cross-Battery Assessment, Third Edition
by Dawn P. Flanagan, Samuel O. Ortiz, and Vincent C. Alfonso

Essentials of DAS-II® Assessment
by Ron Dumont, John O. Willis, and Colin D. Elliott

Essentials of Dyslexia Assessment and Intervention
by Nancy Mather and Barbara J. Wendling

Essentials of Evidence-Based Academic Interventions
by Barbara J. Wendling and Nancy Mather

Essentials of Executive Functions Assessment
by George McCloskey and Lisa A. Perkins

Essentials of Forensic Psychological Assessment, Second Edition
by Marc J. Ackerman

Essentials of Gifted Assessment
by Steven I. Pfeiffer

Essentials of IDEA for Assessment Professionals
by Guy McBride, Ron Dumont, and John O. Willis

Essentials of Individual Achievement Assessment
by Douglas K. Smith

Essentials of Intellectual Disability Assessment and Identification
by Alan W. Brue and Linda Wilmshurst

Essentials of KABC-II Assessment
by Alan S. Kaufman, Elizabeth O. Lichtenberger, Elaine Fletcher-Janzen, and Nadeen L. Kaufman *Essentials of KTEA™- 3 and WIAT®-III Assessment*
by Kristina C. Breaux and Elizabeth O. Lichtenberger

Essentials of MCMI®- IV Assessment
by Seth D. Grossman and Blaise Amendolace

Essentials of Millon™ Inventories Assessment, Third Edition
by Stephen Strack

Essentials of MMPI-A™ Assessment
by Robert P. Archer and Radhika Krishnamurthy

Essentials of MMPI-2® Assessment, Second Edition
by David S. Nichols

Essentials of Myers-Briggs Type Indicator® Assessment, Second Edition
by Naomi L. Quenk

Essentials of NEPSY®- II Assessment
by Sally L. Kemp and Marit Korkman

Essentials of Neuropsychological Assessment, Second Edition
by Nancy Hebben and William Milberg

Essentials of Nonverbal Assessment
by Steve McCallum, Bruce Bracken, and John Wasserman

Essentials of PAI® Assessment
by Leslie C. Morey

Essentials of Planning, Selecting, and Tailoring Interventions for Unique Learners
by Jennifer T. Mascolo, Vincent C. Alfonso, and Dawn P. Flanagan

Essentials of Processing Assessment, Second Edition
by Milton J. Dehn

Essentials of Psychological Assessment Supervision
by A. Jordan Wright

Essentials of Psychological Tele-Assessment
by A. Jordan Wright and Susan Engi Raiford

Essentials of Psychological Testing, Second Edition
by Susana Urbina

Essentials of Response to Intervention
by Amanda M. VanDerHeyden and Matthew K. Burns

Essentials of Rorschach® Assessment
by Tara Rose, Michael P. Maloney, and Nancy
Kaser-Boyd

*Essentials of Rorschach Assessment: Comprehensive System
and R-PAS*
by Jessica R. Gurley

*Essentials of School Neuropsychological Assessment,
Third Edition*
by Daniel C. Miller and Denise E. Maricle

*Essentials of Social Emotional Learning (SEL): The
Complete Guide for School Practitioners*
by Donna Black

*Essentials of Specific Learning Disability Identification,
Second Edition*
by Vincent C. Alfonso and Dawn P. Flanagan
*Essentials of Stanford-Binet Intelligence Scales (SB5)
Assessment*
by Gale H. Roid and R. Andrew Barram

*Essentials of TAT and Other Storytelling Assessments,
Second Edition*
by Hedwig Teglasi

Essentials of Temperament Assessment
by Diana Joyce

*Essentials of Trauma-Informed Assessment and Interventions
in School and Community Settings*
by Kirby L. Wycoff and Bettina Franzese

Essentials of WAIS®- IV Assessment, Second Edition
by Elizabeth O. Lichtenberger and Alan S. Kaufman

Essentials of WISC®- IV Assessment, Second Edition
by Dawn P. Flanagan and Alan S. Kaufman

Essentials of WISC-V® Assessment
by Dawn P. Flanagan and Vincent C. Alfonso

Essentials of WISC-V Integrated Assessment
by Susan Engi Raiford

Essentials of WJIV® Cognitive Abilities Assessment
by Fredrick A. Schrank, Scott L. Decker, and John M.
Garruto

Essentials of WJIV® Tests of Achievement
by Nancy Mather and Barbara J. Wendling

Essentials of WMS®- IV Assessment
by Lisa Whipple Drozdick, James A. Holdnack, and
Robin C. Hilsabeck

Essentials of WNV™ Assessment
by Kimberly A. Brunnert, Jack A. Naglieri, and Steven T.
Hardy-Braz

Essentials of Working Memory Assessment and Intervention
by Milton J. Dehn

Essentials of WPPSI™- IV Assessment
by Susan Engi Raiford and Diane L. Coalson

Essentials of WRAML2 and TOMAL-2 Assessment
by Wayne Adams and Cecil R. Reynolds

Essentials of Treatment Planning, Second Edition
by Mark E. Maruish

Essentials of the California Verbal Learning Test
by Thomas J. Farrer and Lisa Whipple Drozdick

Essentials

of Bayley™-4 Assessment

Vincent C. Alfonso

Joseph R. Engler

Andrea D. Turner

WILEY

Registered Office(s)
John Wiley & Sons, Inc., 111 River Street, Hoboken, NJ 07030, USA

Editorial Office
111 River Street, Hoboken, NJ 07030, USA
For details of our global editorial offices, customer services, and more information about Wiley products visit us at www.wiley.com.
Wiley also publishes its books in a variety of electronic formats and by print-on-demand. Some content that appears in standard print versions of this book may not be available in other formats.

Library of Congress Cataloging-in-Publication Data
Names: Alfonso, Vincent C., author.
Title: Essentials of Bayley™–4 assessment /
  Vincent C. Alfonso, Joseph R. Engler, Andrea D. Turner.
Description: First Edition. | Hoboken, NJ : John Wiley & Sons, [2021] |
  Series: Essentials of Psychological Assessment | Includes
  bibliographical references and index. | Contents: Foreword: Bayley-4
  Assessment at a Glance -- Overview of the Bayley-4 -- How to Administer
  the Bayley-4 -- How to Score the Bayley-4 -- How to Interpret the
  Bayley-4 -- Clinical Applications of the Bayley-4 -- Technical Review
  Including the Strengths and Limitations of Bayley-4 -- Illustrative Case
  Examples and Reports -- The Bayley-4 on Q-global.
Identifiers: LCCN 2021021052 (print) | LCCN 2021021053 (ebook) | ISBN
  9781119696018 (Paperback) | ISBN 9781119696056 (PDF) | ISBN
  9781119696032 (ePub)
Subjects: LCSH: Bayley Scales of Infant Development. | Child
  development--Testing. | Infants--Development--Testing.
Classification: LCC RJ51.D48 A44 2021 (print) | LCC RJ51.D48 (ebook) |
  DDC 153.9/4000832--dc23
LC record available at https://lccn.loc.gov/2021021052
LC ebook record available at https://lccn.loc.gov/2021021053
Cover image: © Greg Kuchik/Getty Images
Cover design by Wiley

Set in 10/12.5 Adobe Garamond Pro by Integra Software Services Pvt. Ltd, Pondicherry, India

SKY10031968_121421

The year 2020 was one that most of us would like to forget for myriad reasons. Indeed, it was filled with great suffering, tragedy, and loss. In recognition and memory of all those who became sick, unemployed, lonely, desperate, and of course those who perished as a result of COVID-19, I dedicate this volume. And to all infants and toddlers that they may grow, develop, and thrive in a safe, healthy, and prosperous world.

V.C.A.

First and foremost, I dedicate this book to the most influential person on my development. On January 23, 2020 I lost my mom (Debbie Engler) unexpectedly. I miss her every day, but feel her unconditional love and support in all aspects of my life. To my beautiful wife, Calissa, you brighten the world with your smile and I am happy to share this journey with you. To my beautiful children, Siena and Elin, you bring me more joy than you will ever know. I am blessed to call you mine, and am excited to see what your future holds.

J.R.E.

To my love, Israel, who is my champion in all things and has always understood me at a deeper level than anyone else; I am in awe of the miracle evolution of our family and I'm privileged to share in this life with you. To Dr. Robin Gurwitch and Vicki Cook, I will forever be grateful to you for introducing me to assessment of young children and setting me on a career path filled with laughter and toys. And to all of the children and families I've worked with over the years, you have been the true teachers on my professional journey.

A.D.T.

CONTENTS

	Acknowledgments	xi
	About the Authors	xiii
	Series Preface	xv
	Foreword	xvii
	Essentials of Bayley™–4 Assessment	xix
One	Overview of the Bayley–4	1
Two	How to Administer the Bayley–4	91
Three	How to Score the Bayley–4	135
Four	How to Interpret the Bayley–4	163
Five	Clinical Applications of the Bayley–4	185
Six	Technical Review Including the Strengths and Limitations of the Bayley–4	205

Seven   Illustrative Case Examples and Reports   225

Eight   The Bayley–4 on Q-global by Andre C. Lane (reproduced by permission of Elsevier)   247

Index   269

ACKNOWLEDGMENTS

We would like to acknowledge several people for their special and extraordinary contributions in producing this volume. The first group of people to whom we want to express our deepest appreciation comes from John Wiley & Sons (Wiley) and the first person is Darren Lalonde, Acquisitions Editor, for supporting us through the contract and publication process. The second person from Wiley is Monica Rogers, Associate Managing Editor, for working with us through the publication process, especially when COVID-19 became a challenge none of us expected, impacting life the way it did and continuing to do so. We would also like to recognize Christina Weyrauch and Janane Sivakumar for their assistance in completing the publication process.

The second group comes from Pearson. Several individuals gave of their time to engage in ZOOM conversations and discuss the various Bayley Scales with us. Drs. Larry Weiss, James Gyurke, and Glen Aylward (all of whom were associated with either the Psychological Corporation or Pearson) provided rich and useful information about Dr. Bayley, her venerable scales, and the process of publishing the Bayley–4. A special word of thanks to Dr. Aylward who communicated with us via email for months, answering our questions, providing support, and sharing his sense of humor. Of course we recognize him for his kind and beautiful words in the foreword of this volume. Two additional individuals from Pearson also deserve our gratitude. Andre C. Lane, Associate Research Director at Pearson, who graciously allowed us to reproduce his chapter *The Bayley–4 on Q-global* from another book and Shelley Hughes, Product Manager for Bayley–4 at Pearson, who provided us with many materials, waived licensing fees, and supported our work to the end.

The third group is not a group, but a person. Yet, given all that she did to assist us in producing this volume she very well could be considered a group! Miriam Carlson, a graduate student assistant, worked tirelessly in providing us with articles, reference lists, feedback on drafts, and levity that was needed throughout the process. In addition, Miriam never frowned, said no to a request, or complained. We offer her our deepest gratitude and hope she is proud of her contributions.

ABOUT THE AUTHORS

Vincent C. Alfonso, Joseph R. Engler, and Andrea D. Turner
Gonzaga University and Pearson Assessments

Vincent C. Alfonso, PhD is Professor in and Former Dean of the School of Education at Gonzaga University in Spokane, Washington. He also served as Interim Dean of the Ferkauf Graduate School of Psychology at Yeshiva University and Professor in and Associate Dean of the Graduate School of Education, Fordham University, New York City. He is past president of Division 16 (School Psychology) of the American Psychological Association (APA), and Fellow of Divisions 16, 5, and 43 of the APA. He is also Fellow of the Association for Psychological Science. In February 2014, he received the *Outstanding Contributions to Training* award from the Trainers of School Psychologists and in August 2017, he received the *Jack Bardon Distinguished Service Award* from Division 16 of the APA. Dr. Alfonso has published scholarly work for nearly 30 years and most recently he co-edited *Healthy Development in Young Children: Evidence-based Interventions for Early Education* published by the APA and *Psychoeducational Assessment of Preschool Children* (5th Edition) published by Routledge.

Joseph R. Engler, PhD is an Associate Professor and Director of School Psychology at Gonzaga University in Spokane, Washington. Dr. Engler received his BA at Minot State University and his PhD at The University of South Dakota. Dr. Engler began his professional career in Tooele, Utah and remains active in the profession through advocacy and leadership at the local, state, and national level. His research interests include preschool assessment, critical evaluation of psychometric tests, and parental involvement.

Andrea D. Turner, PhD is a licensed psychologist and research director for Pearson Clinical Assessment and is a primary developer of cognitive and ability tests including the various Wechsler Scales. She has more than 20 years of experience in university clinic, community mental health, private practice, and private agency settings providing individual and group therapy and assessment services for children and young adults. Dr. Turner has provided early childhood mental health consultation to Part C and Head Start programs and consultation regarding children with developmental disabilities for public schools. She served as president and board member of the Kansas Association for Infant and Early Childhood Mental Health. Her specialties include infant and early childhood mental health consultation and assessment, and treatment and assessment of developmental disabilities.

I n the *Essentials of Psychological Assessment Series*, we have attempted to provide the reader with books that deliver key practical information in the most efficient and accessible manner. Many books in the series feature specific *topics* in a variety of domains, such as specific learning disabilities, social-emotional learning, neuropsychological assessment, cross-battery assessment, and adaptive behavior assessment. Books in this category are intended for professionals in psychology and education – and for graduate students in these or related disciplines – who are involved with any aspect of assessment and intervention. A second category of books in this series, such as *Essentials of Bayley^{TM}–4 Assessment*, is devoted to a single test. Books in this category offer a concise yet thorough review of an instrument, with special attention given to the details of administration, scoring, interpretation, application, and tips for best practice of the test. Students can rely on series books in both categories for a clear and concise overview of the important assessment tools and key topics in which they must become proficient to practice skillfully, efficiently, and ethically in their chosen fields. Experienced clinicians will feel equally at home with this series in their efforts to remain on the cutting edge of new research and new instruments (including revisions of old ones) in an array of diverse fields.

Wherever feasible, visual cues highlighting key points are utilized alongside systematic, step-by-step guidelines. Chapters are focused and succinct. Topics are organized for an easy understanding of the essential material related to a particular test or topic. Theory and research are continually woven into the fabric of each book, but always to enhance the practical application of the material, rather than to sidetrack or overwhelm readers. With this series, we aim to challenge and assist readers interested in psychological assessment to aspire to the highest level of competency by arming them with the tools they need for knowledgeable, informed practice. We have long been advocates of "intelligent" testing – the notion that numbers are meaningless unless they are brought to life by the clinical acumen and expertise of examiners. Assessment must be used to make a difference in the child's life or the adult's life or why bother to test? All books in the series – whether devoted to specific tests or general topics – are consistent with this credo. We want this series to help our readers, novice and veteran alike, to benefit from the intelligent assessment approaches of the authors of each book.

In *Essentials of Bayley™–4 Assessment*, the authors accomplish the complex task of providing all the needed information to administer, score, and interpret this venerable developmental assessment. However, they surpass the usual content of test-based volumes in the *Essentials of Psychological Assessment Series* by providing readers with a clearly written history of early childhood assessment, including an appendix listing more than 200 instruments used with young children; a tribute to the underappreciated Dr. Nancy Bayley; and a thorough review of all four editions of the Bayley Scales.

In addition, the esteemed authors provide a systematic review and evaluation of quantitative and qualitative characteristics, not only for those practitioners who are interested in these "data," but for those practitioners who know how to integrate test performance interpretation based on the strengths and limitations of the instrument. Infant, toddler, and preschooler case studies from different perspectives offer graduate students, novice practitioners, and seasoned practitioners examples of how to write reports that convey important clinical and technical information in a reader-friendly manner. The last chapter in the volume addresses digital administration of the Bayley–4 via Q-interactive and is very helpful for practitioners who select this administration method.

All told, *Essentials of Bayley™–4 Assessment* delivers a thorough, clinical, and technical treatise on the gold standard in the field of early childhood assessment in a highly readable manner that should be received well by practitioners from multiple disciplines across the experience continuum. Kudos to Alfonso, Engler, and Turner for gifting us this volume!

Alan S. Kaufman, PhD, and
Nadeen L. Kaufman, EdD
Series Editors
Yale Child Study Center
Yale University School of Medicine

I am honored that the authors of this volume of the *Essentials* series invited me to write the Foreword. I must admit that when I participated in a conference call with Dr. Vinny Alfonso, lead author of this volume, and Dr. Larry Weiss, retired Vice President of Global Research & Development for Pearson Assessment, I was a bit leery as to how this book differed from my recently published *Bayley 4: Clinical Use and Interpretation*. Dr. Alfonso quickly allayed my concerns and also convinced me that he is a persuasive guy. Seriously though, it became apparent that our views on infant and toddler assessment are very similar and the two books would complement each other or could stand alone.

Essentials of Bayley™–4 Assessment is timely and addresses basic considerations and principles applicable to testing young children. The history of the various editions of the Bayley is presented as background. This is followed by administration, scoring, and interpretation of the test. The technical review (Chapter 6) has a unique rating checklist of desirable qualities that should be contained in tests and the authors apply this to the Bayley–4. The authors present a fair, balanced review of the Bayley–4, indicating strengths and limitations. They do not simply endorse a new test just because it is new; rather, the authors methodically evaluate if the test has improved normative data, contains new constructs, if increased ease in administration and decreased time for administration are evident, and if special clinical groups were included. The overall format is well planned and economical. I view *Essentials* as a sophisticated "how to" reference.

This book provides a sound foundation for the Bayley–4 and addresses current advances in infant assessment. It would be appropriate as a graduate-level testing resource and could then be supplemented by the applied *Clinical Use and Interpretation* volume to round out a course in infant and toddler testing. This would fill a gap in the testing curriculum and enable evaluators to become more effective and accurate in their assessments.

The authors accurately emphasize that testing infants and young children is significantly different than evaluating older children, adolescents, or adults. A thread that runs throughout the volume is that there is a major difference between a technician and a practitioner, and this difference is particularly critical when working with young children. As the authors infer, practitioners must read the situation and behaviors of the child *and* the caregiver, possess keen observational skills in order to detect subtle behaviors, know when to take a break due to flagging motivation in the child, and not to jump to conclusions without considering all available data. These skills are developed by experience—not by simply reading a manual. Nonetheless, combining *Essentials* with hands-on experience is an excellent way to enhance this skill set.

Glen P. Aylward, PhD, ABPP
Author, *Bayley–4*

ESSENTIALS OF BAYLEY™–4 ASSESSMENT BAYLEY–4 AT A GLANCE

Vincent C. Alfonso, Joseph R. Engler, and Andrea D. Turner
Gonzaga University and Pearson Assessments

One of our mentors, Dr. Bruce Bracken, wrote recently that it is common for scholars to write or edit books but relatively uncommon for such scholarly works to reach multiple editions (Alfonso et al., 2020, p. xxii). That sentiment is as applicable to assessments as it is to books, and so it is with the *Bayley Scales of Infant and Toddler Development–Fourth Edition* (Bayley–4; Bayley & Aylward, 2019). In several ways, the Bayley–4 maintains the standard-setting qualities of previous editions yet is clearly an improvement and arguably the best option for the assessment of infants and toddlers. For example, the Bayley–4 has five comprehensive scales, excellent quantitative and qualitative characteristics, helpful clinical and caregiver-friendly materials, and multiple uses. Similar to other volumes in the *Essentials* assessment series, we provide an overview of the Bayley–4, include detailed chapters on administration and scoring, provide interpretive guidelines, discuss clinical applications, evaluate the quantitative and qualitative characteristics, and offer three case examples and reports. In addition, we include a chapter on Q-global® written by Andre C. Lane (2020) and published in Glen Aylward's (2020) volume *Bayley–4 Clinical Use and Interpretation.*

In the overview chapter we try to educate practitioners, especially new practitioners, on the history and importance of early childhood assessment. We note that early childhood assessment is relatively new in the United States and requires additional education, training, and experience (e.g., Alfonso et al., 2020). Indeed, it was only in 2000 that the American Psychological Association (APA) recognized the Society of Pediatric Psychology as Division 54 of the APA.[1] Although the National Association of School Psychologists has a pediatric school psychology special interest group, there are less than 250 members in that group out of nearly 25,000 total members.[2] In a recent survey by Lockwood and Farmer (2019), assessment of infants and toddlers received limited emphasis or was not covered by 49 and 16%, respectively, of cognitive assessment course instructors in the United States. Finally, Schmitt and colleagues (Schmitt et al., 2020) investigated pediatric topic publication trends in five school psychology journals from 2002 to 2019 and stated, "Current trends highlight a need for future empirical articles related to assessment and, particularly, school-based intervention for non-ADHD pediatric health conditions" (p. 171). The overview chapter also includes a tribute to Dr. Nancy Bayley, a summary of the Bayley Scales from 1969 to 2019, a summary of our review of the quantitative and qualitative characteristics of the Bayley–4, and an appendix with basic information on nearly 200 infant and toddler assessments and screeners.

Chapters 2 and 3 address in detail, administration and scoring of the Bayley–4. For example, Chapter 2 highlights preparation for developmental assessment, administration formats, administration times, test materials, item types, administration guidelines, assessment of children with disabilities, managing unusual or problem behaviors during testing, and tele-practice. Chapter 3 highlights available scores, general scoring procedures, scoring responses on the paper record form, social-emotional and adaptive behavior scoring and analysis, and scoring responses on Q-global. These chapters have multiple call-outs such as *don't forgets*, *cautions*, and *rapid references*, along with many figures and tables to assist the practitioner in learning the ins and outs of Bayley–4 administration and scoring.

We explain in Chapter 4 that early childhood assessment and evaluation are markedly different from school-aged or adolescent assessment and evaluation. As such, we provide an integrated model of Bayley–4 assessment performance, a discussion of theoretical underpinnings and assessment content, and multiple examples of interpretive statements especially regarding quantitative interpretation of the young child's performance. Chapter 5 addresses clinical applications of the Bayley–4 as a screening tool, as a progress monitoring tool, and as a diagnostic tool. We review and discuss in detail the Bayley–4 Screening Test and Autism Spectrum Disorder Checklist, utility of growth scale values, and utility of the Bayley–4 in diagnosing children with various developmental disabilities and disorders.

In Chapter 6 we explain our evaluation of the quantitative and qualitative characteristics of the Bayley–4 that is summarized in Chapter 1. This is an extensive evaluation emphasizing the strengths and limitations of the Bayley–4 in the context of developmental assessment and should be read by all practitioners, as the information therein provides clear assistance in understanding and interpreting the young child's performance. Chapter 7 includes three unique case examples and reports highlighting the utility of the Bayley–4 in assessing infants and toddlers. Chapter 8 covers Q-global in detail for practitioners who prefer digital administration of the Bayley–4.

Some final comments pertain to how honored and appreciative we are to be afforded the opportunity to write this volume. The three of us are in awe of the clinical brilliance of Drs. Bayley and Aylward and are incredibly passionate about early childhood assessment and intervention. We are particularly grateful to Drs. Susie E. Raiford and Alan S. Kaufman, two of our most respected mentors and colleagues, for having confidence in us to prepare this treatise on the gold standard in infant and toddler assessment. We hope that practitioners enjoy reading the *Essentials of Bayley™–4 Assessment* as much as we enjoyed preparing it for them.

NOTES

1 Retrieved from https://societyofpediatricpsychology.org/significant_milestones.
2 Retrieved from http://communities.nasponline.org/communities/
community-home?CommunityKey=11e5aab8-5218-4269-a634-3cdabcf15a6f.

REFERENCES

Alfonso, V. C., Bracken, B. A., & Nagle, R. J. (Eds.). (2020). *Psychoeducational assessment of preschool children* (5th ed.). https://doi.org/10.4324/9780429054099

Alfonso, V. C., Ruby, S., Wissel, A. M., & Davari, J. (2020). School psychologists in early childhood settings. In F. C. Worrell, T. L. Hughes, & D. D. Dixson (Eds.), *The Cambridge handbook of applied school psychology* (pp. 579–597). Cambridge University Press.

Aylward, G. P. (2020). *Bayley 4 clinical use and interpretation*. Academic Press.

Bayley, N., & Aylward, G. P. (2019). *Bayley Scales of Infant and Toddler Development* (4th ed.). Pearson.

Lane, A. C. (2020). The Bayley–4 on Q-global. In G. P. Aylward, *Bayley 4 clinical use and interpretation* (pp. 113–135). Elsevier.

Lockwood, A. B., & Farmer, R. L. (2019). The cognitive assessment course: Two decades later. *Psychology in the Schools, 57*(2), 265–283. https://doi.org/10.1002/pits.2229

Schmitt, A., Wodrich, D. L., & Lorenzi-Quigley, L. (2020). Current status of pediatric topics in five school psychology journals: Publication trends between 2002-2019. *School Psychology, 35*(3), 171–178. https://dx.doi.org/10.1037/spq0000346

One

OVERVIEW OF THE BAYLEY–4

Vincent C. Alfonso, Joseph R. Engler, and Andrea D. Turner
Gonzaga University and Pearson Assessments

ASSESSING INFANT AND TODDLER DEVELOPMENT

It is important to have a context from which to understand the main focus of this volume, which, of course, is the *Bayley Scales of Infant and Toddler Development–Fourth Edition* (Bayley–4; Bayley & Aylward, 2019a). As such, we begin with a brief history of infant and toddler development by using several sources of information including Black and Matula (2000), Goodman (1990), and Kelley and Surbeck (2007). Additionally, Sattler (2018a) has a very useful summary of the historical milestones on intellectual and developmental assessment. The interested reader is encouraged to review these sources as well as others to gain a thorough understanding of the history of infant and toddler assessment. Next, we highlight the importance of infant and toddler assessment, state the purposes of early childhood assessment, and list the typical developmental domains assessed. Finally, we provide a summary list of nearly 200 infant and toddler assessments as a resource; that summary list is found in the Appendix.

BRIEF HISTORY OF INFANT AND TODDLER ASSESSMENT[1]

Many practitioners, especially those new to the assessment of infants and toddlers, may believe practitioners have been assessing young children for a long time, yet the history of early childhood assessment including infants, toddlers, and preschoolers is only about 200 years old (Kelley & Surbeck, 2007). Influences on early childhood assessment include dozens of individuals, but a few in

---

particular are worth mentioning. For example, the precursor to early childhood assessment and developmental psychology may be attributed to the naturalistic observations of Johann Heinrich Pestalozzi in the 18th century and G. Stanley Hall, who is regarded as the father of developmental psychology and was the first president of the American Psychological Association (APA; Black & Matula, 2000). In the latter part of the 19th century, Sir Francis Galton, a cousin to Charles Darwin, constructed "tests of memory, motor, and sensory functions to differentiate between high and low achievers" (Kelley & Surbeck, 2007, p. 4). As a result, Galton became known as the father of mental testing. Perhaps the most famous early contributor to the practice of early childhood assessment, especially the assessment of mental ability or intelligence, was Alfred Binet, who, with Theodore Simon, created the Binet–Simon Scale for measuring the intelligence of school children (Binet & Simon, 1905). It was translated into English from French by Henry Goddard (a student of G. Stanley Hall) who also believed in the importance of early diagnosis, systematic testing, and special placements for school-aged students who evidenced learning difficulties (Kelley & Surbeck, 2007). The Binet–Simon Scale became the template for most, if not all, intelligence and cognitive batteries to the present day.

The child study movement of the early 1900s, that saw a proliferation of funding, studies, and assessments of school-aged children focusing on intelligence, memory, perception, emotion, personality, and motivation, influenced early childhood psychologists to begin paying attention to infants, toddlers, and preschoolers (Black & Matula, 2000; Kelley & Surbeck, 2007). Among the most famous and influential early childhood (infant) psychologists was Arnold Gesell who was also a pediatrician by training. Some refer to him as the grandfather of infant assessment (Goodman, 1990). According to Black and Matula (2000), Gesell, who was greatly influenced by Charles Darwin, "compiled a schedule of tasks for *infants ages* 4, 6, 9, 12, and 18 months of age and 2, 3, 4, and 5 years of age" (Gesell, 1925a, p. 3). These Developmental Schedules continued to be used for decades in various circles, especially by medical personnel (Goodman, 1990), and influenced the first infant intelligence tests such as the *Cattell Infant Intelligence Scale* (Cattell, 1940), *Griffiths Mental Development Scale for Testing Babies from Birth to Two Years* (Griffiths, 1951), and *Bayley Scales of Infant Development* (Bayley, 1969). Black and Matula (2000) state, "These early assessments were designed to catalog an infant's level of development at various ages and to establish normative data" (p. 4). They did not predict future functioning as many thought they would, which called into question their utility (Goodman, 1990).

In the past 50 years, several factors or variables influenced the importance of early childhood assessment as well as the proliferation of measures or instruments to accomplish the task of reliable and valid assessment. Perhaps the most salient are the following, as cited in Black and Matula (2000): (a) many premature and medically challenged infants are surviving, which typically necessitates assessment, (b) infant assessments are needed to determine if infants are developing at an expected rate or evidencing a developmental

> **DON'T FORGET 1.1**
>
> Two of the most influential educational initiatives in the history of the United States were Head Start and early intervention via public laws.

delay, (c) whether young children meet the criteria for early intervention services, and (d) whether early intervention is effective in improving their rate of development. The next section of this chapter addresses directly the importance of infant and toddler assessment. We end this section with a brief discussion of two of the most influential educational initiatives in the history of the United States; namely, Head Start and early intervention (via public laws).

Head Start and its younger sibling, Early Head Start, are arguably the most successful early childhood programs of the past 57 and 25 years, respectively, especially when services they provide continue for years after children begin the programs. In short, these programs are designed to provide high-quality early childhood education and care that have a positive impact on young children's, especially those from low-income households, cognitive, language, and social development (Raines et al., 2020). The roots of Head Start[2] date back to 1965 when President Lyndon B. Johnson declared war on poverty. Drs. Robert Cooke and Edward Zigler were instrumental in launching Head Start, which established performance standards in 1975 and began offering full-day and full-year services in 1998. In 2007, the Improving Head Start for the School Readiness Act was reauthorized. Several provisions were included in this act to ensure the delivery of high-quality early childhood education and care. In the years that followed, additional changes were made to Head Start and Early Head Start including the Designation Renewal System and revised Program Performance Standards. The Head Start Program serves more than 1 million children and families each year and since 1965 has served more than 36 million children and families. It is administered by the Administration for Children and Families in the Department of Health and Human Services.

A series of public laws passed between 1975 and 2004 guaranteed all students (and children) a free and appropriate public education, or FAPE, and an Individualized Education Program, or IEP, for students identified with a disability that would address their specific educational needs (McBride et al., 2011). The first of these public laws, called The Education of the Handicapped Act (EHA), was passed in 1975, went into effect in 1977, and ensured special education and related services to students with disabilities between the ages of 5 and 21 years. Effectively, the EHA, or Public Law [PL] 94-142, addressed the needs of school-aged students. In 1986 PL 99-457, the Education of the Handicapped Act Amendments, was passed and required states to provide FAPE to children with disabilities aged 3–5 years. PL 99-457 also included Part H, the Handicapped Infants and Toddlers Program, which "established incentives for states to develop services for infants and toddlers with special needs" (Nagle et al., 2020, p. 3). Typically, services could be rendered when an infant assessment revealed developmental delays in cognitive, physical, communication, social or emotional, and/or adaptive development (Black & Matula, 2000). Infants diagnosed with a physical or mental condition who had a high probability to result in developmental delay were also included.

In 1990, PL 101-476 renamed the original act (i.e., the EHA) the Individuals with Disabilities Education Act or IDEA and in 1991 PL 102-119 (Individuals with Disabilities Education Act Amendments of 1991) included developmental delay as a classification option for children with disabilities between the ages of 3 and 5 years. The IDEA was reauthorized in 1997 (PL 105-17) and extended the classification of developmental delay to the age of 9 years. Then in 2004, the IDEA was renamed the Individuals with Disabilities Education Improvement Act (IDEIA; PL 108-446). Part B, Section 619 of the IDEIA incorporated previous amendments ensuring free and appropriate special education services for preschoolers aged 3 to 5 years and continued to allow states to use developmental delay as a classification category for individuals up to the age of 9 years (Alfonso et al., in press; Raines et al., 2020). Again, areas of developmental delay included cognitive, communication, social or emotional, and/or adaptive domains. Part C of IDEIA continued to encourage states to develop and provide comprehensive early intervention services for infants and toddlers with disabilities and their families, emphasized providing care in the home and in community settings, and mandated family involvement in the evaluation and intervention process (Alfonso et al., in press; Raines et al., 2020).

According to Part C of IDEIA, young children (i.e., birth to age 3 years) eligible for early intervention services are those who demonstrate delays via a reliable and valid assessment, already have diagnosed conditions associated with future developmental delay, or are "at-risk" for a disability (Roberts & Kennert, 2018). IDEIA also emphasized transitional services from Part C to Part B programs for preschoolers as well as a focus on scientifically-based academic and behavioral interventions, including early literacy interventions. Part C also required family directed assessment and an Individualized Family Service Plan, or IFSP, to address resources, priorities, and concerns of the family as well as the identification of supports and services necessary to assist the family in meeting the developmental needs of their child (Alfonso et al., in press; Lipkin & Okamoto, 2015).

Finally, in 2015, PL 107-110 or the No Child Left Behind Act, which has its roots in the original Elementary and Secondary Education Act of 1965 (PL 89-10), was replaced by the Every Student Succeeds Act (ESSA; PL 114-95). The ESSA expanded access to high-quality early learning with the particular goal of reaching children who are disadvantaged or have high needs. It also includes funding to improve the coordination, quality, and access to early childhood education.

IMPORTANCE OF ASSESSING INFANT AND TODDLER DEVELOPMENT

There are few guarantees in life and perhaps even fewer facts or truths in psychology or education. However, in the past few decades research and myriad studies have demonstrated the benefits of early childhood education and early intervention (Alfonso, Ruby et al., 2020; Guralnick, 1997; Hughes & Quinn, 2020; Raines et al., 2020; Ramey & Ramey, 1998, 2004; Ramey et al., 2014; Redden et al., 2001, 1999; Schweinhart & Weikart, 1998; Trohanis, 2008; Zigler & Muenchow, 1992). Moreover, this fact or truth seems to resonate with individuals from all walks of life, political parties, and professions who engage in working with young children (e.g., Division for Early Childhood [DEC] of the Council for Exceptional Children, Division for Early Childhood, 2014; National Association for the Education of Young Children [NAEYC], National Association of School Psychologists, 2015; Public Laws 99–457, 101–476, 105–117, and 108–446).

The importance of early childhood education and early intervention, together with major advances in pre-natal care, pediatric medicine, neuro-psychology, and neuroimaging, have highlighted the need for reliable and valid assessment of infants and toddlers (e.g., Aylward, 2010, 2020; Brito et al., 2019; Kelley & Surbeck, 2007; McCloskey et al., 2020; Snow & Van Hemel, 2008). Many scholars, researchers, and organizations believe there are several purposes of infant and toddler assessment. For example, Nagle et al. (2020) integrated other sources such as NAEYC, DEC, and individual scholarly works to summarize the major purposes, which they state are the following: (a) screening, (b) diagnosis and eligibility determination, (c) individual program planning and monitoring, and (d) program evaluation.

> **DON'T FORGET 1.2**
>
> The major purposes of infant and toddler assessment include screening, diagnosis and eligibility determination, individual program planning and monitoring, and program evaluation.

Typical domains of development requiring assessment include cognitive abilities and processes, motor skills, speech and language skills, social-emotional behavior, and adaptive behavior (Alfonso et al., 2020; Alfonso, Engler et al., 2020; Bellman et al., 2013; Brassard & Boehm, 2007; NAEYC, 2020; National Research Council, 2008). Additional domains to assess include intrauterine (prenatal and perinatal), physical, parenting and parenting stress, and play. The last domain, play, is particularly important to assess as there is ample evidence regarding the benefits of play on the young child's developing brain, social interactions, and cognitive functioning (e.g., Kelly-Vance & Ryalls, 2020).

Indeed, the Bayley–4, the newest edition of the venerable Bayley Scales, may be used for the following purposes: (a) to identify children with developmental delay, (b) research related to individual program planning and monitoring and program evaluation, and (c) to monitor a child's developmental progress. The first and third purposes are accomplished with the Bayley–4 by assessing the young child's cognitive, language, motor, social-emotional, and adaptive behavior functioning.

> **DON'T FORGET 1.3**
> ....
> The Bayley–4 provides information on a young child's cognitive, language, motor, social-emotional, and adaptive behavior functioning.

INFANT AND TODDLER ASSESSMENTS

Black and Matula (2000) provided a brief overview of 11 infant developmental assessments and cautioned readers that the quality of normative data varied and that readers should review test manuals to determine the psychometric quality of these assessments as well as their suitability (qualitative characteristics) for young children. Here, in the Appendix, we provide a list of nearly 200 infant and toddler developmental assessments including screening instruments dating as far back as 1916 to the present time. It is clear that the sheer number of assessments available for young children has increased greatly, which is perhaps an indirect testament to the importance and growing practice of assessing young children. Indeed, according to Kelley and Surbeck (2007), "More than 200 assessment instruments were constructed and published in the years 1960–1980" (p. 14). These assessments cover a variety of developmental domains including those stated earlier (i.e., cognitive, motor, speech and language, social-emotional behavior, and adaptive behavior).

Space limitations preclude a discussion or even a brief description of these assessments. However, we refer readers to Tables 1.3 to 1.5 later in this chapter and to

Chapter 6 for criteria to evaluate infant and toddler assessments and our evaluation of the Bayley–4, respectively. These tables and text can assist new practitioners who are interested in reviewing and evaluating assessments used with young children. In addition, the readers may find Alfonso et al. (2018), Bracken et al. (1998), Brassard and Boehm (2007), Engler and Alfonso (2020), Floyd et al. (2015), Lidz (2002), Monsma et al. (2020), Mowder et al. (2009), Nuttall et al. (1999), and Terjesen and colleagues (Terjesen et al., 2019), to name a few, as useful scholarly works in their deliberations regarding selection of a psychometrically sound and suitable assessment of young children.

> ## CAUTION 1.1
> ....
> Given the variability regarding the psychometric soundness and suitability of assessments for young children, practitioners should review the quantitative and qualitative characteristics of the assessment before employing it.

HISTORY AND DEVELOPMENT OF THE BAYLEY SCALES

In the sections that follow, we provide a brief biography of Dr. Nancy Bayley as a tribute to her lifelong accomplishments and contributions to developmental psychology, young children and their families, and society as a whole. Next we discuss the first three Bayley Scales (Bayley, 1969, 1993, 2006) to give readers a sense of the timeline of these venerable scales as well as the improvements that took place from edition to edition. This section concludes with information regarding the development of the Bayley–4.

BRIEF BIOGRAPHY OF DR. NANCY BAYLEY[3]

It is not an understatement to claim that Dr. Nancy Bayley was one of the most prolific authors, test developers, and erudite developmental psychologists in the United States and perhaps the world. A review of Rapid Reference 1.1 demonstrates this clearly and, in fact, may underestimate her accomplishments and contributions. She is, without doubt, one of the few premier female test developers in psychology who was recognized in certain circles; however, her name and illustrious career are not known to many professionals who do not work with young children. Here we provide a brief biography of Dr. Bayley, highlighting her accomplishments and contributions, before exploring the history and development of the Bayley Scales, now of course in its 4th edition.

Dr. Bayley was the third of five children and was born on September 28, 1899 to Prudence Cooper and Frederick W. Bayley in Dalles, Oregon. She died from respiratory failure at 95 years of age in Carmel, California in 1994.

≡ *Rapid Reference 1.1*

Summary of Dr. Bayley's Accomplishments and Contributions to Developmental Psychology

- Published *The California First Year Mental Scale* in 1933 and *The California Infant Scale of Motor Development* in 1936
- Published *Mental Growth During the First Three Years* in 1933
- Served as head of child development in the Laboratory of Psychology at the National Institute of Mental Health in Bethesda, Maryland, in 1954
- Served as president of the Society for Research in Child Development from 1961 to 1963
- Received the Distinguished Scientific Contribution Award of the American Psychological Association in 1966. She was the first woman to receive this honor.
- Published the Bayley Scales of Infant Development in 1969
- Received the G. Stanley Hall Award for distinguished contributions to developmental psychology in 1971 and the Gold Medal Award of the American Psychological Association in 1982
- Served as an examiner for the American Board of Professional Examiners in Professional Psychology
- Served as representative from the Division on Developmental Psychology to the Council of Representatives of the American Psychological Association
- Published more than 200 scholarly works
- Referenced 316 times between 1983 and 1991
- Contributed to research in the areas of growth and skeletal maturation, body build and androgyny, issues of measurement and methodology, and motor and mental development

Sources: Lipsitt and Eichorn (1990), Rosenblith (1992)

Although she was often sick as a child, she completed elementary and secondary school. Then she attended the University of Washington where she planned to study to be an English teacher. Rather than becoming an English teacher, she became interested in psychology after taking a course with E. B. Guthrie. Thereafter, she earned her bachelor's and master's degrees in psychology in 1922 and 1924, respectively. She served as a research assistant at the University's Gatzert Foundation for Child Welfare and her master's thesis involved the construction of performance tests for preschool children. Dr. Bayley continued her education at the University of Iowa where she earned her PhD in psychology and became greatly interested in studying young children, especially infants and toddlers. Her dissertation research involved studying children's fears using the galvanic skin response.

Although she taught at the University of Wyoming for two years, her strong interest in young children, motivation to conduct research, and clinical acumen led her to the Institute for Child Welfare, which is now the Institute of Human Development. After an invitation from Harold E. Jones at the University of California, Berkeley in 1928 she quickly engaged in her first and still very impressive research project called the Berkeley Growth Study (Bayley & Schaefer, 1964). She married John R. Reid in 1929 whom she met at Berkeley. It was at the Institute for Human Development that Dr. Bayley worked on and published *The California First Year Mental Scale* and *The California Infant Scale of Motor Development* in 1933 and 1936, respectively, as well as *Mental Growth During the First Three Years* in 1933, a landmark publication in developmental psychology. The aforementioned scales would be the foundation of the *Bayley Scales of Infant Development* (BSID) published in 1969.

Dr. Bayley held professor posts at Berkeley, Stanford University, and the University of Maryland. In addition, she became chief of the section on Child Development at the National Institute of Mental Health (NIMH) in Bethesda, Maryland in 1954 where she worked on the National Collaborative Perinatal Project, a study of 50,000 children from birth to age eight years. The study examined neurological and psychological disorders, including cerebral palsy and intellectual disability. She held the chief position at the NIMH for 10 years while maintaining a research position at Berkeley and was an administrator of the Harold E. Jones Child Study Center of the Institute of Human Development. Dr. Bayley retired from the University of California, Berkeley in 1968 only to complete the BSID that quickly became the gold standard instrument for assessing young children's mental and motor functioning (Sattler, 2018b). In 1966, she was the first woman to receive the Distinguished Scientific Contribution Award from the APA. Two excellent sources of information regarding Dr. Bayley are Lipsitt and Eichorn (1990) and Rosenblith (1992). Finally, we had the opportunity to speak with Drs. James Gyurke, Larry Weiss, and Glen Aylward prior to writing this volume. They were instrumental in revising the Bayley Scales over the years and either interacted with or were very familiar with Dr. Bayley's works. Rapid Reference 1.2 has testimonials from them in a tribute to Dr. Bayley and the Bayley Scales.

≡ Rapid Reference 1.2

Testimonials to Dr. Bayley and The Bayley Scales

- I met with her the night before she passed away and she was very frail. She had extraordinary powers of observation and normal child development. Dr. Bayley was a master clinician as she would sit for hours and observe children. At the time I worked on revising the original Bayley Scales, it was the most important work I did.

  Dr. James Gyurke, Psychological Corporation

(Continued)

- Tests in the field had become very psychometric, but when going back in time, test authors were master practitioners such as Dr. Nancy Bayley. The clinician versus technician continues today and that is why we "begged" Dr. Glen Aylward to author the Bayley–4. We wanted a balance between a clinical tool while maintaining psychometric rigor. We needed the touch of a master clinician and respected scholar.

Dr. Larry Weiss, Pearson Clinical Assessment

- Dr. Bayley could obtain child information as they left the office! She was meticulous in all she did including her 20 pages of notes on selecting the size of the blocks for the test. "I am honored to be the author of the Bayley–4 and to carry on the tradition set forth by Nancy Bayley of providing the reference standard for infant and toddler assessment" (Aylward, 2020, p. xiii).

Dr. Glen Aylward, Author, Bayley–4

Sources: Aylward (2020); Drs. Gyurke, Weiss, and Aylward (personal communications, December 7, 10, 2020)

BAYLEY SCALES (BAYLEY, 1969, 1993, 2006)

Although the original BSID was published in 1969[4], Dr. Bayley already had been involved working with and researching young children for more than 30 years! Effectively, the BSID was "a derivative of several theoretically eclectic scales of infant development and a broad cross-section of infant and child research" (Bayley, 2006, p. 1). According to Black and Matula (2000), the BSID had its foundation in *The California First-Year Mental Scale* (Bayley, 1933), *The California Preschool Mental Scale* (Jaffa, 1934), and *The California Infant Scale of Motor Development* (Bayley, 1936). The resultant BSID sampled the widest array of mental and motor abilities on a developmental assessment at the time, was theoretically eclectic, became the first large-scale standardized, norm-referenced assessment of these abilities, and included the Infant Behavior Record (IBR), which was based upon observations during the assessment and completed after testing (Aylward, 1997; Whatley, 1987).

The BSID assessed infants between the ages of 2 and 30 months of age via items that were "arranged in ordinal sequence of increasing difficulty, representing the maturation of abilities in cognitive and motor development" (Black & Matula, 2000, p. 10). Two standard scores were available on the BSID; namely, the Mental Development Index or MDI from the Mental Scale that assessed sensory-perceptual abilities, object constancy, memory, learning and problem-solving ability, communication and verbal skills, and early abstracting ability and the Psychomotor Development Index or PDI from the Motor Scale that assessed gross and fine motor skills and control of the body (Whatley, 1987). These scores had a mean of 100 and standard deviation of 16. The IBR was used to describe the young child's behavior relative to same-aged children and focused on "the child's social orientation, emotional tone, object orientation, attention span, goal directedness, interest focus, energy, overall evaluation of the child's performance, and representativeness of test performance" (Whatley, 1987, p. 39). Select characteristics of the BSID including, but not limited to, names of scales, items per scale, administration time, strengths, and limitations are found in Table 1.1. Rapid Reference 1.3 lists comprehensive sources on the development of the various Bayley Scales.

As noted in Table 1.1, the BSID norms had become outdated, some test materials were no longer relevant, and research indicated a need for greater reliability and validity of the scales. Thus, the *Bayley Scales of Infant Development–Second Edition* (BSID–II; Bayley, 1993) "was designed to update the normative data, to expand the age range to 1 to 42 months, to incorporate research-based items that demonstrate predictive validity, to update the stimulus materials, to conduct reliability and validity studies, to report data from clinical populations of children, and to ensure a standardized assessment of children's mental and motor performance" (Black & Matula, 2000, p. 10) (see Table 1.1). The BSID–II standardization sample included 1,700 infants between 1 and 42 months of age with one hundred infants (50 females and 50 males) in each of 17 age groups. According to Black and Matula (2000), "The sample was stratified according to the 1988 update of the U.S. census by race/ethnicity, parent education and geographic region. To be included in the normative sample, infants had to be full term (36 to 42 weeks gestation) with birth weight appropriate for gestational age, have no significant medical complications, no disabilities, and not be receiving treatment or intervention for disabilities" (pp. 15–16).

The structure of the BSID–II was very similar to that of the BSID in that it included the Mental and Motor Scales that yielded an MDI and PDI, respectively. However, the standard deviation of these scales changed from 16 to 15, which was the standard deviation of many other developmental and cognitive batteries at the time and currently. The IBR became the Behavior Rating Scale or BRS and "was completely revised to increase the reliability of the Scale and to facilitate scoring and interpretation" (Bayley, 1993, p. 2). It is completed by the practitioner and includes information from the child's caregiver and observations by the practitioner (Anastasi & Urbina, 1997). Factors on the BRS included Attention/Arousal and Motor Quality for infants between 1 and 5 months and Orientation/Engagement, Emotional Regulation, and Motor Quality for infants between 6 and 42 months. Black and Matula (2000) indicated "raw scores are converted to percentiles for each factor within each age group. A total raw score

Table 1.1 Select Characteristics of the Bayley Scales from 1969 to 2019

Characteristic	Bayley Scales of Infant Development (BSID)	Bayley Scales of Infant Development–Second Edition (BSID–II)	Bayley Scales of Infant and Toddler Development–Third Edition (Bayley–III)	Bayley Scales of Infant and Toddler Development–Fourth Edition (Bayley–4)
Author(s) and Year of Publication	Nancy Bayley (1969)	Nancy Bayley (1993)	Nancy Bayley (2006)	Nancy Bayley and Glen P. Aylward (2019a)
Original and Revision Goals	– Developmental assessment versus an intelligence test – Provide an assessment of a child's current developmental status in comparison with normatively based expectations – Flexible administration format into a standardized procedure – Item administration was to be influenced by the child's age, temperament, and success rate – Use of a modified power sequence for item administration	– Update the normative data – Expand age range from 1 to 42 months – Improve content coverage using research-based items with demonstrated predictive validity – Modernize items using materials that facilitate infection control, reduce gender and racial bias, and are attractive to young children – Conduct reliability and validity studies and explore the factor structure of the Mental and Motor Scales and the Behavior Rating Scale – Collect data on clinical populations of children	– Update normative sample and clinical studies – Provide normative data from five scales - Cognitive, Language, Motor, Social-Emotional, and Adaptive – Updated reliability and validity studies – Modernize items such as playful, engaging toys and activities that encourage interaction – Provide greater content coverage – Optional training materials and software-based scoring assistant	– Update normative sample and clinical studies – Simplify administration and reduce administration time – Improve content coverage – Improve clinical utility – Updated reliability and validity studies – Digital delivery, scoring, and reporting via Q-global – Updated content based on research and user feedback

Scales (Number of Items)	Mental (163)
	Motor (81)
	Infant Behavior Record (30)
		Mental (178)
		Motor (111)
		Behavior Rating (30)
			Cognitive (91)
			Language (97)
			  – Receptive Communication (49)
			  – Expressive Communication (48)
			Motor (138)
			  – Fine Motor (66)
			  – Gross Motor (72)
			Social-Emotional Scale (35)
			Adaptive Behavior (241)
			  – Conceptual – Communication (25)
			  – Conceptual – Functional Pre-Academics (23)
			  – Conceptual – Self-Direction (25)
			  – Practical – Community Use (22)
			  – Practical – Home Living (25)
			  – Practical – Health and Safety (24)
			  – Practical – Self-Care (24)
			  – Social – Leisure (22)
			  – Social – Social (24)
			  – Motor (27)
				Cognitive (81)
				Language (79)
				  – Receptive Communication (42)
				  – Expressive Communication (37)
				Motor (104)
				  – Fine Motor (46)
				  – Gross Motor (58)
				Social-Emotional Scale (35)
				Adaptive Behavior (120)
				  – Communication – Receptive (23)
				  – Communication – Expressive (28)
				  – Daily Living Skills – Personal (30)
				  – Socialization – Interpersonal Relationships (20)
				  – Socialization – Play and Leisure (19)

(Continued)

Table 1.1 (Continued)

Characteristic	BSID	BSID–II	Bayley–III	Bayley–4
Administration Time	45–60 minutes depending on child's age	30–60 minutes depending on child's age	50–90 minutes depending on child's age	30–70 minutes depending on child's age
Scores	– Mental Development Index (standard score) – Psychomotor Development Index (standard score)	– Mental Development Index (standard score) – Psychomotor Development Index (standard score) – Percentile ranks – Developmental age equivalents	– Scaled – Standard – Percentile ranks – Confidence intervals – Developmental age equivalents – Growth	– Scaled – Standard – Percentile ranks – Confidence intervals – Developmental age equivalents – Growth scale values – Percent delay
Optional Digital Administration	None	None	None, but included software-based scoring and reporting assistant as well as a PDA administration tool	Yes, including Web-based administration, scoring, and reporting via Q-global
Included Caregiver Report	No	No	Yes	Yes
Theoretical Underpinnings	No particular theory; eclectic	No particular theory; eclectic	No particular theory; eclectic	Integrated neuro-environmental synthesis model of development

Included Children with Clinical Diagnoses in the Normative Sample	No	No	Yes	No, for the most part. However, 34 children with Down syndrome were included in the normative sample to increase the variance at the lower extreme of the normal distribution.
Included Guidance to Adjust for Prematurity	Yes	Yes	Yes	Yes
Included Accommodations and Modifications to Describe Adaptations to Testing Situations	No	Yes	Yes	Yes
Included Developmental Risk Indicators	No	No	Yes	Yes
Encouraged Parent/Caregiver to Be Included in the Testing Process	Qualified Yes	Qualified Yes	Yes	Yes

(Continued)

Table 1.1 (Continued)

Characteristic	BSID	BSID–II	Bayley–III	Bayley–4
Reported Major Strengths	– Sampled the widest array of mental and motor abilities on a developmental assessment at the time – Included the Infant Behavior Record to describe behavior during testing – Evidence for clinical utility and measurement integrity via test–retest reliability, item analyses, and standardization procedures – Videotapes for use in training examiners available through The Psychological Corporation, and training films rented from the Extension Media Center, University of California, Berkeley	– Replacement of the Infant Behavior Rating form with the Behavior Rating Scale – Inclusion of circumscribed item sets – Excellent construct validity – Strong psychometric properties for the MDI and PDI – The use of facets attemps to provide information on Motor, Cognitive, Language, and Social Scales – Record forms included comprehensive information that facilitated learning how to administer items – Most materials were attractive, well-designed, safe, and appealing to young children – Supportive research on the reliability and validity of the BSID–II	– Included two manuals, a more user-friendly stimulus book, bright, colorful, engaging materials, a less heavy test kit, and a separate and complete parent report – Made available a training video – Allowed for software-based scoring and reporting and a PDA administration tool – Item scoring was more straightforward and manageable and allows for more efficient calculation of the raw score – Provided norms at 10-day intervals for very young children and included growth scores – The majority of the stated goals of the revision process were attained – Included five scales and did a commendable job of separating the assessment of cognitive and language functioning – Factorial invariance across cultures – Useful in cognitive and language assessment of individuals with autism spectrum disorder – Several exemplary psychometric properties and research conducted during development and subsequently	– Maintains the scales that are necessary for identifying and diagnosing developmental delays in young children – Inclusion of polytomous scoring – Incorporates caregivers in the assessment process by using Caregiver Questions – Several exemplary psychometric properties especially for the Cognitive, Language, and Motor Scales – Contains attractive materials with manipulatives that are engaging for young children, limited expressive and receptive language requirements on subtests not assessing language, and opportunities to teach tasks

Reported Major Limitations				
	– No circumscribed item sets – Basal and ceiling of 10 consecutive passes and failures, respectively – The factor structure varied across ages, but there is very limited predictability from 3 to 24 months – Limited predictive validity evidence and questionable sensitivity to identifying language delay – Low test–retest reliability, lack of interpretive guidance, and questionable subscores – Norms became outdated, yet no revision until 1993	– Did not provide: separate scores for facets or domains, diagnostic information, or standard scores <50 – Use of item sets became confusing with infants who had atypical development – Did not provide information about the infant's skills in the five areas of development identified by IDEA 97 – Included weak coverage of the social facet—only three items beyond 4-month level – Did not include evidence of predictive validity – Did not provide guidelines for adaptation of the BSID–II for use in other languages or with infants from other cultures	– Included some questionable psychometric properties such as reliability and floors at the youngest ages and norm shifts – No evidence provided to demonstrate predictive validity and accuracy or how intervention provision was improved as a result of administering the Bayley–III – No test-retest reliability data reported for the Social-Emotional Scale – No intercorrelations reported for factors – Some research questioned the Bayley–III's sensitivity to identifying developmental delay and severe disability	– Test authors did not provide a confirmatory factor analysis to support the overall structure of the Bayley–4, but used the Bayley–III confirmatory factor analysis data – More limited to assessing young children at the lower level of functioning – Test–retest characteristics are questionable at best – Replacement materials are very expensive and cannot be purchased individually

(Continued)

Table 1.1 (Continued)

Characteristic	BSID	BSID–II	Bayley–III	Bayley–4
		– Minimal guidelines on using BSID–II to evaluate infants with disabilities – The test kit was very heavy and awkward to carry – There were no training materials or training criteria to ensure the test is administered appropriately – Some research questioned the validity of the mental and motor scales of the BSID-II		

Sources: Albers and Grieve (2007); Alfonso, Engler et al. (this volume); Alfonso et al. (2005); Anastasi and Urbina (1997); Anderson and Burnett (2017); Anderson et al. (2010); Aylward (2013); Aylward and Zhu (2019c); Bayley (1969, 1993, 2006c); Bayley and Alyward (2019c); Black and Matula (2000); Bos (2013); Bradley-Johnson and Johnson (2007); Burns et al. (1992); Campbell et al. (1986); Cook et al. (1989); Crowe et al. (1987); Damarin (1979); Flanagan and Alfonso (1995); Gagnon and Nagle (2000); Gauthier et al. (1999); Glenn et al. (2001); Goldstein et al. (1995); Hack et al. (2005); Hua et al. (2019); Jary et al. (2013); Johnson et al. (2014); Leguire and Fellows (1990); Lennon et al. (2008); Lowe et al. (2012); Manandhar et al. (2016); Matula et al. (1997); McClain et al. (2000); Milne et al. (2012); Moore et al. (2012); Nellis and Gridley (1994); Pendergast et al. (2018); Provost et al. (2004); Rademeyer and Jacklin (2013); Ranjitkar et al. (2018); Robertson et al. (2010); Ross and Lawson (1997); Reuner et al. (2013); Sattler (2018b); Siegel et al. (1995); Snyder and Sheehan (1992); Tobin and Hoff (2007); Torras-Mañá et al. (2014, 2016); Velikos et al. (2015); Venn (2007); Vohr et al. (2012); Washington et al. (1998); Weiss et al. (2010); Whatley (1987).

≡ *Rapid Reference 1.3*

Comprehensive Sources on the Various Bayley Scales

Bayley Scales of Infant Development (Bayley, 1969)

Bayley, N. (1933). *The California First-Year Mental Scale.* Berkeley: University of California Press.

Bayley, N. (1936). *The California Infant Scale of Motor Development.* Berkeley: University of California Press.

Bayley, N. (1969). *The Bayley Scales of Infant Development: Manual.* Psychological Corporation.

Damarin, F. (1979). Bayley Scales of Infant Development. In O. K. Buros (Ed.), *Eighth Mental Measurements Yearbook* (Vol. 1). Gryphon Press.

Rhodes, L., Bayley, N., & Yow, B. C. (1984). *Supplement to the manual for the Bayley Scales of Infant Development.* San Antonio, TX: The Psychological Corporation.

Bayley Scales of Infant Development–Second Edition (Bayley, 1993)

Bayley, N. (1993). *Bayley Scales of Infant Development* (2nd ed.): *Manual.* Psychological Corporation.

Black, M. M., & Matula, K. (2000). *Essentials of Bayley Scales of Infant Development–II assessment.* Hoboken, NJ: John Wiley & Sons.

Nellis, L., & Gridley, B. E. (1994). Review of the Bayley Scales of Infant Development (2nd ed.), *Journal of School Psychology, 32,* 201–209.

Bayley Scales of Infant and Toddler Development–Third Edition (Bayley, 2006a)

Albers, C. A., & Grieve, A. J. (2007). Test Review: Bayley, N. (2006). Bayley Scales of Infant and Toddler Development – (3rd ed.). San Antonio, TX: Harcourt Assessment. *Journal of Psychoeducational Assessment, 25*(2), 180–190. https://doi.org/10.1177/0734282906297199

Bayley, N. (2006a). *Bayley Scales of Infant and Toddler Development* (3rd ed.). Pearson.

Bayley, N. (2006b). *Bayley Scales of Infant Development* (3rd ed.): *Administration manual.* Pearson.

Bayley, N. (2006c). *Bayley Scales of Infant Development* (3rd ed): *Technical manual.* Pearson.

Tobin, R. M., & Hoff, K. E. (2007). [Test review of Bayley Scales of Infant and Toddler Development–Third Edition]. In K. F. Geisinger, R. A. Spies, J. F. Carlson, & B. S. Plake (Eds.), *The seventeenth mental measurements yearbook.* Retrieved from http://marketplace.unl.edu/buros

Venn, J. J. (2007). [Test review of Bayley Scales of Infant and Toddler Development–Third Edition]. In K. F. Geisinger, R. A. Spies, J. F. Carlson, & B. S. Plake (Eds.), *The seventeenth mental measurements yearbook.* Retrieved from http://marketplace.unl.edu/buros

(Continued)

Weiss, L. G., Oakland, T., & Aylward, G. (2010). *Bayley–III clinical use and interpretation*. Academic Press.

Bayley Scales of Infant and Toddler Development–Fourth Edition (Bayley & Aylward, 2019a)

Aylward, G. P. (2020). *Bayley 4 clinical use and interpretation*. Academic Press.
Bayley, N., & Aylward, G. P. (2019b). *Bayley Scales of Infant and Toddler Development* (4th ed.): *Administration manual*. Pearson.
Bayley, N., & Aylward, G. P. (2019c). *Bayley Scales of Infant and Toddler Development* (4th ed.): *Technical manual*. Pearson.
Bayley, N., & Aylward, G. P. (2019d). *Bayley Scales of Infant and Toddler Development* (4th ed): *Screening test manual*. Pearson.

can also be converted to a percentile by age group to provide an overall assessment of the infant's behavior" (pp. 14–15).

The BSID–II Mental and Motor Scales included many items retained from the BSID, new Mental Scale items that measured perceptual development, problem solving, number concepts, language and personal/social development, and new Motor Scale items that measured quality of movement, sensory integration, and perceptual-motor integration (Bayley, 1993; Black & Matula, 2000). In addition, the BSID–II included item sets to address criticisms of the BSID basal and ceiling rules and confusion regarding where to begin the test (see Table 1.1). These item sets, which were arranged according to chronological age, included series of items that increased in difficulty. Although somewhat novel at the time and a welcome change from the BSID, item sets were criticized greatly (see Chapter 5, Black & Matula, 2000 and Table 1.1). Table 1.1 and Rapid Reference 1.3 provide additional information and comprehensive sources on the BSID–II, respectively.

Some 13 years later, the *Bayley Scales of Infant and Toddler Development–Third Edition* (Bayley–III; Bayley, 2006a) was published "to improve the quality and to enhance the utility of the instrument" (Bayley, 2006b, p. 1) and to assess the developmental functioning of infants and toddlers between 1 and 42 months. In many ways, the Bayley–III maintained the gold standard qualities of its predecessor, such as several exemplary psychometric properties, sampling of important young children's abilities and processes, and attractive/appealing materials to engage young children. There were, however, several major changes or revisions to the BSID–II that are noteworthy. For example, the Bayley–III was comprised of five distinct scales including the traditional Mental (renamed Cognitive) and

Motor Scales, a Language Scale, a Social-Emotional Scale, and an Adaptive Behavior Scale. Including five distinct scales was done, in part, to be consistent with federal and professional standards as well as to provide practitioners with a greater or broader understanding of a young child's strengths and weaknesses (Pinon, 2010). The Social-Emotional Scale items were derived from the *Greenspan Social-Emotional Growth Chart: A Screening Questionnaire for Infants and Young Children* (Greenspan, 2004) and the Adaptive Behavior Scale was derived from the Parent/Primary Caregiver Form for ages 0–5 of the *Adaptive Behavior Assessment System* (2nd ed.) or ABAS–II (Harrison & Oakland, 2003). These latter two scales replaced the BRS on the BSID–II. A Behavior Observation Inventory was added to the Bayley–III to assess the child's behavior during testing and how it related to the child's behavior at home. The Bayley–III also included a Caregiver Report that highlighted the child's strengths and weaknesses, provided an explanation of what was measured, and listed suggestions to promote skill development (Pinon, 2010).

The MDI and PDI did not appear on the Bayley–III. In addition, the Language and Motor Scales were divided into subscales, namely, Receptive and Expressive Communication for the Language Scale and Fine and Gross Motor for the Motor Scale. The Cognitive Scale did not have subtests because it "assesses a uniform construct" (Pinon, 2010, p. 19) and items did not require a verbal response. The standardization sample for the Cognitive, Language, and Motor Scales of the Bayley–III included 1,700 children with 100 infants in each of 17 age groups (Bayley, 2006c). Stratification variables included age, sex, parent education level, race/ethnicity, and geographic region. Details regarding the standardization of the Social-Emotional Scale and Adaptive Behavior Scale are found in Bayley (2006c).

The Cognitive, Language, and Motor Scales as well as the domains of the ABAS–II had a mean of 100 and standard deviation of 15. Subscales of the Language and Motor Scales, skill areas of the Social-Emotional Scale, and the ABAS–II had a mean of 10 and standard deviation of 3. The Cognitive Scale also had a scaled score associated with it. Space limitations preclude detailed information regarding item development of the Bayley–III Cognitive, Language, and Motor Scales. However, it is noteworthy that 45 Mental Scale items were deleted, 22 Motor Scale items were deleted, 19 new items were added to the Cognitive Scale, 59 new items were added to the Language Scale, and 22 new items were added to the Motor Scale. Most of the other items on these three scales were either retained as they were on the BSID–II or modified. Item development for the Social-Emotional and Adaptive Behavior Scales is described in Bayley (2006c).

Finally, considerable effort was made to strengthen the psychometric qualities of the instrument, improve its clinical utility, simplify administration procedures, and update item administration and stimulus materials on the Bayley–III (Bayley, 2006b). Table 1.1 and Rapid Reference 1.3 provide additional information and comprehensive sources on the Bayley–III, respectively.

BAYLEY–4 (BAYLEY & AYLWARD, 2019A)

In 2019, NCS Pearson published the Bayley–4 with Nancy Bayley and Glen P. Aylward as the authors of this long-awaited revision of the gold standard in the assessment of young children. Dr. Larry Weiss, former Vice President of Global Research and Development for Pearson Clinical Assessment, proudly tells the story of how he landed Dr. Glen P. Aylward as an author of the Bayley–4 and "the perfect person to assume the legacy of Nancy Bayley" (Aylward, 2020, p. xi). Indeed, Dr. Aylward had been working with children for decades, authored myriad publications, developed the *Bayley Infant Neurodevelopmental Screener* (BINS; Aylward, 1995), and contributed to the development of the BSID–II and Bayley–III (Aylward, 2020). He has been gracious to communicate with us to ensure that we provide a complete, meaningful, helpful, and honest volume on the Bayley–4.

In this section we cover the Bayley–4 revision goals, structure, and description of scales and subtests. In subsequent sections of this chapter we provide a summary of the quantitative and qualitative characteristics of the Bayley–4 as well as some final comments on this recently published instrument. Chapters 2 and 3 provide a thorough coverage of administration and scoring, respectively, while Chapter 4 covers interpretation, Chapter 5 addresses clinical applications, Chapter 6 discusses our evaluation of the Bayley–4, Chapter 7 includes several case examples and reports, and Chapter 8 discusses the Bayley–4 on Q-global.

Revision Goals

There were seven revision goals for the Bayley–4 and they are discussed in Bayley and Aylward (2019c). Rapid Reference 1.4 lists these goals and Chapter 6 provides our evaluation of how well the goals were met. Three of these goals warrant mention here. First, in our communications with Dr. Aylward, he said he was most proud of the polytomous scoring approach because it provides valuable

≣ Rapid Reference 1.4

Revision Goals of the Bayley–4

- Maintain the basic qualities and format of the Bayley–III
- Develop a polytomous scoring approach to differentiate mastery, emergence, and absence of a skill
- Include caregivers in the evaluation process
- Reduce test time and simplify administration
- Improve content coverage of the subtests across ages
- Improve diagnostic sensitivity and clinical utility of the instrument
- Update the normative data

Source: Bayley and Aylward (2019c).

information regarding developmental delay versus deficit (G. P. Aylward, personal communication, December 10, 2020; Aylward, 2020). The second goal worthy of mention here is including caregivers in the evaluation process because not only do caregivers provide valuable information about what the child can and cannot do, but having them involved maintains the caregiver bond during a novel experience with unfamiliar adults.

The third revision goal worthy of mention is improving content coverage of the subtests across the ages. In short, the Bayley Scales have been atheoretical until the Bayley–4. The latest incarnation of the Bayley Scales, especially the Cognitive, Language, and Motor Scales, are based on an integrated neuro-environmental synthesis model of development explicated clearly and thoroughly in Aylward (2020). For example, Aylward discusses canalization, neuronal plasticity, epigenetics, components of the environment, and disruption and insult. We believe it is incumbent for users of the Bayley–4 to read Aylward's discussion as well as other sources to keep up-to-date with advances in neuroanatomy, neuropsychology, and the interplay of genetics and environmental influences.

Structure

The Bayley–4 has the same scales and subtests as the Bayley–III (i.e., Cognitive, Language [comprised of the Receptive and Expressive Communication subtests], Motor [comprised of the Fine and Gross Motor subtests], Social-Emotional, and Adaptive Behavior). The structure of the Bayley–4 is depicted in Figure 1.1. There are many abbreviations used throughout the Bayley–4 materials and thus they are included in Table 1.2.

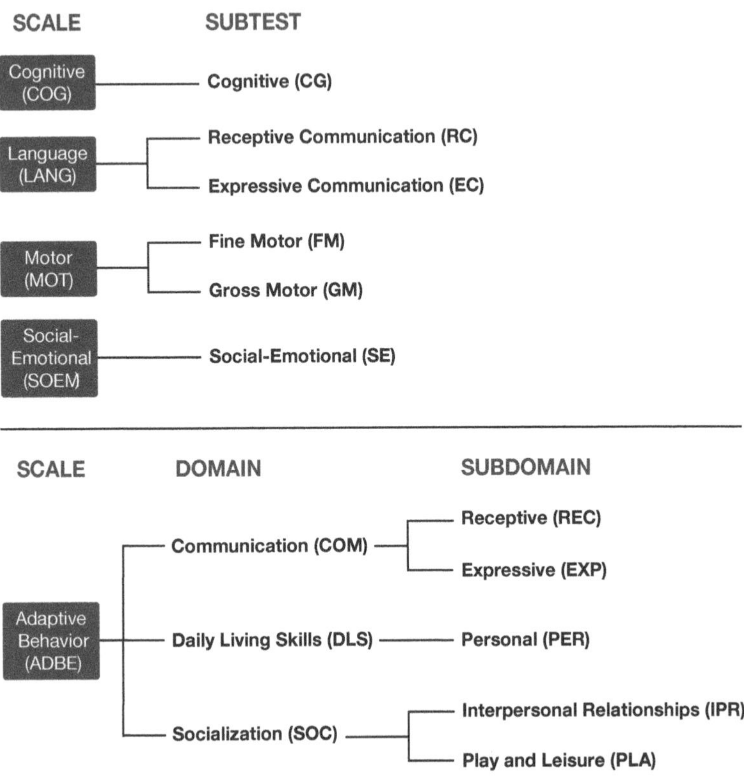

Figure 1.1   Bayley–4 Test Structure.
Note: From Bayley Scales of Infant and Toddler Development, Fourth Edition (Bayley™–4). Copyright © 2019 NCS Pearson, Inc. Reproduced with permission. All rights reserved.

CAUTION 1.2

Be mindful that the Bayley–4 Cognitive, Language, and Motor Scales were standardized together; the Social-Emotional and Adaptive Behavior Scales were standardized separately from the Cognitive, Language, and Motor Scales and from each other.

It is important to note that the Cognitive, Language, and Motor Scales were standardized together (see Table 1.4 and Chapter 6 for details) and are similar to the same-named scales on the Bayley–III. The Social-Emotional Scale was derived from the *Greenspan Social-Emotional Growth Chart: A Screening Questionnaire for Infants and Young Children* (Greenspan, 2004) and remains "unchanged from the Bayley–III" (Bayley & Aylward, 2019c). The Adaptive Behavior Scale is no longer a derivative of the ABAS–II (Harrison & Oakland, 2003) as on the

Table 1.2   Bayley–4 Abbreviations

Scale subtest	Abbreviation	Scale domain subdomain	Abbreviation
Cognitive	COG	**Adaptive Behavior**	ADBE
Cognitive	CG	Communication	COM
Language	LANG	Receptive	REC
Receptive Communication	RC	Expressive	EXP
Expressive Communication	EC	Daily living skills	DLS
Motor	MOT	Personal	PER
Fine motor	FM	Socialization	SOC
Gross motor	GM	Interpersonal Relationships	IPR
Social-Emotional	SOME	Play and Leisure	PLA
Social-Emotional	SE		
Score	**Abbreviation**		
Social-Emotional Sensory processing	SP		

Bayley–III, but is a derivative of the *Vineland Adaptive Behavior Scales* (3rd ed.), *Comprehensive Parent/Caregiver Form* (Vineland-3; Sparrow et al., 2016).

Brief Description of the Scales, Subtests, Domains, Subdomains, Caregiver Report, and Behavior Observation Inventory

According to Bayley and Aylward (2019c), the Cognitive Scale of the Bayley–4 assesses various abilities and processes including "sensorimotor development, exploration and manipulation, object relatedness, concept formation, memory, precursors to executive function, and other cognitive processing aspects" (p. 4) such as counting, cardinality, and play via 81 items. This scale retained most items from the Bayley–III, but deleted 18 from that edition for a variety of reasons, such as items exhibiting high correlations or too complex to administer and included 8 new items to provide greater discrimination at the lower end of functioning (Aylward, 2020). Additional details regarding the developmental nature and increasing complexity of items on the Cognitive Scale are found in Chapter 3 of Aylward (2020).

The Language Scale of the Bayley–4 assesses preverbal behaviors, vocabulary development, vocabulary related to morphological development, understanding of morphological markers, social referencing, and verbal comprehension via the 49-item Receptive Communication subtest. Fifteen items from the Bayley–III were deleted from the Bayley–4 because of difficulty scoring and redundancy among other reasons (Aylward, 2020), and two new items were added. In addition, six Cognitive Scale items were included on the Receptive Communication subtest. The Expressive Communication subtest of the Language Scale assesses vocalizations (e.g., cooing, babbling), gesturing, and speaking via 48 items. Thirteen items from the Bayley–III were deleted from the Bayley–4 and two new items were added. Although the Cognitive and Language Scales are separate on the Bayley–4, as they were on the Bayley–III, Aylward (2020) cautions practitioners that items on each scale are not independent. That is, some Cognitive Scale items involve language (especially receptive language skills) and some Language Scale items tap higher level cognitive functioning (such as learning and applying concepts). Indeed, these two scales are correlated across the ages at .72.

As stated earlier, the Motor Scale is comprised of the Fine and Gross motor subtests. The Fine Motor subtest is comprised of 46 items assessing or involving prehension, visual perception, perceptual-motor integration, motor planning, motor speed, distal maturation, cognition, and size of the infant's hands (Aylward, 2020; Bayley & Aylward, 2019c). Twenty-five items from the Bayley–III Fine Motor subtest were deleted from the Bayley–4 (Bayley & Aylward, 2019c) and five new items were added to the Fine Motor subtest "to lower test floors at specific ages" (Aylward, 2020, p. 53). The Gross Motor subtest is comprised of 58 items assessing or involving head control, trunk control, locomotion, motor planning, static positioning, dynamic movement, and neuro-developmental characteristics (Aylward, 2020; Bayley & Aylward, 2019c). According to Aylward (2020), gross motor functioning and "abilities are affected by the infant's size, weight, coordination, ability to deal with antigravity input, strength, and maturation" (p. 53). Twenty items from the Bayley–III Gross Motor subtest were deleted from the Bayley–4 and seven new items were added (Bayley & Aylward, 2019c) to tap primitive reflexes, protective reflexes, rolling from stomach to back, and jumping off the floor (Aylward, 2020). Although written about the Bayley–III Motor Scale, Case-Smith and Alexander (2010) provide one of the best treatises on fine and gross motor assessment and interpretation of infants and toddlers.

The Social-Emotional Scale of the Bayley–4 is comprised of 35 items that tap self-regulation and interest in the world, communication needs, engaging others and establishing relationships, using emotions in an interactive, purposeful manner, and using emotional signals or gestures to solve problems (Bayley & Aylward, 2019c; Greenspan, 2004). This scale or questionnaire is completed by the primary caregiver and provides information on a child's emotional milestones by age. For example, very young infants (0–5 months) typically begin to self-regulate, show increasing interest in the world, and engage in relationships. Infants between the ages of 6–14 months typically progress from using emotions in an interactive, purposeful manner to using emotional signals or gestures to communicate. Toddlers between the ages of 15 and 42 months progress from using emotional signals or gestures to solve problems, to using symbols or ideas to communicate intentions or feelings, to using symbols or ideas to communicate more than basic needs, and then to creating bridges between emotions and ideas (Greenspan, 2004).

The final scale on the Bayley–4 is the 120 item Adaptive Behavior Scale composed of select items and skill areas of the Vineland-3 and is completed by the primary caregiver. There are three domains on the Adaptive Behavior Scale including Communication, Daily Living Skills, and Socialization. These domains have subdomains including Receptive and Expressive (Communication), Personal (Daily Living Skills), and Interpersonal Relations and Play and Leisure (Socialization). According to Bayley and Aylward (2019c), "Fifty-one items were retained from the Receptive and Expressive subdomains to compose the Communication Domain item set, 30 items from the Personal subdomain compose the Daily Living Skills domain, and 39 items were retained from the Interpersonal Relationships and Play and Leisure subdomains for the Socialization domain" (p. 17). Interested readers are encouraged to see Bayley and Aylward (2019c) for details regarding item selection. The Adaptive Behavior Scale measures what a child does as well as what the child may be able to do (but does not necessarily do with any regularity). Aylward (2020) adds that "adaptive behavior reflects what the child typically does in daily interactions with the environment; if the toddler has the capacity to do a task but does not do it routinely, this behavior is not considered adaptive" (p. 62). Measurement of adaptive behavior (which is modifiable) is important for most young children, but is critical for young children suspected of intellectual disability (American Association on Intellectual and Developmental Disabilities, 2010; American Psychiatric Association, 2013; Brue & Wilmshurst, 2016).

As on the Bayley–III, the Cognitive, Language, Motor, and Social-Emotional Scales as well as the domains of the Adaptive Behavior Scale have a mean of 100 and standard deviation of 15. Subtests of the Language and Motor Scales and subdomains of the Adaptive Behavior Scale have a mean of 10 and standard

> ## DON'T FORGET 1.5
>
> The Cognitive, Language, Motor, and Social-Emotional Scales as well as the domains of the Adaptive Behavior Scale have a mean of 100 and standard deviation of 15. Subtests of the Language and Motor Scales and subdomains of the Adaptive Behavior Scale have a mean of 10 and standard deviation of 3. The Cognitive and Social-Emotional Scales also have scaled scores associated with them.

deviation of 3. The Cognitive and Social-Emotional Scales also have scaled scores associated with them. Interpretation of young children's performance and ratings by primary caregivers on the Bayley–4 is discussed in depth in Chapter 4, but is informed greatly by the quantitative and qualitative characteristics of the test, which are addressed next in summary form and in detail in Chapter 6.

As with the Bayley–III, the Bayley–4 includes a Caregiver Report (CR) and Behavior Observation Inventory (BOI). The CR should be provided routinely to the primary caregiver (Aylward, 2020). This report consists of information regarding the nature of the Bayley–4 and what it measures, a description of the child's test results, and activities for the caregiver to work on with the child. The BOI, found on the last page of the Bayley–4 Record Form, includes 13 items, characteristics, or behaviors on which the practitioner and parent or caregiver rate the child. However, the practitioner rates the child on behavior evidenced during testing and the parent or caregiver rates the child's everyday behavior. All 13 behaviors are rated as not at all typical (never or rarely), somewhat typical (some of the time), or typical (most of the time). An example behavior is *explores objects in the environment*. The practitioner rates the child's exploration during testing and the parent or caregiver rates the child's exploration on a daily basis. The CR and BOI are valuable tools for communicating test performance and behavior, respectively, with parents and other caregivers. Rapid Reference 1.5 provides basic information on the Bayley–4 and its publisher.

QUANTITATIVE CHARACTERISTICS OF THE BAYLEY–4

In this section we provide a summary of our evaluation of the quantitative characteristics of the Bayley–4 using Engler and Alfonso's (2020) criteria for evaluating the adequacy of the quantitative characteristics of early childhood measures. These criteria have been evolving for more than 25 years after Flanagan and Alfonso (1995) expanded upon Bracken's (1987) seminal work on the technical adequacy of preschool instruments. Table 1.3 includes the criteria we used to evaluate the standardization, reliability, floors and ceilings, item gradients, and validity of the Bayley–4.

Table 1.4 provides our evaluation of these quantitative characteristics. As can be seen in this table, many of the quantitative characteristics for the Cognitive,

---

≡ Rapid Reference 1.5

Bayley Scales of Infant and Toddler Development (4th ed.)

Authors: Nancy Bayley, PhD and Glen P. Aylward, PhD, ABPP

Publication Date: September 2019

Scales: Cognitive, Language, Motor, Social-Emotional, and Adaptive Behavior

Age Range: 16 days to 42 months

Administration Time: 30 to 70 minutes (depending on the child's age)

Qualifications of Examiners: Qualification level B. Examiners should have training and experience in administering and interpreting standardized assessments with infants and toddlers. Typically, examiners have training at the masters or doctoral level and supervised experience, in accordance with guidelines from the American Psychological Association, the American Educational Research Association, and the National Council on Measurement in Education. For more information on Pearson's qualification policies please click on the following link: Qualification Policy or https://www.pearsonassessments.com/professional-assessments/ordering/how-toorder/qualifications/qualifications-policy.html.

Publisher: Pearson
Phone: +1 (800) 627-7271
Fax: +1 (800) 232-1223
PearsonAssessments.com

Price: Complete Kit (Digital) $1,050.70; Complete Kit $1,168.50
To learn more please visit PearsonAssessments.com/Bayley4

Language, and Motor Scales of the Bayley–4 were rated good or adequate. For example, we rated the recency of the normative data, item gradients, and validity evidence of these scales as good. In addition, we rated the scale floors and ceilings as adequate. Our ratings of the Social-Emotional Scale varied greatly from good to inadequate, with many quantitative characteristics rated inadequate. For example, recency of normative data and item gradients were rated good whereas all test–retest reliability characteristics were rated inadequate because no data were reported in Greenspan (2004). Finally, our ratings of the quantitative characteristics of the Adaptive Behavior Scale were somewhat lower in general. For example, most characteristics were rated adequate or inadequate including subdomain floors and ceilings and test-retest reliability.

Table 1.3   Criteria for Evaluating the Adequacy of the Quantitative Characteristics of Early Childhood Measures

Quantitative Characteristic	Criteria	Evaluative Classification
Standardization[a]		
Size of normative group and number of participants		
	200 persons per each one-year interval and at least at each age/grade interval, 2000 persons overall	Good
	100 persons per each one-year interval and at least 1,000 persons overall	Adequate
	Neither criterion above is met	Inadequate
Recency of normative data		
	Collected in 2012 or later	Good
	Collected between 2002 and 2011	Adequate
	Collected in 2001 or earlier	Inadequate
Age divisions of norm tables		
	One to two months	Good
	Three to four months	Adequate
	Greater than four months	Inadequate
Match of the demographic characteristics of the normative group to the U.S. population (e.g., gender, race) with SES included	Normative group represents the U.S. population on five or more important demographic variables	Good
	Normative group represents the U.S. population on three or four important demographic variables with SES included	Adequate
	Neither criterion is met	Inadequate

Criterion	Standard	Rating
Reliability		
Internal consistency reliability coefficient (subtests and composites)	Greater than or equal to .90 (≥ .90)	Good
	.80 to .89	Adequate
	Less than .80 (< .80)	Inadequate
Test–retest reliability coefficient (composites only)	Greater than or equal to .90 (≥ .90)	Good
	.80 to .89	Adequate
	Less than .80 (< .80)	Inadequate
Test-retest reliability coefficient (tests only)	Greater than or equal to .80 (≥.80)	Adequate
	Less than .80 (< .80)	Inadequate
Test–retest sample		
Size and representativeness of test–retest sample	Sample contains at least 100 participants and represents the U.S. population on at least five or more demographic variables	Good
	Sample contains at least 50 participants and represents the U.S. population on three or four demographic variables	Adequate
	Neither criterion is met	Inadequate

(Continued)

Table 1.3 (Continued)

Quantitative Characteristic	Criteria	Evaluative Classification
Age range of the test-retest sample	Spans no more than a 1-year interval	Good
	Spans no more than 2 years	Adequate
	Spans more than 2 years or extends beyond the preschool age range (i.e., 2–5 years), regardless of interval size	Inadequate
Length of test–retest interval[b]	Interval ≤ 3 months	Good
	Interval > 3 and ≤ 6 months	Adequate
	Interval > 6 months	Inadequate
Test Floors Subtests[c]	Raw score of 1 is associated with a standard score greater than 2 standard deviations below the normative mean	Adequate
	Raw score of 1 is associated with a standard score less than or equal to 2 standard deviations below the normative mean	Inadequate
Composites[d]	Composite standard score greater than 2 standard deviations below the normative mean	Adequate
	Composite standard score less than or equal to 2 standard deviations below the normative mean	Inadequate

Ceilings		
Subtests[e]	Highest raw score obtained is associate with a standard score greater than 2 standard deviations above the normative mean	Adequate
	Highest raw score is associated with a standard score less than or equal to 2 standard deviations above the normative mean	Inadequate
Composites[f]	Composite standard score greater than 2 standard deviations above the normative mean	Adequate
	Composite standard score less than or equal to 2 standard deviations above the normative mean	Inadequate
Item gradients[g]		
Item gradient violations	No item gradient violations occur *or* all item gradient violations are between 2 and 3 standard deviations below the normative mean *or* the total number of violations is < 5% across the age range of the test	Good
	All item gradient violations occur between 1 and 3 standard deviations below the normative mean *or* the total number of violations is $\geq 5\% \leq 15\%$ across the age range of the test	Adequate
	All or any portion of item gradient violations occur between the mean and 1 standard deviation below the normative mean *or* the total number of violations is > 15% across the age range of the test	Inadequate

(Continued)

Table 1.3 (Continued)

Quantitative Characteristic	Criteria	Evaluative Classification
Validity[h] Presence and quality of specific forms of validity evidences	5 or 6 forms of validity evidence and the authors' evaluation of available data	Good
	4 forms of validity evidence and the authors' evaluation of available data	Adequate
	< 4 forms of validity evidence and the authors' evaluation of available data	Inadequate

[a]An overall rating is obtained as follows: Good = All Goods; Adequate = Goods and Adequates; Inadequate = Goods and/or Adequates, and Inadequates.
[b]The criteria presented here regarding the length of the test–retest interval differ from traditional criteria used with school-age children because young children's abilities change rapidly.
[c]Assuming a scale having a mean of 100 and a standard deviation of 15, a raw score of 1 that is associated with a standard score of ≤ 69 would constitute an adequate floor.
[d]Floors are calculated based on the aggregate of the subtest raw scores that comprise the composites, where one item per subtest is scored correctly.
[e]Assuming a scale having a mean of 100 and a standard deviation of 15, the highest raw score possible is associated with a standard score ≥ 131 would constitute an adequate ceiling.
[f]Ceilings are calculated based on the aggregate of the subtest raw scores that comprise the composites, where all items in a subtest are scored correctly.
[g]An item gradient is defined as the increase in standard score points associated with a one-point increase in raw score values. An item gradient violation occurs when a one-point increase in raw score points is associated with a standard score increase of greater than one third of a standard deviation (Bracken, 1987). [h]The standards for validity in the 2014 publication *Standards for Educational and Psychological Testing* differ from those in the 1999 publication of the same name. Most notably, in the 2014 publication there is one overarching standard or guiding principle for validity with 25 standards subsumed under three clusters. The third cluster, namely, Specific Forms of Validity Evidence, has 15 of the 25 standards subsumed under 6 forms of validity evidence. These six forms of validity evidence are akin to the five sources of validity evidence found in the 1999 publication and in earlier versions of this table. Ratings of "Good" or "Adequate" were made only when the available validity evidence was reviewed positively by the authors and corroborated by other reviews in the extant literature. Note: From Psychoeducational Assessment of Preschool Children (5th ed.). Copyright © 2020 Taylor and Francis Group LLC. Reproduced with permission of The Licensor through PLSclear.
Note: From Psychoeducational Assessment of Preschool Children (5th ed.). Copyright © 2020 Taylor and Francis Group LLC. Reproduced with permission of The Licensor through PLSclear.

Chapter 6 provides a detailed explanation for our ratings, a summary of the Bayley–4 quantitative strengths and limitations, and recommendations for future research. Overall, the Bayley–4 Cognitive, Language, and Motor Scales are psychometrically sound and maintain the strong reputation of previous Bayley Scales. Given the weak psychometric rigor of the Social-Emotional Scale, practitioners should not make any diagnostic decisions based on ratings of young children's social-emotional functioning. The Adaptive Behavior Scale is sound, for the most part, but practitioners should be informed of its limitations when interpreting young children's performance.

> **CAUTION 1.3**
>
> Given the limited psychometric rigor of the Social-Emotional Scale, practitioners should not make any diagnostic decisions based on ratings of young children's social-emotional functioning.

QUALITATIVE CHARACTERISTICS OF THE BAYLEY–4

In some respects the qualitative characteristics of an instrument designed to assess young children's development are more important than the quantitative characteristics because it is incumbent upon the clinician to engage the young child for an extended period of time in order to obtain reliable and valid test performance results. Bracken and Theodore (2020) discusses at length the challenges of assessing and testing young children. For example, they state that young children, by their very nature, are distracted, impulsive, have limited attention spans, and do not communicate well, making it difficult to obtain reliable and valid results. In addition, the inexperienced practitioner may express anxiety, doubt, and lack of confidence in the testing environment that may unduly have a negative effect on the young child's performance. Thus, it is critical that early childhood instruments are attractive, engaging, appealing, and easy to administer to young children. As a result the practitioner, young child, and caregiver can be relatively confident that test results reflect what the young child can and cannot do (i.e., validity).

Engler and Alfonso (2020) described several qualitative characteristics of early childhood measures such as attractiveness of test materials, efficient administration procedures, and suitability of test directions for young children and applied them to preschool cognitive tests. Here, we review those characteristics as they apply to the Bayley–4 and determine whether the Bayley–4 Cognitive, Language, and Motor Scales meet the "criteria." We did not review the Social-Emotional and Adaptive Behavior Scales as the qualitative characteristics were not readily applicable.

Our review and evaluation of the qualitative characteristics indicated that the Bayley–4 Cognitive, Language, and Motor Scales met the "criteria" for 7 of the 10 characteristics (see Table 1.5). For example, these scales incorporate attractive test materials, efficient administration procedures, and limited language demands

Table 1.4 Evaluation of the Quantitative Characteristics of the Bayley–4

Standardization	Bayley–4 Scale				
	Cognitive	Language	Motor	Social-Emotional	Adaptive Behavior
Normative Group	Adequate	Adequate	Adequate	Inadequate	Inadequate
Recency of Normative Data	Good	Good	Good	Good	Good
Age Divisions of Normative Tables	Adequate to Good	Adequate to Good	Adequate to Good	Inadequate to Good	Inadequate to Good
Match of Demographic Data to U.S. Population	Adequate	Adequate	Adequate	Adequate	Adequate
Reliability					
Internal Consistency (Scales and Subtests or Domains and Subdomains)	Good	Inadequate to Good	Adequate to Good	Inadequate to Good	Adequate to Good
Test-Retest Reliability (Scales or Domains)	Adequate	Adequate	Inadequate to Adequate	Inadequate	Inadequate to Adequate
Test–Retest Reliability (Subtests or Subdomains)	Not applicable	Inadequate to Adequate	Inadequate to Adequate	Not applicable	Inadequate to Adequate

Test–Retest Sample					
Size/Representativeness of Sample	Good	Good	Good	Inadequate	Adequate
Age Range of Sample	Inadequate	Inadequate	Inadequate	Inadequate	Inadequate
Length of Interval	Good	Good	Good	Inadequate	Good
Floors					
Subtests or Subdomains	Not applicable	Inadequate to Adequate	Inadequate to Adequate	Not applicable	Inadequate to Adequate
Scales or Domains	Adequate	Adequate	Adequate	Adequate	Adequate
Ceilings					
Subtests or Subdomains	Not applicable	Inadequate to Adequate	Inadequate to Adequate	Not applicable	Inadequate to Adequate
Scales or Domains	Adequate	Adequate	Adequate	Inadequate to Adequate	Adequate
Item Gradient					
Violations	Good	Good	Good	Good	Good
Validity					
Presence and Quality of Evidence	Good	Good	Good	Inadequate	Adequate

Note: Ratings are based upon the criteria set forth in Table 1.2.

Table 1.5 Evaluation of the Qualitative Characteristics of the Bayley–4

Qualitative Characteristic	Bayley–4 Scale				
	Cognitive	Language	Motor	Social-Emotional	Adaptive Behavior
Attractive Test Materials (e.g., manipulatives, colorful test materials)	✓	✓	✓	N/A	N/A
Efficient Administration Procedures (e.g., alternates verbal/nonverbal subtests, begins tasks with stimulating task)	✓	✓	✓	N/A	N/A
Limited Expressive Language Requirement Unless Assessing Language (e.g., majority of tasks require one- or two-word response, and/or gestures)	✓	✓	✓	N/A	N/A
Incorporates Nonverbal Score(s) Unless Assessing Language				N/A	N/A
Limited Receptive Language Requirements Unless Assessing Language	✓	✓	✓	N/A	N/A
Directions are Suitable for Young Children	✓	✓	✓	N/A	N/A
Includes Opportunities to "Teach Task" (e.g., uses sample items, includes multiple trials, provides demonstrations)	✓	✓	✓	N/A	N/A
Includes Alternative Stopping Rules	✓	✓	✓	N/A	N/A
Translation or Adaptation Available in Other Languages				N/A	N/A
Appropriate Degree of Language Demands and Cultural Loading				N/A	N/A

Note. A checkmark indicates that the authors deemed this qualitative characteristic as being met. Certain qualitative characteristics are more subjective in nature than other characteristics; therefore, readers are encouraged to review early childhood measures independently using the above criteria. N/A = not applicable because these scales are rating scales responded to by the child's caregiver. They are not administered directly to children and are included here for completeness.

unless language is assessed directly. Conversely, these scales are not available in other languages and there are no data on cultural loadings of items or tasks. Chapter 6 provides a detailed explanation for our ratings and a summary of the Bayley–4 qualitative strengths and limitations.

SUMMARY OF BAYLEY–4 OVERVIEW

In the first sections of this chapter we provided information on the history and importance of infant and toddler assessment as well as a rather long list of infant and toddler instruments for the interested reader. Then, via a brief biography of Dr. Nancy Bayley, we attempted to give readers a sense of what she contributed to developmental psychology, the assessment of infants and toddlers, and psychology in general. We also attempted to provide readers with an understanding of the history and development of all editions of the Bayley Scales, concluding with the Bayley–4. Finally, we reviewed and offered our evaluation of the quantitative and qualitative characteristics of the Bayley–4.

TEST YOURSELF

1. **Infant and toddler assessment has been a practice for about how many years?**
   a) 200
   b) 300
   c) 400
   d) 500
2. **Two of the most influential educational initiatives in the history of the United States were:**
   a) Universal prekindergarten and special education
   b) Head Start and special education
   c) General education and special education
   d) Head Start and early intervention
3. **The major purposes of infant and toddler assessment are the following except:**
   a) Screening
   b) Determining career interests
   c) Individual program planning and monitoring
   d) Diagnosing and eligibility determination
4. **The Bayley–4 may be used for the following except:**
   a) Assessing young children's current developmental functioning
   b) Progress monitoring
   c) Providing parents with helpful information regarding their young children
   d) Predicting future cognitive functioning

5. **The original Bayley Scales of Infant Development set the standard for infant assessment because it:**
   a) Sampled the widest array of mental and motor abilities on a developmental assessment at the time
   b) Included a large standardization sample
   c) Included the Infant Behavior Record to describe behavior during testing
   d) All of the above
6. **All editions of the Bayley Scales included the following except:**
   a) Hundreds of items
   b) Many appealing stimuli
   c) Polytomous scoring
   d) Impressive quantitative characteristics
7. **The following statements are true regarding the Bayley–4 Cognitive Scale except:**
   a) It is based on the Cattell–Horn–Carroll Theory of Cognitive Abilities
   b) It is comprised of 81 items
   c) It has items that tap sensorimotor development, exploration and manipulation, object relatedness, among other skills
   d) For the most part, it does not involve verbal responses from the child
8. **Quantitative characteristics of early childhood assessments include all of the following except:**
   a) Reliability
   b) Attractive test materials
   c) Floors and ceilings
   d) Item gradients
9. **Qualitative characteristics of early childhood assessments include the following:**
   a) Attractive test materials
   b) Opportunities to teach the task
   c) Limited language demands unless assessing language
   d) All of the above
10. **The Bayley–4 has exemplary quantitative and qualitative characteristics except for which of the following:**
    a) Reliability of the Cognitive, Language, and Motor Scales
    b) Item gradients of all scales
    c) Test–retest reliability characteristics of the Social-Emotional Scale
    d) Validity of the Cognitive, Language, and Motor Scales

Answers: 1. (a); 2. (d); 3. (b); 4. (d); 5. (d); 6. (c); 7. (a); 8. (b); 9. (d); 10. (c).

REFERENCES

Achenbach, T. (1997). *Caregiver-Teacher Report Form: Manual.* Achenbach System of Empirically Based Assessment.

Achenbach, T., & Rescorla, L. (2000). *Achenbach System of Empirically Based Assessment, Preschool Module: Manual.* Achenbach System of Empirically Based Assessment.

Albers, C. A., & Grieve, A. J. (2007). Test Review: Bayley, N. (2006). Bayley Scales of Infant and Toddler Development (3rd ed.). San Antonio, TX: Harcourt Assessment. *Journal of Psychoeducational Assessment, 25*(2), 180–190. Retrieved from https://doi.org/10.1177/0734282906297199

Alfonso, V. C., Bracken, B. A., & Nagle, R. J. (Eds.) (2020). *Psychoeducational assessment of preschool children* (5th ed.). Routledge. Retrieved from https://doi.org/10.4324/9780429054099

Alfonso, V. C., Engler, J. R., & Lepore, J. C. C. (2020). Assessing and evaluating young children: Developmental domains and methods. In V. C. Alfonso & G. J. DuPaul (Eds.), *Healthy development in young children: Evidence-based interventions for early education* (pp. 13–44). American Psychological Association. Retrieved from https://doi.org/10.1037/0000197-002

Alfonso, V. C., Engler, J. R., & Stavrou, E. (in press). Assessment of preschoolers and school readiness. In L. A. Theodore, B. A. Bracken, & M. A. Bray (Eds.), *School psychology desk reference.* Oxford University Press.

Alfonso, V. C., Ruby, S., Wissel, A. M., & Davari, J. (2020). School psychologists in early childhood settings. In F. C. Worrell, T. L. Hughes, & D. D. Dixson (Eds.), *The Cambridge handbook of applied school psychology* (pp. 579–597). Cambridge University Press.

Alfonso, V. C., Russo, P. M., Fortugno, D. A., & Rader, D. E. (2005). Critical review of the Bayley Scales of Infant Development (2nd ed.): Implications for assessing young children with developmental delays. *The School Psychologist, 59*(2), 67–73.

Alfonso, V. C., Shanock, A., Muldoon, D., Benway, N., & Oades-Sese, G. (2018). *Psychometric integrity of preschool speech/language tests: Implications for diagnosis and progress monitoring of treatment.* [Poster presentation]. Association for Psychological Science, San Francisco, California, United States.

Alpern, G. D. (2020). *Developmental Profile* (4th ed.). Western Psychological Services.

Alpern, G. D., Boll, T. J., & Shearer, M. (1986). *The Developmental Profile II: Manual.* Western Psychological Services.

Alpern, G. D., Boll, T. J., & Shearer, M. (2007). *Developmental Profile* (3rd ed.). Western Psychological Services.

Als, H., Tronick, E., Lester, B. M., & Brazelton, T. B. (1977). The Brazelton Neonatal Behavioral Assessment Scale (BNBAS). *Journal of Abnormal Child Psychology, 5*(3), 215–231. Retrieved from https://doi.org/10.1007/BF00913693

American Association on Intellectual and Developmental Disabilities. (2010). *Intellectual and Developmental Disabilities, 48*(4), 307–309. Retrieved from https://doi.org/10.1352/1934-9556-48.4.307

American Psychiatric Association. (2013). *Diagnostic and statistical manual of mental disorders* (5th ed.). Retrieved from https://doi.org/10.1176/appi.books.9780890425596

Ammer, J. J., & Bangs, T. E. (2000). *Birth to Three Assessment and Intervention System* (2nd ed.). Pro-Ed.

Anastasi, A., & Urbina, S. (1997). *Psychological testing* (7th ed.). Prentice Hall/Pearson Education.

Anderson, P. J., & Burnett, A. (2017). Assessing developmental delay in early childhood – concerns with the Bayley–III scales. *The Clinical Neuropsychologist, 31*(2), 371–381. Retrieved from https://doi.org/10.1080/13854046.2016.1216518

Anderson, P. J., De Luca, C. R., Hutchinson, E., Roberts, G., Doyle, L. W., & Victorian Infant Collaborative Group. (2010). Underestimation of developmental delay by the new Bayley–III Scale. *Archives of Pediatrics & Adolescent Medicine, 164*(4), 352–356. Retrieved from https://doi.org/10.1001/archpediatrics.2010.20

Apfel, N. H., & Provence, S. (2001). *Infant-Toddler and Family Instrument.* Brookes Publishing Company.

Aylward. G. P. (1995). *Bayley Infant Neurodevelopmental Screener.* Psychological Corporation.

Aylward, G. P. (1997). Conceptual issues in developmental screening and assessment. *Journal of Developmental and Behavioral Pediatrics, 18*(5), 340–349. Retrieved from https://doi.org/10.1097/00004703-199710000-00010

Aylward, G. P. (2010). Methodological considerations in neurodevelopmental outcome studies of infants born prematurely. In C. Nosarti, R. Murray, & M. Hack, *Neurodevelopmental outcomes of preterm birth from childhood to adult life* (pp. 164–175). Cambridge University Press. Retrieved from https://doi.org/10.1017/CBO9780511712166

Aylward, G. P. (2013). Continuing issues with the Bayley–III: Where to go from here. *Journal of Developmental and Behavioral Pediatrics, 34*(9), 697–701.

Aylward, G. P. (2020). *Bayley–4 clinical use and interpretation.* Academic Press.

Aylward, G. P., & Zhu, J. J. (2019). *The Bayley Scales: Clarification for clinicians and researchers.* NCS Pearson. Retrieved from https://www.pearsonassessments. com/content/dam/school/global/clinical/us/assets/Bayley–4/Bayley–4-technical-report.pdf

Bangs, T. E. (1986). *Birth to Three Assessment and Intervention System.* Riverside Publishing.

Bankson, N. W. (1990). *Bankson Language Screening Test* (2nd ed.). Pro-Ed.

Baron-Cohen, S., Allen, J., & Gillberg, C. (1992). Can autism be detected at 18 months? The needle, the haystack, and the CHAT. *The British Journal of Psychiatry: The Journal of Mental Science, 161,* 839–843. Retrieved from https://doi.org/10.1192/bjp.161.6.839

Bayley, N. (1933). *The California First-Year Mental Scale.* University of California Press.

Bayley, N. (1936). *The California Infant Scale of Motor Development.* University of California Press.

Bayley, N. (1969). *The Bayley Scales of Infant Development: Manual.* Psychological Corporation.

Bayley, N. (1993). *Bayley Scales of Infant Development* (2nd ed.): *Manual.* Psychological Corporation.

Bayley, N. (2006a). *Bayley Scales of Infant and Toddler Development* (3rd ed.). Pearson.

Bayley, N. (2006b). *Bayley Scales of Infant Development* (3rd ed.): *Administration manual.* Pearson.

Bayley, N. (2006c). *Bayley Scales of Infant Development* (3rd ed): *Technical manual.* Pearson.

Bayley, N., & Aylward, G. P. (2019a). *Bayley Scales of Infant and Toddler Development* (4th ed.). Pearson.

Bayley, N., & Aylward, G. P. (2019b). *Bayley Scales of Infant and Toddler Development* (4th ed.): *Administration manual.* Pearson.

Bayley, N., & Aylward, G. P. (2019c). *Bayley Scales of Infant and Toddler Development* (4th ed.): *Technical manual.* Pearson.

Bayley, N., & Aylward, G. P. (2019d). *Bayley Scales of Infant and Toddler Development* (4th ed.): *Screening test manual.* Pearson.

Bayley, N., & Schaefer, E. S. (1964). Correlations of maternal and child behaviors with the development of mental abilities. *Monographs of the Society for Research in Child Development, 29*(6), 97. Retrieved from https://doi.org/10.2307/1165805

Beery, K. E. (1989). *Developmental Test of Visual-Motor Integration* (3rd rev.). Modern Curriculum Press.

Beery, K. E., Buktenica, N. A., & Beery, N. A. (2010). *Beery-Buktenica Developmental Test of Visual-Motor Integration* (6th ed.): *Manual.* Pearson.

Behar, L., & Stringfield, S. (1974). *Preschool Behavior Questionnaire: Scale and Manual.* Learning Institute of North Carolina.

Bellman, M., Byrne, O., & Sege, R. (2013). Developmental assessment of children. *British Medical Journal, 346.* https://doi.org/10.1136/bmj.e8687

Binet, A., & Simon, T. (1905). New methods for the diagnosis of the intellectual level of subnormals. In H. H. Goddard (Ed.), *Development of intelligence in children (The Binet-Simon Scale).* Williams & Wilkins.

Black, M., & Matula, K. (2000). *Essentials of Bayley Scales of Infant Development-II assessment.* John Wiley & Sons.

Blank, M., Rose, S. A., & Berlin, L. J. (2003). *Preschool Language Assessment Instrument* (2nd ed.): *Examiner's manual.* Pro-Ed.

Boehm, A. E. (2001). *Boehm Test of Basic Concepts Preschool: Examiner's manual.* Pearson.

Bos, A. F. (2013). Bayley–II or Bayley–III: What do the scores tell us? *Developmental Medicine & Child Neurology, 55*(11), 978–979. Retrieved from https://doi.org/doi:10.1111/dmcn.12234

Bracken, B. A. (1987). Limitations of preschool instruments and standards for minimal levels of technical adequacy. *Journal of Psychoeducational Assessment, 5*(4), 313–326. Retrieved from https://doi.org/10.1177/073428298700500402

Bracken, B. A. (1984). *Bracken Basic Concept Scale: Examiner's manual.* Psychological Corporation.

Bracken, B. A. (1998). *Bracken Basic Concept Scale, Revised.* Psychological Corporation.

Bracken, B. A. (2006a). *Bracken Basic Concept Scale* (3rd ed.), *Receptive: Examiner's manual.* Pearson.

Bracken, B. A. (2006b). *Bracken Basic Concept Scale, Expressive: Examiner's manual.* Pearson.

Bracken, B. A. (2007). *Bracken School Readiness Assessment* (3rd ed.): *Manual.* Pearson.

Bracken, B. A., Keith, L. K., & Walker, K. C. (1998). Assessment of preschool behavior and social-emotional functioning: A review of thirteen third-party instruments. *Journal of Psychoeducational Assessment, 16*(2), 153–169. https://doi.org/10.1177/073428299801600204

Bracken, B. A., & Theodore, L. A. (2020). Observation of preschool children's assessment-related behaviors. In V. C. Alfonso, B. A. Bracken, & R. J. Nagle (Eds.), *Psychoeducational Assessment of Preschool Children* (5th ed., pp. 32–54). Routledge.

Bradley-Johnson, S., & Johnson, C. M. (2001). *Cognitive Abilities Scale* (2nd ed.). Pro-Ed.

Bradley-Johnson, S., & Johnson, C. M. (2007). Infant and toddler cognitive assessment. In B. A. Bracken & R. J. Nagle (Eds.), *Psychoeducational assessment of preschool children* (4th ed., pp. 325–357). Lawrence Erlbaum Associates Publishers.

Bradley-Johnson, S., Johnson, C. M., Connard, P., Arick, J. R., & Krug, D. A. (2018). *Assessment for Persons Profoundly or Severely Impaired* (2nd ed.): *Examiner's manual.* Western Psychological Services.

Brassard, M. R., & Boehm, A. E. (2007). Assessment of emotional development and behavior problems. In *Preschool assessment: Principles and practices* (pp.508–576). Guilford Press.

Bricker, D., Capt, B., & Pretti-Frontczak, K. (2002). *Assessment, Evaluation, and Programming System for Infants and Children* (2nd ed.). Brookes Publishing.

Brigance, A. (1990). *Brigance Early Preschool Screen.* Curriculum Associates.

Brigance, A. (1992). *Brigance K & 1 Screen,* (3rd ed.). Curriculum Associates.

Brigance, A. (1985). *Brigance Preschool Screen.* Curriculum Associates.

Brigance, A., & French, B. (2013). *Brigance Early Childhood Screens III: Technical manual.* Curriculum Associates.

Briggs-Gowan, M. J., & Carter, A. S. (1998). *Infant-Toddler Social & Emotional Assessment, Revised.* Yale University and the University of Massachusetts, Boston.

Briggs-Gowan, M. J., Carter, A. S., Irwin, J. R., Wachtel, K., & Cicchetti, D. V. (2004). The Brief Infant-Toddler Social and Emotional Assessment: Screening for social-emotional problems and delays in competence. *Journal of Pediatric Psychology, 29*(2), 143–155. Retrieved from https://doi.org/10.1093/jpepsy/jsh017

Brito, N. H., Fifer, W. P., Amso, D., Barr, R., Bell, M. A., Calkins, S., Flynn, A., Montgomery-Downs, H. E., Oakes, L. M., Richards, J. E., Samuelson, L. M., & Colombo, J. (2019). Beyond the Bayley: Neurocognitive assessments of development during infancy and toddlerhood. *Developmental Neuropsychology, 44*(2), 220–247. Retrieved from https://doi.org/10.1080/87565641.2018.1564310

Brown, T. E. (1996). *Brown Attention-Deficit Disorder Scales.* Pearson.

Brown, T. E. (2001). *Brown Attention-Deficit Disorder Scales* (2nd ed.). Pearson.

Brown, T. E. (2018). *Brown Attention-Deficit Disorder Scales* (3rd ed.). Pearson.

Brue, A. W., & Wilmshurst, L. (2016). *Essentials of intellectual disability assessment and identification.* John Wiley & Sons.

Bruinicks, R. H., Woodcock, R. W., Weatherman, R. F., & Hill, B. K. (1984). *Scales of Independent Behavior.* DLM Teaching Resources.

Bruininks, R. K., Woodcock, R. W., Weatherman, R. F., & Hill, B. K. (1996). *Scales of Independent Behavior, Revised.* Riverside Publishing.

Burns, W. J., Burns, K. A., & Kabacoff, R. I. (1992). Item and factor analyses of the Bayley Scales of Infant Development. *Advances in Infancy Research, 7,* 199–214.

Bzoch, K. R., & League, R. (1991). *Receptive-Expressive Emergent Language Scale: Examiner's manual.* Pro-Ed.

Bzoch, K. R., League, R., & Brown, V. L. (2003). *Receptive-Expressive Emergent Language Test* (3rd ed.): *Examiner's manual.* Pro-Ed.

Bzoch, K. R., League, R., & Brown, V. L. (2020). *Receptive-Expressive Emergent Language Test* (4th ed.): *Examiner's manual.* Pro-Ed.

California Institute for Mental Health. (2000). Mental Health Screening Tool (MHST 0-5). Retrieved from https://www.cibhs.org/sites/main/files/file-attachments/screeningtool5-adult_1.pdf

Campbell, S. K., Siegel, E., Parr, C. A., & Ramey, C. T. (1986). Evidence for the need to renorm the Bayley Scales of Infant Development based on the performance of a population-based sample of 12-month-old infants. *Topics in Early Childhood Special Education, 6*(2), 83–96. Retrieved from https://doi.org/10.1177/027112148600600208

Capute, A. J., & Accardo, P. J. (1996). *Clinical Adaptive Test/Clinical Linguistic Auditory Milestone scale.* Brookes Publishing.

Carey, W. B., McDevitt, S. C., Fullard, W., Medoff-Cooper, B., & Hegvik, R. L. (2007). *Carey Temperament Scales: Manual.* Behavioral-Developmental Initiatives.

Carrow-Woolfolk, E. (1974). *Carrow Elicited Language Inventory.* Learning Concepts.

Carrow-Woolfolk, E. (1985). *Test for Auditory Comprehension of Language, Revised: Examiner's manual.* DLM Teaching Resources.

Carrow-Woolfolk, E. (2011). *Oral and Written Language Scales* (2nd ed.): *Manual.* Pearson.

Carter, A. S., & Briggs-Gowan, M. (2004). *The Infant-Toddler and Brief Infant Toddler Social Emotional Assessment.* Psychology Corporation.

Case-Smith, J., & Alexander, H. (2010). The Bayley–III motor scale. In L. G. Weiss, T. Oakland, & G. P. Aylward (Eds.), *Bayley–III clinical use and interpretation* (pp. 77–146). Elsevier. Retrieved from https://doi.org/10.1016/b978-0-12-374177-6.10004-2

Cattell, P. (1940). *Cattell Infant Intelligence Scale.* Psychological Corporation.

Centers for Disease Control and Prevention. (2019). *Child development positive parenting tips|CDC.* U.S. Department of Health and Human Services. Retrieved from https://www.cdc.gov/ncbddd/childdevelopment/positiveparenting/index.html

Conners, C. K. (2009). *Conners Early Childhood: Manual.* Multi-Health Systems.

Constantino, J. N., & Gruber, C. P. (2012). *Social Responsiveness Scale* (2nd ed.). Western Psychological Services.

Cook, M. J., Holder-Brown, L., Johnson, L. J., & Kilgo, J. L. (1989). An examination of the stability of the Bayley Scales of Infant Development with high-risk infants. *Journal of Early Intervention, 13*(1), 45–49. Retrieved from https://doi.org/10.1177/105381518901300106

Crowe, T. K., Deitz, J. C., & Bennett, F. C. (1987). The relationship between the Bayley Scales of Infant Development and preschool gross motor and cognitive performance. *The American Journal of Occupational Therapy, 41*(6), 374–378. Retrieved from https://doi.org/10.5014/ajot.41.6.374

Crumrine, L., & Lonegan, H. (1999). *Pre-Literacy Skills Screening.* Pro-Ed.

Damarin, F. (1979). Bayley Scales of Infant Development. In O. K. Buros (Ed.), *Eighth Mental Measurements Yearbook* (Vol. *1*). Gryphon Press.

DeGangi, G., Poisson, S., Sickel, R., & Wiener, A. S. (1995). *Infant-Toddler Symptom Checklist.* Pearson.

Division for Early Childhood. (2014). DEC recommended practices in early intervention/early childhood special education 2014. http://www.dec-sped.org/recommendedpractices

Dunn, D. D. (2018). *Peabody Picture Vocabulary Test* (5th ed.). Pearson.

Dykes, M. K., & Mruzek, D. W. (2012). *Developmental Assessment for Individuals with Severe Disabilities* (3rd ed.): *Examiner's manual.* Pro-Ed.

Early Childhood Learning and Knowledge Center (ECLKC). (2019). *Head start timeline.* U.S. Department of Health & Human Services. Retrieved from https://eclkc.ohs.acf.hhs.gov/about-us/article/head-start-timeline

Ehrler, D. J., & McGhee, R. L. (2008). *Primary Test of Nonverbal Intelligence: Examiner's manual.* Western Psychological Services.

Elementary and Secondary Education Act, 20 U.S.C. 2701 *et seq.* (1965). https://www2.ed.gov/about/offices/list/oii/nonpublic/eseareauth.pdf

Elliott, C. D. (1990). *Differential Ability Scales.* Psychological Corporation.

Elliott, C. D. (2007). *Differential Ability Scales* (2nd ed.): *Manual.* Pearson.

Emde, R. N., Wolf, D. P., & Oppenheim, D. (2003). *MacArthur Story Stem Battery.* Oxford University Press.

Engler, J. R., & Alfonso, V. C. (2020). Cognitive assessment of preschool children. In V. C. Alfonso, B. B. Bracken, & R. J. Nagle (Eds.), *Psychoeducational assessment of preschool children* (5th ed., pp. 226–249). Routledge. Retrieved from https://doi.org/10.4324/9780429054099

Every Student Succeeds Act, 20 U.S.C. § 6301 (2015). https://www.congress.gov/bill/114th-congress/senate-bill/1177

Eyberg, S., & Pincus, D. (1999). *Eyberg Child Behavior Inventory & Sutter-Eyberg Student Behavior Inventory, Revised: Manual.* Psychological Assessment Resources.

Fantuzzo, J. W., Coolahan, K. C., Mendez, J. L., McDermott, P. A., & Sutton-Smith, B. (1998). *Penn Interactive Peer Play Scale.* Elsevier Science (Firm).

Fewell, R., & Langley, M. B. (1984). *Developmental Activities Screening Inventory* (2nd ed.). Pro-Ed.

Finello, K. M., & Poulsen, M. K. (2018). *Behavioral Assessment of Baby's Emotional and Social Style.* WestEd.

Flanagan, D. P., & Alfonso, V. C. (1995). A critical review of the technical characteristics of new and recently revised intelligence tests for preschool children. *Journal of Psychoeducational Assessment, 13*(1), 66–90. Retrieved from https://doi.org/10.1177/073428299501300105

Floyd, R. G., Shands, E. I., Alfonso, V. C., Phillips, J. F., Autry, B. K., Mosteller, J. A., Skinner, M., & Irby, S. (2015). A systematic review and psychometric evaluation of adaptive behavior scales and recommendations for practice. *Journal of Applied School Psychology, 31*(1), 83–113. Retrieved from https://doi.org/10.1080/15377903.2014.979384

Fluharty, N. B. (2000). *Fluharty Preschool Speech and Language Screening Test* (2nd ed.): *Examiner's manual.* Pro-Ed.

Folio, M. R., & Fewell, R. R. (2000). *Peabody Developmental Motor Scales* (2nd ed.): *Manual.* Pearson.

Foster, R., Giddan, J. J., & Stark, J. (1973). *Assessment of Children's Language Comprehension: Manual.* Consulting Psychologists Press.

Frankenburg, W. K., & Dodds, J. B. (1967). The Denver Developmental Screening Test. *The Journal of Pediatrics, 71*(2), 181–191. Retrieved from https://doi.org/10.1016/S0022-3476(67)80070-2

Frankenburg, W. K., Doods, J., Archer, P., & Bresnick, B. (1990). *Denver Developmental Screening* (2nd ed.): *Manual.* Denver Developmental Materials.

Frankenburg, W. K., Fandel, A., Sciarillo, W., & Burgess, D. (1981). The newly abbreviated and revised Denver Developmental Screening Test. *Journal of Pediatrics, 99,* 995–999.

Frankenburg, W. K., Goldstein, A. D., & Camp, B. W. (1971). The revised Denver Developmental Screening Test: Its accuracy as a screening instrument.

The Journal of Pediatrics, 79(6), 988–995. Retrieved from https://doi.org/10.1016/s0022-3476(71)80195-6

Fudala, J. B., & Reynolds, W. M. (1986). *Arizona Articulation Proficiency Scale Manual and Picture Test Cards.* Western Psychological Services.

Gadow, K., & Sprafkin, J. (1997). *ADHD Symptom Checklist-4: Manual.* Checkmate Plus.

Gadow, K. D., & Sprafkin, J. (2000). *Early Childhood Inventory* (3rd ed.). Prentice Hall.

Gadow, K. D., & Sprafkin, J. (2010). *Early Childhood Inventory* (4th ed.). Checkmate Plus.

Gadow, K. D., & Sprafkin, J. (2014). *Early Childhood Inventory* (5th ed.). Checkmate Plus.

Gagnon, S. G., & Nagle, R. J. (2000). Comparison of the revised and original versions of the Bayley Scales of Infant Development. *School Psychology International, 21*(3), 293–305. https://doi.org/10.1177/0143034300213006

Gardner, M. F. (1985). *Receptive One-Word Picture Vocabulary Test.* Academic Therapy Publications.

Gardner, M. F. (1990). *Expressive One-Word Picture Vocabulary Test, Revised.* Academic Therapy Publication.

Gardner, M. F. (1995). *Test of Visual Motor Skills Revised: Manual.* Psychological and Educational Publications.

Gauthier, S. M., Bauer, C. R., Messinger, D. S., & Closius, J. M. (1999). The Bayley Scales of Infant Development-II: Where to start? *Journal of Developmental and Behavioral Pediatrics, 20*(2), 75–79. Retrieved from https://doi.org/10.1097/00004703-199904000-00001

Geffner, D., & Goldman, R. (2010). *Auditory Skills Assessment: Manual.* Pearson.

Gesell, A. (1925a). *The Mental Growth of the Preschool Child.* Macmillan.

Gesell, A. (1925b). *Gesell developmental schedules.* Stoelting.

Gesell, A., & Amatruda, C. (1941). *Gesell Developmental Schedules.* Psychological Corporation.

Gilliam, J. E. (2001). *Gilliam Asperger's Disorder Scale: Examiner's manual.* Western Psychological Services.

Gilliam, J. E. (2005). *Gilliam Autism Rating Scale* (2nd ed.): *Examiner's manual.* Pro-Ed.

Ginsburg, H. P., & Baroody, A. J. (2003). *Test of Eearly Mathematics Ability* (3rd ed.): *Examiner's manual.* Pro-Ed.

Glascoe, F. P. (2002). The Brigance Infant and Toddler Screen: Standardization and validation. *Journal of Developmental and Behavioral Pediatrics: JDBP,*

23(3), 145–150. Retrieved from https://doi.org/10.1097/00004703-200206000-00003

Glascoe, F. P. (2012). *Parents' Evaluation of Developmental Status*. PEDStest.com.

Glenn, S., Dayus, B., Cunningham, C., & Horgan, M. (2001). Mastery motivation in children with Down syndrome. *Down Syndrome: Research & Practice, 7*(2), 52–59. Rerieved from https://doi.org/10.3104/reports.114

Goldman, R., & Fristoe, M. (2000). *Goldman-Fristoe Test of Articulation* (2nd ed.): *Manual.* Pearson.

Goldstein, D. J., Fogle, E. E., Wieber, J. L., & O'Shea, T. M. (1995). Comparison of the Bayley Scales of Infant Development (2nd ed.) and the Bayley Scales of Infant Development with premature infants. *Journal of Psychoeducational Assessment, 13*(4), 391–396. Retrieved from https://doi.org/10.1177/073428299501300406

Good, R. H., & Kaminski, R. A. (Eds.). (2002). *Dynamic Indicators of Basic Early Literacy Skills* (6th ed.). Institute for the Development of Educational Achievement.

Goodman, J. F. (1990). Infant intelligence: Do we, can we, should we assess it? In C. R. Reynolds & R. W. Kamphaus (Eds.), *Handbook of psychological and Educational Assessment* (pp. 183–204). Guilford Press.

Goodman, R. (1997). The Strengths and Difficulties Questionnaire: A research note. *Journal of Child Psychology and Psychiatry, 38*(5), 581–586. Retrieved from https://doi.org/10.1111/j.1469-7610.1997.tb01545.x

Greenspan, S. I. (2004). *Greenspan Social-Emotional Growth Chart: A Screening Questionnaire for Infants and Young Children: Manual.* Psychological Corporation.

Greenspan, S. I., DeGangi, G. A., & Wieder, S. (2001). *The Functional Emotional Assessment Scale.* Interdisciplinary Council on Developmental and Learning Disorders.

Gresham, F. M., & Elliot, S. N. (1990). *Social Skills Rating System: Manual.* American Guidance Service.

Gresham, F. M., & Elliot, S. N. (2008). *Social Skills Improvement System Rating Scales: Manual.* Pearson.

Griffiths, R. (1951). *The Griffiths Mental Development Scale for Testing Babies from Birth to Two Years.* Child Development Research Centre.

Griffiths, R. (1967). *Griffiths Mental Developmental Scale.* University of London Press.

Guralnick, M. J. (Ed.) (1997). *The effectiveness of early intervention.* Brookes.

Hack, M., Taylor, H. G., Drotar, D., Schluchter, M., Cartar, L., Wilson-Costello, D., Klein, N., Friedman, H., Mercuri-Minich, N., & Morrow, M. (2005). Poor predictive validity of the Bayley Scales of Infant Development for cognitive function of extremely low birth weight children at school age. *Pediatrics, 116*(2), 333–341. Retrieved from https://doi.org/10.1542/peds.2005-0173

Hammill, D., & Bryant, B. (1991). *Detroit Test of Learning Aptitude–Primary* (2nd ed.). Pro-Ed.

Hammill, D., & Bryant, B. (2005). *Detroit Test of Learning Aptitude–Primary* (3rd ed.): *Examiner's manual.* Pro-Ed.

Harrison, P., Kaufman, A., Kaufman, N., Bruininks, R., Rynders, J., Ilmer, S., Sparrow, S., & Cicchetti, D. (1990). *Early Screening Profiles: Manual.* Pearson.

Harrison, P. L., & Oakland, T. (2000). *Adaptive Behavior Assessment System.* Psychological Corporation.

Harrison, P. L., & Oakland, T. (2003). *Adaptive Behavior Assessment System* (2nd ed.). Psychological Corporation.

Harrison, P. L., & Oakland, T. (2015). *Adaptive Behavior Assessment System* (3rd ed.): *Manual.* Pearson.

Hedrick, D. L., Prather, E. M., & Tobin, A. R. (1975). *Sequenced Inventory of Communication Development, Revised.* Western Psychological Services.

Hedrick, D. L., Prather, E. M., & Tobin, A. R. (1984). *Sequenced Inventory of Communication Development.* University of Washington Press.

High/Scope Educational Research Foundation. (2003). *Preschool Child Observation Record* (2nd ed.). High/Scope Press.

Hiskey, M. S. (1966). *Hiskey-Nebraska Test of Learning Aptitude.* Union College Press.

Hoover, H. D., Hieronymous, A. N., Frisbie, D. A., & Dunbar, S. B. (1996). *Iowa Test of Basic Skills: Administration manual.* Riverside.

Howes, C., & Matheson, C. C. (1992). *Revised Peer Play Scale.* American Psychological Association.

Hresko, W., Reid, D. K., & Hammill, D. D. (1991). *Test of Early Language Development* (2nd ed.). Pro-Ed.

Hresko, W. P., Reid, D. K., & Hammill, D. D. (1999). *Test of Early Language Development* (3rd ed.): *Manual.* Pearson.

Hresko, W. P., Reid, D. K., & Hammill, D. D. (2018). *Test of Early Language Development* (4th ed.): *Manual.* Pro-Ed.

Hua, J., Li, Y., Ye, K., Ma, Y., Lin, S., Gu, G., & Du, W. (2019). The reliability and validity of Bayley–III cognitive scale in China's male and female children.

Early Human Development, 129, 71–78. Retrieved from https://doi.org/10.1016/j.earlhumdev.2019.01.01

Huer, M. B., & Miller, L. (2011). *Test of Early Communication and Emerging Language: Examiner's manual.* Pro-Ed.

Hughes, T. L., & Quinn, C. V. (2020). Working with young children living in stressful environments. In V. C. Alfonso & G. J. DuPaul (Eds.), *Healthy development in young children: Evidence-based interventions for early education* (pp. 297–315). American Psychological Association. Retrieved from https://doi.org/10.1037/0

Ilg, F. L., & Ames, L. B. (1972). *Gesell School Readiness Test.* Harper & Row.

Individuals with Disabilities Education Improvement Act, Pub. L. 108–446, 118 Stat. 2647 (2004).

Ireton, H. (1988). *Preschool Developmental Inventory: Manual.* Behavior Science System.

Ireton, H. (1992). *Child Development Inventories: Manual.* Behavior Science Systems.

Ireton, H. (1994). *Infant Development Inventory.* Behavior Science Systems.

Ireton, H. (2006). *Infant Developmental Inventory: Manual.* Behavior Science Systems.

Jaffa, A. S. (1934). *The California Preschool Mental Scale, Form A.* University of California Press.

Jary, S., Whitelaw, A., Walløe, L., & Thoresen, M. (2013). Comparison of Bayley-2 and Bayley-3 scores at 18 months in term infants following neonatal encephalopathy and therapeutic hypothermia. *Developmental Medicine and Child Neurology, 55*(11), 1053–1059. Retrieved from https://doi.org/10.1111/dmcn.12208

Jensen, S. L. (2012). *Early Functional Communication Profile: Manual.* Western Psychological Services.

Johnson, S., Moore, T., & Marlow, N. (2014). Using the Bayley–III to assess neurodevelopmental delay: Which cut-off should be used? *Pediatric Research, 75*(5), 670–674. https://doi.org/10.1038/pr.2014.10

Kaufman, A. S., & Kaufman, N. L. (1983). *Kaufman Assessment Battery for Children: Interpretive manual.* American Guidance Service.

Kaufman, A. S., & Kaufman, N. L. (1993). *Kaufman Survey of Early Academic and Language Skills: Manual.* Pearson.

Kaufman, A. S., & Kaufman, N. L. (2004). *Kaufman Assessment Battery for Children* (2nd ed.): *Manual.* Pearson.

Kaufman, A. S., & Kaufman, N. L. (2018). *Kaufman Assessment Battery for Children* (2nd ed., Normative Update): *Manual.* Pearson.

Kaufman, N. L. (1995). *Kaufman Speech Praxis Test for Children: Manual.* Wayne State University Press.

Kelley, M. F., & Surbeck, E. (2007). History of preschool assessment. In B. A. Bracken & R. Nagle (Eds.), *Psychoeducational assessment of preschool children* (4th ed., pp. 3–28). Lawrence Erlbaum Associates Publishers.

Kelly-Vance, L., & Ryalls, B. O. (2020). Play-based approaches to preschool assessment. In V. C. Alfonso, B. B. Bracken, & R. J. Nagle (Eds.), *Psychoeducational assessment of preschool children* (5th ed.). Routledge. Retrieved from https://doi.org/10.4324/9780429054099

Knobloch, H., Stevens, F., & Malone, A. S. (1980). *Gesell Developmental Schedules*. Harper and Row.

Korkman, M., Kirk, U., & Kemp, S. (1998). *NEPSY: Manual*. Pearson.

Korkman, M., Kirk, U., & Kemp, S. (2007). *NEPSY* (2nd ed.): *Manual*. Pearson.

Krug, D. A., Arick, J. R., & Almond, P. (1993). *Autism Screening Instrument for Educational Planning* (2nd ed.): *Manual*. Pro-Ed.

LaFreniere, P. J., & Dumas, J. E. (1995). *Social Competence and Behavior Evaluation Preschool Edition: Examiner's manual*. Western Psychological Services.

Lambert, N. M., Windmiller, M., Tharinger, D., & Cole, L. (1981). *AAMD Adaptive Behavior Scale School Edition: Manual*. Publishers Test Service.

Langley, M. B., Fewell, R., & Maddox, T. (2010). *Cognitive Assessment of Young Children: Examiner's manual*. Pro-Ed.

LeBuffe, P. A., & Naglieri, J. A. (1999). *The Devereux Early Childhood Assessment*. Kaplan Press.

LeBuffe, P. A., & Naglieri, J. A. (2002). *Devereux Early Childhood Assessment Clinical Form*. Kaplan Press.

Lee, L. L. (1971). *Northwestern Syntax Screening Test*. University Press.

Leguire, L. E., & Fellows, R. R. (1990). Time to renorm the Bayley. *Review: Rehabilitation and Education for Blindness and Visual Impairment, 22*(1), 7–12.

Lennon, E. M., Gardner, J. M., Karmel, B. Z., & Flory, M. J. (2008). Bayley Scales of Infant Development. In J. B. Benson & M. M. Haith (Eds.), *Language, memory, and cognition in infancy and early childhood* (pp. 37–48). Academic Press.

Lewis, N. P., & Khan, L. M. (2002). *Khan-Lewis Phonological Analysis* (2nd ed.). *Manual*. Pearson.

Lidz, C. S. (2002). *Early childhood assessment*. John Wiley & Sons.

Linder, T. (2008). *Transdisciplinary Play-Based Assessment, Second Edition: Manual*. Brookes Publishing.

Lipkin, P. H., & Okamoto, J. K. (2015). The Individuals with Disabilities Education Act (IDEA) for children with special educational needs. *Pediatrics, 136*(6), e1650 - e1662. https://doi.org/10.1542/peds.2015-34.

Lippke, B., Dickey, S., Selmar, J., & Soder, A. (1997). *Photo Articulation Test, Third Edition: Manual.* Pro-Ed.

Lipsitt, L. P. & Eichorn, D. H. (1990). Nancy Bayley (1899 –). In A. N. O' Connell & N. F. Russo (Eds.), *Women in psychology: A bio-bibliographic sourcebook.* Greenwood Press.

Lord, C., Rutter, M., DiLavore, P. C., Risi, S., Gotham, K., Bishop, S. L., Luystr, R. J., & Guthrie, W. (2012). *Autism Diagnostic Observation Schedule* (2nd ed.): *Manual.* Pearson.

Lowe, J. R., Erickson, S. J., Schrader, R., & Duncan, A. F. (2012). Comparison of the Bayley II mental developmental index and the Bayley III cognitive scale: Are we measuring the same thing? *Acta Paediatrica, 101*(2), 55–58. Retrieved from https://doi.org/10.1111/j.1651-2227.2011.02517.x

Lowe, M., & Costello, A. J. (1988). *Symbolic Play Test* (2nd ed.). GL Assessment.

Manandhar, S. R., Dulal, S., Manandhar, D. S., Saville, N., & Prost, A. (2016). Acceptability and reliability of the Bayley Scales of Infant Development III cognitive and motor scales among children in Makwanpur. *Journal of Nepal Health Research Council, 14*(32), 47–50.

Marcott, A. (2009). *Evaluating Acquired Skills in Communication* (3rd ed.): *Examiner's manual.* Pro-Ed.

Mardell, C. M., & Goldenberg, D. S. (2011). *Developmental Indicators for the Assessment of Learning* (4th ed.): *Manual.* Pearson.

Mardell-Czudnowski, C. D., & Goldenberg, D. S. (1983). *Developmental Indicators for the Assessment of Learning, Revised.* Childcraft Education.

Mardell-Czudnowski, C., & Goldenberg, D. S. (1990). *Developmental Indicators of the Assessment of Learning, Revised.* American Guidance Service.

Mardell-Czudnowski, C., & Goldenberg, D. S. (1998). *Developmental Indicators for the Assessment of Learning* (3rd ed.). American Guidance Services.

Martin, N. A. (2010). *Test of Visual-Motor Skills* (3rd ed.): *Manual.* Western Psychological Services.

Martin, R. P. (1988). *The Temperament Assessment Battery for Children.* Clinical Psychology Publishing.

Matula, K., Gyurke, J. S., & Aylward, G. P. (1997). Bayley Scales-II. *Journal of Developmental and Behavioral Pediatrics, 18*(2), 112–113. Retrieved from https://doi.org/10.1097/00004703-199704000-00008

McBride, G., Dumont, R., & Willis, J. O. (2011). *Essentials of IDEA for assessment professionals.* John Wiley & Sons.

McCarney, S. B., & Arthaud, T. J. (2004). *Attention Deficit Disorders Evaluation Scale* (3rd ed.). Howthorne Educational Services. Retrieved from https://www.silvereye.com.au/documents/sample_pages/prod3308.pdf

McCarthy, D. (1972). *The McCarthy Scales of Children's Abilities*. Psychological Corporation.

McClain, C., Provost, B., & Crowe, T. K. (2000). Motor development of two-year-old typically developing Native American children on the Bayley Scales of Infant Development II motor scale. *Pediatric Physical Therapy, 12*(3), 108–113.

McCloskey, G., Petry, B., McIntosh, L., Kelly, J., & Filacheck, J. (2020). Neuropsychological assessment pf preschool children. In V. C. Alfonso, B. B. Bracken, & R. J. Nagle (Eds.), *Psychoeducational assessment of preschool children* (5th ed., pp. 375–398). Routledge. Retrieved from https://doi.org/10.4324/9780429054099

McConaughy, S. H., & Achenbach, T. M. (2004). *Test Observation Form (TOF): Manual*. University of Vermont, Research Center for Children, Youth, & Families.

McGhee, R. L., Ehrler, D. J., & DiSimoni, F. (2007). *Token Test for Children* (2nd ed.): *Examiner's manual*. Pro-Ed.

McGuire, J., & Richman, N. (1988). *Preschool Behavior Checklist*. Academic Therapy. Publications.

Meadow, K. P. (1983). *Meadow/Kendall Social-Emotional Assessment Inventories for Deaf and Hearing: Revised manual*. Pre-College Programs.

Meisels, S. J., Jablon, J. R., Marsden, D. B., Dichtelmiller, M. L., & Dorfman, A. B. (2001). *The Work Sampling System* (4th ed.). Pearson Early Learning.

Meisels, S. J., & Marsden, D. B. (2019). *Early Screening Inventory* (3rd ed.). Pearson.

Meisels, S. J., Marsden, D. B., Dombro, A. M., Weston, D. R., & Jewkes, A. M. (2003). *The Ounce Scale: Manual*. Pearson.

Meisels, S. J., Marsden, D. B., Wiske, M. S., & Henderson, L. W. (1997). *The Early Screening Inventory Revised*. Pearson.

Merrell, K. W. (1994). *Preschool and Kindergarten Behavior Scales: Manual*. Clinical Psychology Publishing.

Merrell, K. W. (2003). *Preschool and Kindergarten Behavior Scales* (2nd ed.): *Examiner's manual*. Pro-Ed.

Milani-Comparetti, A., & Gidoni, E. (1967). Routine developmental examination in normal and retarded children. *Developmental Medicine & Child Neurology, 9*(5), 631–638. Retrieved from https://doi.org/10.1111/j.1469-8749.1967.tb02335.x

Miller, L. J. (1988). *Miller Assessment for Preschoolers*. Western Psychological Services.

Miller, L. J. (1993). *FirstSTEP: Screening Test for Evaluating Preschoolers*. Pearson.

Milne, S., McDonald, J., & Comino, E. J. (2012). The use of the Bayley Scales of Infant and Toddler Development III with clinical populations: A preliminary exploration. *Physical & Occupational Therapy in Pediatrics, 32*(1), 24–33. Retrieved from https://doi.org/10.3109/01942638.2011.592572

Monsma, E. V., Miedema, S. T., Brian, A. S., & Williams, H. G. (2020). Assessment of gross motor development in preschool children. In V. C. Alfonso, B. B. Bracken, & R. J. Nagle (Eds.), *Psychoeducational assessment of preschool children* (5th ed., pp. 283–319). Routledge.

Moore, T., Johnson, S., Haider, S., Hennessy, E., & Marlow, N. (2012). Relationship between test scores using the second and third editions of the Bayley Scales in extremely preterm children. *The Journal of Pediatrics, 160*(4), 553–558. Retrieved from https://doi.org/10.1016/j.jpeds.2011.09.047

Mowder, B. A., Rubinson, F., & Yasik, A. E. (Eds). (2009). *Evidence-based practice in infant and early childhood psychology.* John Wiley & Sons.

Mullen, E. M. (1995). *Mullen Scales of Early Learning, AGS Edition.* American Guidance Service.

Nagle, R. J., Gagnon, S. G., & Kidder-Ashley, P. (2020). Issues in preschool assessment. In V. C. Alfonso, B. B. Bracken, & R. J. Nagle (Eds.), *Psychoeducational assessment of preschool children* (5th ed., pp. 3–31). Routledge.

National Association for the Education of Young Children. (2020). Retrieved from http://www.naeyc.org

National Association of School Psychologists. (2015). *Early childhood services: Promoting positive outcomes for young children [Position statement].*

National Research Council. (2008). *Early childhood assessment: Why, what, and how.* The National Academies Press. Retrieved from https://doi.org/10.17226/12446

Nehring, A. D., Nehring, E. F., Bruni, J. R., & Randolph, P. L. (1992). *Learning Accomplishment Profile-Diagnostic Standardized Assessment.* Kaplan Press.

Neisworth, J. T., Bagnato, S. J., Salvia, J., & Hunt, F. M. (1999). *Temperament and Atypical Behavior Scale: Manual.* Brookes Publishing.

Nellis, L., & Gridley, B. E. (1994). Review of the Bayley Scales of Infant Development (2nd ed.). *Journal of School Psychology, 32*(2), 201–209. https://doi.org/10.1016/0022-4405(94)90011-6

Newborg, J. (1984). *Battelle Developmental Inventory.* Riverside Publishing.

Newborg, J. (2004). *Battelle Developmental Inventory* (2nd ed.). Riverside Publishing.

Newborg, J. (2020). *Battelle Developmental Inventory* (3rd ed.). Riverside Insights.

Nihira, K., Foster, R., Shellhaas, M., & Leland, H. (1974). *AAMD Adaptive Behavior Scale.* American Association on Mental Deficiency.

No Child Left Behind Act of 2001, Pub. L. No. 107-110, § 101, 115 Stat. 1425 (2002). https://www.govinfo.gov/content/pkg/PLAW-107publ110/pdf/PLAW-107publ110.pdf

Nurss, J. R., & McGauvran, M. E. (1995). *Metropolitan Readiness Test* (6th ed.). Harcourt Brace.

Nuttall, E. V. E., Romero, I. E., & Kalesnik, J. E. (1999). *Assessing and screening preschoolers: Psychological and educational dimensions*. Allyn & Bacon.

Office of Head Start. (2019). *History of Head Start*. U.S. Department of Health & Human Services. https://www.acf.hhs.gov/ohs/about/history-head-start

Ostrov, J. M. (2005). *Early Childhood Play Project: Observational coding manual*. Department of Psychology.

Parham, L. D., & Ecker, C. (2010). *Sensory Processing Measure–Preschool: Manual*. Western Psychological Services.

Pendergast, K. (1969). *Photo Articulation Test*. International Printers.

Pendergast, L. L., Schaefer, B. A., Murray-Kolb, L. E., Svensen, E., Shrestha, R., Rasheed, M. A., Scharf, R. J., Kosek, M., Vasquez, A. O., Maphula, A., Costa, H., Rasmussen, Z. A., Yousafzai, A., Tofail, F., Seidman, J. C., & Network Investigators, M. A. L.-E. D. (2018). Assessing development across cultures: Invariance of the Bayley–III Scales across seven international MAL-ED sites. *School Psychology Quarterly, 33*(4), 604–614. Retrieved from https://doi.org/10.1037/spq0000264

Pinon (2010). Theoretical background and structure of the Bayley Scales of Infant Development (3rd ed.). In L. G. Weiss, T. Oakland, & G. P. Aylward (Eds.), *Bayley–III clinical use and interpretation* (pp. 1–28). Academic Press.

Provence, S., Erikson, J., Vater, S., Pruett, K., Rosinia, J., & Palmeri, S. (2016). *Infant-Toddler Developmental Assessment* (2nd ed.): *Manual*. Pro-Ed.

Provost, B., Heimerl, S., McClain, C., Kim, N. H., Lopez, B. R., & Kodituwakku, P. (2004). Concurrent validity of the Bayley Scales of Infant Development II Motor Scale and the Peabody Developmental Motor Scales-2 in children with developmental delays. *Pediatric Physical Therapy, 16*(3), 149–156. Retrieved from https://doi.org/10.1097/01.PEP.0000136005.41585.FE

Rademeyer, V., & Jacklin, L. (2013). A study to evaluate the performance of black South African urban infants on the Bayley Scales of Infant Development III. *South African Journal of Child Health, 7*(2), 54–59.

Raines, T. C., Malone, C. M., Beidleman, L. M., & Bowman, N. (2020). National policies and laws affecting children's health and education. In V. C. Alfonso & G. J. DuPaul (Eds.), *Healthy development in young children: Evidence-based interventions for early education* (pp. 319–336). American Psychological Association. Retrieved from https://doi.org/10.1037/0000197-016

Ramey, C. T., & Ramey, S. L. (1998). Prevention of intellectual disabilities: Early interventions to improve cognitive development. *Preventive Medicine, 27*(2), 224–232. https://doi.org/10.1006/pmed.1998.0279

Ramey, C. T., & Ramey, S. L. (2004). Early learning and school readiness: Can early intervention make a difference? *Merrill-Palmer Quarterly, 50*(4), 471–491. Retrieved from https://doi.org/10.1353/mpq.2004.0034

Ramey, C. T., Sparling, J. J., & Ramey, S. L. (2014). Interventions for students from impoverished environments. In J. T. Mascolo, V. C. Alfonso, & D. P. Flanagan (Eds.), *Essentials of planning, selecting and tailoring interventions for unique learners* (pp. 415–448). John Wiley & Sons.

Ranjitkar, S., Kvestad, I., Strand, T. A., Ulak, M., Shrestha, M., Chandyo, R. K., Shrestha, L., & Hysing, M. (2018). Acceptability and reliability of the Bayley Scales of Infant and Toddler Development-III among children in Bhaktapur, Nepal. *Frontiers in Psychology, 9,* 1265. Retrieved from https://doi.org/10.3389/fpsyg.2018.01265.

Redden, S. C., Forness, S. R., Ramey, S. L., Ramey, C. T., Brezausek, C. M., & Kavale, K. A. (2001). Children at risk: Effects of a four-year Head Start transition program on special education identification. *Journal of Child and Family Studies, 10*(2), 255–270. Retrieved from https://doi.org/10.1023/A:1016659710619

Redden, S. C., Forness, S. R., Ramey, S. L., Ramey, C. T., Zima, B. T., Brezausek, C. M., & Kavale, K. A. (1999). Head Start children at third grade: Preliminary special education identification and placement of children with emotional, learning, and related disabilities. *Journal of Child and Family Studies, 8*(3), 285–303. Retrieved from https://doi.org/10.1023/A:1022063228843

Reid, D. M., Hresko, W. P., Hammill, D. D., & Wiltshire, S. (1991). *Test of Early Reading Ability: Deaf or Hard of Hearing.* Pro-Ed.

Reid, D. M., Hresko, W. P., Hammill, D. D., & Wiltshire, S. (2001). *Test of Early Reading Ability* (3rd ed.). Pro-Ed.

Reuner, G., Fields, A. C., Wittke, A., Löpprich, M., & Pietz, J. (2013). Comparison of the developmental tests Bayley–III and Bayley-II in 7-month-old infants born preterm. *European Journal of Pediatrics, 172*(3), 393–400. Retrieved from https://doi.org/10.1007/s00431-012-1902-6

Reuter, J. R., Katoff, L., & Gruber, C. (2000). *Kent Inventory of Developmental Skills.* Western Psychological Services.

Reynell, J., & Gruber, C. (1990). *Reynell Developmental Language Scales: Manual.* Western Psychological Services.

Reynell, J., & Zinkin, P. (1979). *Reynell-Zinkin Scales: Developmental Scales for Young Visually Handicapped Children: Manual.* NFER Publishing Company.

Reynolds, C. R., & Kamphaus, R. W. (1992). *Behavior Assessment System for Children.* American Guidance Service.

Reynolds, C. R., & Kamphaus, R. W. (2004). *Behavior Assessment System for Children* (2nd ed.). Pearson.

Reynolds, C. R., & Kamphaus, R. W. (2007a). *BASC-2 Behavioral and Emotional Screening System: Manual.* Pearson.

Reynolds, C. R., & Kamphaus, R. W. (2007b). *Test of Irregular Word Reading Efficiency: Professional manual.* Psychological Assessment Resources.

Reynolds, C. R., & Kamphaus, R. W. (2015a). *BASC-3 Behavioral and Emotional Screening System: Manual.* Pearson.

Reynolds, C. R., & Kamphaus, R. W. (2015b). *Behavior Assessment System for Children* (3rd ed.). Pearson.

Rhodes, L., Bayley, N., & Yow, B. C. (1984). *Supplement to the manual for the Bayley Scales of Infant Development.* The Psychological Corporation.

Riley, G., & Bakker, K. (2009). *Stuttering Severity Instrument* (4th ed.): *Examiner's manual.* Pro-Ed.

Roberts, H., & Kennert, B. (2018). Primer on special education. In H. Needelman & B. Jackson (Eds.), *Follow-up for NICU graduates.* Springer. Retrieved from https://doi.org/10.1007/978-3-319-73275-6_16

Robertson, C. M., Hendson, L., Biggs, W. S., & Acton, B. V. (2010). Application of the Flynn effect for the Bayley III Scales. *Archives of Pediatrics & Adolescent Medicine, 164*(11), 1072–1073. Retrieved from https://doi.org/10.1001/archpediatrics.2010.199

Robins, D. L., Fein, D., & Barton, M. L. (1999). *Modified Checklist for Autism in Toddlers.* Self-Published.

Roid, G. H. (2005). *Stanford–Binet Intelligence Scales* (5th ed.): *Technical manual.* Pro-Ed.

Roid, G. H., & Miller, L. J. (1997). *Leiter International Performance Scale Revised: Examiner's manual.* Stoelting.

Roid, G. H., & Miller, L. J. (2013). *Leiter International Performance Scale* (3rd ed.). Stoelting.

Roid, G. H., & Sampers, J. L. (2004). *Merrill-Palmer Revised: Manual.* Western Psychological Services.

Rosenblith, J. F. (1992). A singular career: Nancy Bayley. *Developmental Psychology, 28*(5), 747–758. https://doi.org/10.1037/0012-1649.28.5.747

Ross, G., & Lawson, K. (1997). Using the Bayley-II: Unresolved issues in assessing the development of prematurely born children. *Journal of Developmental and Behavioral Pediatrics, 18*(2), 109–111. Retrieved from https://doi.org/10.1097/00004703-199704000-00007

Rutter, M., Bailey, A., & Lord, C. (2003). *Social Communication Questionnaire.* Western Psychological Services.

Rutter, M., LeCouteur, A., & Lord, C. (2003). *Autism Diagnostic Interview Revised: Manual*. Pearson.

Sattler, J. M. (2018a). *Assessment of children: Cognitive foundations and applications* (6th ed.). Author.

Sattler, J. M. (2018b). *Resource guide to accompany assessment of children: Cognitive foundations and applications* (6th ed.). Author.

Schafer, D. S., & Moersch, M. S. (1981). *Developmental Programming for Infants and Young Children*. University of Michigan Press.

Schopler, E., Bourgondien, M. E., Wellman, G. J., & Love, S. R. (2010). *Childhood Autism Rating Scale* (2nd ed.): *Manual*. Pearson.

Schopler, E., Lansing, M., Reichler, R., & Marcus, L. (2005). *Psychoeducational Profile* (3rd ed.): *Manual*. Pro-Ed.

Schopler, E., Reichler, R., & Renner, B. (1988). *The Childhood Autism Rating Scale*. Western Psychological Services.

Schrank, F. A., McGrew, K. S., Mather, N., & Woodcock, R. W. (2014). *Woodcock-Johnson IV*. Riverside Publishing.

Schweinhart, L. J., & Weikart, D. P. (1998). Why curriculum matters in early childhood education. *Educational Leadership, 55*(6), 57.

Secord, W., & Donohue, J. S. (2013). *Clinical Assessment of Articulation and Phonology (2nd ed.): Examiner's manual*. Pro-Ed.

Siegel, B. (2004). *Pervasive Developmental Disorders Screening Test* (2nd ed.). Psychological Corporation/Harcourt Assessment.

Siegel, L. S., Cooper, D. C., Fitzhardinge, P. M., & Ash, A. J. (1995). The use of the Mental Development Index of the Bayley Scale to diagnose language delay in 2-year-old high risk infants. *Infant Behavior & Development, 18*(4), 483–486. Retrieved from https://doi.org/10.1016/0163-6383(95)90037-3

Simeonsson, R. J. (1979). *Carolina Record of Individual Behavior*. Carolina Institute for Research on Early Education of the Handicapped.

Smith, A. J., & Johnson, R. E. (1977). *Smith-Johnson Nonverbal Performance Scale*. Western Psychological Services.

Snow, C. E., & Van Hemel, S. B. (2008). *Early childhood assessment: Why, what, and how*. The National Academies Press.

Snyder, S., & Sheehan, R. (1992). Rasch analysis of the Standardization data of the Bayley Mental Scale of Infant Development. *Diagnostique, 17*(3), 185–194. Retrieved from https://doi.org/10.1177/153450849201700303

Sparrow, S. S., Balla, D. A., & Cicchetti, D. V. (1984). *Vineland Adaptive Behavior Scales*. American Guidance Service.

Sparrow, S. S., Balla, D. A., & Cicchetti, D. V. (1998). *Vineland Social-Emotional Early Childhood Scales*. American Guidance Service.

Sparrow, S. S., Balla, D. A., & Cicchetti, D. V. (2005). *Vineland Adaptive Behavior Scales* (2nd ed.). Pearson.

Sparrow, S. S., Cicchetti, D. V., & Saulnier, C. A. (2016). *Vineland Adaptive Behavior Scales* (3rd ed.): *Manual.* Pearson.

Squires, J., & Bricker, D. (1995). *Ages & Stages Questionnaires.* Brookes Publishing.

Squires, J., & Bricker, D. (2009). *Ages & Stages Questionnaires* (3rd ed.). Brookes Publishing.

Squires, J., Bricker, D., & Twombly, E. (2002). *Ages and Stages Questionnaire: Social–Emotional.* Brookes Publishing.

Squires, J., Bricker, D., & Twombly, E. (2015). *Ages and Stages Questionnaires: Social–Emotional* (2nd ed.). Brookes Publishing.

Squires, J., Potter, L., & Bricker, D. (1999). *Ages and Stages Questionnaires* (2nd ed.). Brookes Publishing.

Stillman, R. (1978). *The Callier-Azusa Scale.* South Central Regional Center for Services to Deaf-Blind Children and Callier Center for Communication Disorders.

Stone, W. L., Coonrod, E. E., & Ousley, O. Y. (2000). Screening Tool for Autism Two-Year-Olds (STAT): Development and preliminary data. *Journal of Autism and Developmental Disorders, 30*(6), 607–612. Retrieved from https://doi.org/10.1023/A:1005647629002

Stone, W. L., & Hogan, K. L. (1993). A structured parent interview for identifying young children with autism. *Journal of Autism and Developmental Disorders, 23*(4), 639–652. Retrieved from https://doi.org/10.1007/BF01046106

Sundberg, M. L. (2014). *Verbal Behavior Milestones Assessment and Placement Program* (2nd ed.). AVB Press.

Terjesen, M. D., Sciutto, M. J., & O'Brien, C. (2019). Behavior rating scales and the assessment of ADHD in early childhood: A review of psychometric properties and scale features. *Perspectives on Early Childhood Psychology and Education, 4*(1), 5–38.

Terman, L. M. (1916). *The measurement of intelligence: An explanation of and a complete guide for the use of the Stanford revision and extension of the Binet-Simon Intelligence Scale.* Houghton Mifflin.

Terman, L. M., & Merrill, M. A. (1937). *Measuring intelligence.* Houghton Mifflin.

Terman, L. M., & Merrill, M. A. (1960). *Stanford-Binet Intelligence Scale: Manual for the Third Revision Form L-M.* Houghton Mifflin.

Terman, L. M., & Merrill, M. A. (1973). *Stanford-Binet Intelligence Scale: Manual for the Third Revision Form L-M, 1973 norms edition.* Houghton Mifflin.

Thorndike, R. L., Hagen, E. P., & Sattler, J. M. (1986). *Stanford-Binet Intelligence Scale* (4th ed.). Riverside Publishing.

Tobin, R. M., & Hoff, K. E. (2007). Test review of Bayley Scales of Infant and Toddler Development. In K. F. Geisinger, R. A. Spies, J. F. Carlson, & B. S. Plake (Eds.), *The seventeenth mental measurements yearbook (3rd ed.)*. Retrieved from http://marketplace.unl.edu/buros

Torras-Mañá, M., Gómez-Morales, A., González-Gimeno, I., Fornieles-Deu, A., & Brun-Gasca, C. (2016). Assessment of cognition and language in the early diagnosis of autism spectrum disorder: Usefulness of the Bayley Scales of Infant and Toddler Development (3rd ed.). *Journal of Intellectual Disability Research, 60*(5), 502–511. Retrieved from https://doi.org/10.1111/jir.12291

Torras-Mañá, M., Guillamón-Valenzuela, M., Ramírez-Mallafré, A., Brun-Gasca, C., & Fornieles-Deu, A. (2014). Usefulness of the Bayley Scales of Infant and Toddler Development, Third Edition in the early diagnosis of language disorder. *Psicothema, 26*(3), 349–356. Retrieved from https://doi.org/10.7334/psicothema2014.29

Trohanis, P. L. (2008). Progress in providing services to young children with special needs and their families: An overview to and update on the implementation of the Individuals with Disabilities Education Act (IDEA). *Journal of Early Intervention, 30*(2), 140–151. Retrieved from https://doi.org/10.1177/1053815107312050

Ulrich, D. A. (2000). *Test of Gross Motor Development* (2nd ed.): *Examiner's manual*. Western Psychological Services.

Uzgiris, I. C., & Hunt, J. M. (1975). *Infant Psychological Developmental Scale*. University of Illinois Press.

Velikos, K., Soubasi, V., Michalettou, I., Sarafidis, K., Nakas, C., Papadopoulou, V., Zafeiriou, D., & Drossou, V. (2015). Bayley–III Scales at 12 months of corrected age in preterm infants: Patterns of developmental performance and correlations to environmental and biological influences. *Research in Developmental Disabilities, 45-46*, 110–119. Retrieved from https://doi.org/10.1016/j.ridd.2015.07.014

Venn, J. J. (2007). Test review of Bayley Scales of Infant and Toddler Development–Third Edition. In K. F. Geisinger, R. A. Spies, J. F. Carlson, & B. S. Plake (Eds.), *The seventeenth mental measurements yearbook*. Buros Institute of Mental Measurements. Retrieved from http://marketplace.unl.edu/buros

Vohr, B. R., Stephens, B. E., Higgins, R. D., Bann, C. M., Hintz, S. R., Das, A., Newman, J. E., Peralta-Carcelen, M., Yolton, K., Dusick, A. M., Evans, P. W., Goldstein, R. F., Ehrenkranz, R. A., Pappas, A., Adams-Chapman, I., Wilson-Costello, D. E., Bauer, C. R., Bodnar, A., Heyne, R. J., Vaucher, Y. E., Dillard, R. G., Acarregui, M. J., McGowan, E. C., Myers, G.J., Fuller, J., & Eunice Kennedy Shriver National Institute of Child Health and Human

Development Neonatal Research Network. (2012). Are outcomes of extremely preterm infants improving? Impact of Bayley assessment on outcomes. *The Journal of Pediatrics, 161*(2), 222–228. Retrieved from https://doi.org/10.1016/j.jpeds.2012.01.057

Voress, J. K., Maddox, T., & Hammill, D. D. (2012). *Developmental Assessment of Young Children* (2nd ed.). Pearson.

Vort Corporation (1999). *Hawaii Early Learning Profiles, Strands Preschool Version.* Author.

Wagner, R. K., Torgesen, J. K., & Rashotte, C. A. (1999). *Test of Early Language Development* (3rd ed.). Western Psychological Services.

Walker, H. M., Severson, H. H., & Feil, E. G. (1995). *The Early Screening Project.* Sopris West.

Washington, K., Scott, D. T., Johnson, K. A., Wendel, S., & Hay, A. E. (1998). The Bayley Scales of Infant Development-II and children with developmental delays: A clinical perspective. *Journal of Developmental and Behavioral Pediatrics, 19*(5), 346–349. Retrieved from https://doi.org/10.1097/00004703-199810000-00005

Wechsler, D. (1967). *Wechsler Preschool and Primary Scales of Intelligence.* Psychological Corporation.

Wechsler, D. (1989). *Wechsler Preschool and Primary Scale of Intelligence, Revised.* Psychological Corporation.

Wechsler, D. (2002). *Wechsler Preschool and Primary Scale of Intelligence* (3rd ed.). Psychological Corporation.

Wechsler, D. (2012). *Wechsler Preschool and Primary Scale of Intelligence* (4th ed.). Psychological Corporation.

Weiss, L. G., Oakland, T., & Aylward, G. (2010). *Bayley–III clinical use and interpretation.* Academic Press.

Werner, E., & Kresheck, J. (1983). *Structured Photographic Expressive Language Test: Preschool.* Janelle Publications.

Westby, C. E. (1991). A scale for assessing children's pretend play. In C. E. Schaefer, K. Gitlin, A. Sandgrund, & C. Schaefer (Eds.), *Play diagnosis and assessment* (pp. 131–161). John Wiley & Sons.

Westby, C. E. (2000). A scale for assessing children's play. In K. Gitlin-Weiner, A. Sandgrund, & C. Schaefer (Eds.), *Play diagnosis and assessment* (pp. 15–57). John Wiley & Sons.

Wetherby, A. M., & Prizant, B. M. (2002). *Communication and Symbolic Behavior Scales: Developmental Profile.* Brookes Publishing.

Whatley, J. L. (1987). Bayley Scales of Infant Development. In D. J. Keyser & R. C. Sweetland (Eds.), *Test critiques* (Vol. 6, pp. 38–47). Test Corporation of America.

Wiig, E. H., Secord, W. A., & Semel, E. M. (1992). *Clinical Evaluation of Language Fundamentals, Preschool.* Psychological Corporation.

Wiig, E., Secord, W. A., & Semel, E. M. (2004). *Clinical Evaluation of Language Fundamentals, Preschool* (2nd ed.). Harcourt Assessment.

Wiig, E. H., Secord, W. A., & Semel, E. (2020). . *Clinical Evaluation of Language Fundamentals, Preschool* (3rd ed.): *Manual.* Psychological Corporation.

Williams, K. T. (2007). *Expressive Vocabulary Test (2nd ed.): Manual.* Pearson.

Wirt, R. D., Lachar, D., Klinedinst, J. E., Seat, P. D., & Broen, W. E. (1977). *Multidimensional evaluation of child personality: A manual for the Personality Inventory for Children.* Western Psychological Services.

Wong, V., Hui, L. H., Lee, W. C., Leung, L. S., Ho, P. K., Lau, W. L., Fung, C. W., & Chung, B. (2004). A modified screening tool for autism (Checklist for Autism in Toddlers [CHAT-23]) for Chinese children. *Pediatrics, 114*(2), e166–e176. Retrieved from https://doi.org/10.1542/peds.114.2.e166

Woodcock, R. W., & Johnson, M. B. (1977). *Woodcock-Johnson Psychoeducational Battery.* Teaching Resources Corporation.

Woodcock, R. W., & Johnson, M. B. (1989). *Woodcock-Johnson Psychoeducational Battery, Revised.* Riverside.

Woodcock, R. W., McGrew, K. S., & Mather, N. (2001). *Woodcock–Johnson III.* Riverside.

Zeitlin, S. (1985). *Coping Inventory: A Measure of Adaptive Behavior.* Scholastic Testing Service.

Zeitlin, S., Williamson, G. G., & Szczepanski, M. (1988). *Early Coping Inventory.* Scholastic Testing Service.

Zigler, E. F., & Muenchow, S. (1992). *Head Start: The inside story of America's most successful educational experiment.* Basic Books.

Zimmerman, I. R., Steiner, V. G., & Pond, R. E. (2011). *Preschool Language Scales* (5th ed.): *Manual.* Pearson.

Appendix

INFANT AND TODDLER ASSESSMENTS INCLUDING SCREENING ASSESSMENTS

Summary of Infant and Toddler Assessments Including Screening Assessments.

Assessment Name	Author(s) (Year of Publication)	Age Range	Developmental Domains or Areas Assessed
American Association on Mental Deficiency Adaptive Behavior Scale	Nihira, Foster, Shellhaus, and Leland (1974)	3–69 years	Mental, Emotional, Adaptive Behavior, and Developmental Disabilities
American Association on Mental Deficiency Adaptive Behavior Scale, School Edition	Lambert, Windmiller, Tharinger, and Cole (1981)	3 years, 3 months–17 years 2, months	Mental, Emotional, Adaptive Behavior, and Developmental Disabilities
Achenbach System of Empirically Based Assessment Preschool	Achenbach and Rescorla (2000)	1½–5 years	Competencies, Strengths, Adaptive Functioning, Behavioral, Emotional, and Social Problems
Adaptive Behavior Assessment System	Harrison and Oakland (2015, 2003, 2000)	Birth–89 years, 11 months	Adaptive Skills
Attention Deficit Hyperactivity Disorder Symptom Checklist*	Gadow and Sprafkin (1997)	3–18 years	Peer Conflict, Stimulant Side Effects, ADHD (Inattentive Type, Hyperactive–Impulsive Type, and Combined Type), Oppositional Defiant Disorder

(Continued)

Assessment Name	Author(s) (Year of Publication)	Age Range	Developmental Domains or Areas Assessed
Ages and Stages Questionnaires–3rd Edition (ASQ-3) Ages and Stages Questionnaires Social-Emotional– 2nd Edition (ASQ:SE-2) Ages and Stages Questionnaires, Social–Emotional (ASQ-SE) Ages and Stages Questionnaires (ASQ)–2nd Edition Ages and Stages Questionnaires (ASQ)	ASQ:SE & ASQ:SE-2 – Squires, Bricker, and Twombly (2015, 2002) ASQ & ASQ-3 – Squires and Bricker (2009, 1995) ASQ 2nd Edition – Squires, Potter, and Bricker (1999)	ASQ-3: 1–66 months ASQ:SE-2 : 1–72 months ASQ:SE: 42–53 months ASQ 2nd Edition: 4–60 months ASQ: Birth–48 months	ASQ-3: Communication, Motor (Gross & Fine), Problem Solving, and Personal-Social Skills. ASQ:SE-2: Autonomy, Compliance, Adaptive Functioning, Self-Regulation, Affect, Interaction, and Social-Communication. ASQ:SE: Self-Regulation, Compliance, Communication, Adaptive Behavior, Autonomy, Affect, and Interaction ASQ 2nd Edition: Communication, Motor (Gross & Fine), Problem Solving, and Personal-Social
Arizona Articulation Proficiency Scale*	Fudala and Reynolds (1986)	1 year, 6 months–13 years, 11 months	Articulation
Assessment for Persons Profoundly or Severely Impaired Edition*	Bradley-Johnson, Johnson, Connard, Arick, and Krug (2018)	0–24 months	Alertness, Preferences, Problem-Solving Prerequisites, Communication, and Social–Emotional
Assessment of Children's Language Comprehension*	Foster, Giddan, and Stark (1973)	3–6 years, 5 months	Language
Assessment, Evaluation, and Programming System for Infants and Children*	Bricker, Capt, and Pretti-Frontczak (2002)	Birth–6 years	Motor (Gross & Fine), Adaptive, Cognitive, Social Communication, Social Bibliography

Attention Deficit Disorders Evaluation Scale*	McCarney and Arthaud (2004)	Home version, 3–19 years	ADHD (Inattentive Type, Hyperactive–Impulsive Type, and Combined Type)
Auditory Skills Assessment	Geffner and Goldman (2010)	3 years, 6 months –6 years, 11 months	Speech Discrimination, Phonological Awareness, and Non-speech Processing
Autism Diagnostic Interview*	Rutter, LeCouteur, and Lord (2003)	Mental age of 18 months or higher	Communication, Social Development and Play, Repetitive and Restrictive Behaviors, and General Behavior
Autism Diagnostic Observation Schedule*	Lord, Rutter, DiLavore, Risi, Gotham, Bishop, Luyster, and Guthrie (2012)	12 months to adult	Communication and Social Interaction
Autism Screening Instrument for Educational Planning*	Krug, Arick, and Almond (1993)	18 months– adult	Autism Behavior Checklist, Sample of Vocal Behavior, Interaction Assessment, Educational Assessment, and Prognosis of Learning Rate
Bankson Language Screening Test*	Bankson (1990)	3–7 years	Psycholinguistic Skills
Battelle Developmental Inventory	Newborg (2020, 2004, 1984)	Birth–8 years	2004, 1984 – Cognitive, Personal-Social, Adaptive, Motor, and Communication. 2020 – Cognitive, Adaptive, Communication, Social-Emotional, and Motor
Bayley Infant Neurodevelopmental Screener	Aylward (1995)	3–24 months	Neurological, Receptive, and Expressive Functions, Processing, and Mental Activity

(Continued)

Assessment Name	Author(s) (Year of Publication)	Age Range	Developmental Domains or Areas Assessed
Bayley Scales of Infant and Toddler Development – 4th Edition (Bayley–4) and Bayley–4 Screener Bayley Scales of Infant and Toddler Development – 3rd Edition (Bayley–III) Bayley Scales of Infant Development (BSID)	Bayley and Aylward (2019a) Bayley (2006, 1993, 1969)	BSID–II, Bayley–III & Bayley–4: 1–42 months BSID: 2–30 months	Bayley III, Bayley–4, and Bayley–4 Screener: Cognitive, Language (Receptive & Expressive), Motor (Gross & Fine), Social-Emotional, Adaptive Behavior BSID & BSID–II: Mental, Motor, and Behavior
Behavior Assessment System for Children (BASC)	Reynolds and Kamphaus (2015b, 2004, 1992)	2–21 years, 11 months	Behavior
Beery–Buktenica Developmental Test of Visual-Motor Integration*	Beery, Buktenica, and Beery (2010)	Full form: 2–100 years: Short form: 2–7 years	Visual-Motor Integration
Behavioral Assessment of Baby's Emotional and Social Style	Finello and Poulsen (2018)	Birth–3 years	Social-Emotional
[BASC-2] and [BASC-3] Behavioral and Emotional Screening System	Reynolds and Kamphaus (2015a, 2007a)	3–18 years	Behavior and Emotional Strengths and Weaknesses
Birth to Three Assessment and Intervention System–2nd Edition Birth to Three Assessment and Intervention System	Ammer and Bangs (2000) Bangs (1986)	Birth–3 years	Language Comprehension, Language Expression, Nonverbal Thinking, Social/Personal Development, and Motor Development
Boehm Test of Basic Concepts Preschool Edition*	Boehm (2001)	3–5 years, 11 months	Basic Relationship Concepts of Size, Direction, Position, Time, Quantity, Classification, and General

Bracken Basic Concept Scale (3rd ed.), Receptive and Bracken Basic Concept Scale, Expressive Bracken Basic Concept Scale Revised Bracken Basic Concept Scale	Bracken (2006a,b) Bracken (1998) Bracken (1984)	3 years–6 years 11 months 2 years, 6 months–7 years, 11 months 2 years, 4 months–7 years, 11 months	Language Skills and School Readiness
Bracken School Readiness Assessment*	Bracken (2007)	2 years, 6 months–7 years, 11 months	Colors, Letters, Numbers/Counting, Sizes, Comparisons, and Shapes
Brazelton Neonatal Behavioral Assessment Scale	Als, Tronick, Lester, and Brazelton (1977)	Birth–1 month	Habituation, Orientation, Motor Performance, Range of State, State Regulation, Autonomic Regulation, and Abnormal Reflexes.
Brown Attention-Deficit Disorder Scales	Brown (2018, 2001, 1996)	3–18 years	Executive Functioning
Brigance Screens	Brigance and French (2013) Glascoe (2002) Brigance (1992, 1990, 1985)	Birth–5 years	Language (Receptive & Expressive), Motor (Gross & Fine), Academics/Pre-Academics, Self-Help, Social-Emotional Skills
Brief Infant/Toddler Social Emotional Assessment*	Briggs-Gowan, Irwin, Wachtel, Carter, and Cicchetti (2004)	12–36 months	Identify Social-Emotional/Behavioral Problems and Delays in Competence
Callier-Azusa Scale*	Stillman (1978)	Birth–8 years	Motor, Perceptual, Cognitive, Social, Communication and Language Development, and Daily Living Skills

(Continued)

Assessment Name	Author(s) (Year of Publication)	Age Range	Developmental Domains or Areas Assessed
Caregiver–Teacher Report Form	Achenbach (1997)	1 year, 6 months–5 years	Behavior and Emotional Problems
Carey Temperament Scales*	Carey, McDevitt, Medoff-Cooper, Fullard, and Hegvik (2007)	1 month–the end of the 12th year	Temperament (Activity, Biological Regularity, Adaptability, Approach, Intensity, Mood, Persistence, Distractibility, Sensory Threshold)
Carolina Record of Individual Behavior*	Simeonsson (1979)	Birth–6 years	Sensorimotor
Carrow Elicited Language Inventory	Carrow-Woolfolk (1974)	3–7 years, 11 months	Language Skills
Cattell Infant Intelligence Scale	Cattell (1940)	2–30 months	Cognitive
Checklist for Autism in Toddlers	Baron-Cohen, Allen, and Gleeberg (1992)	18 months (with late rescreening(s) as necessary	Gaze monitoring, Pretend Play, Proto-declarative Pointing
Checklist for Autism in Toddlers	Wong, Hui, Lee, Leung, Ho, Lau, Fung, and Chung (2004)	Mental ages 18–24 months	Gaze monitoring, Pretend Play, Proto-declarative Pointing
Child Development Inventories*	Ireton (1992)	15 months–6 years	Social, Self-Help, Motor (Gross & Fine), Expressive Language, Language Comprehension, Letters, and Numbers
Childhood Autism Rating Scale	Schopler, Bourgondien, Wellman, and Love (2010) Schopler, Reichler, and Renner (1988)	2 years and older	Adaptive Skills, Social and Emotional Functioning

Clinical Assessment of Articulation and Phonology*	Secord and Donohue (2013)	2 years, 6 months–11 years, 11 months	Articulation and Phonology
Cognitive Assessment of Young Children	Langley, Fewell, and Maddox (2010)	2 months–5 years, 11 months	Fine Motor Coordination and Planning, Communication and Play, Memory, Reasoning, Perceptual Development, Processing, Classification and Organization, Concept Development, and Practical Knowledge
Cognitive Abilities Scale*	Bradley-Johnson and Johnson (2001)	3 months–3 years, 11 months	Cognitive
Communication and Symbolic Behavior Scales Developmental Profile	Wetherby and Prizant (2002)	Functional communication age of 6–24 months (chronological age from about 6 months to 6 years)	Communication and Language
Conners Early Childhood	Conners (2009)	2–6 years	Attention and Hyperactivity
Coping Inventory: A Measure of Adaptive Behavior	Zeitlin (1985)	3–16 years	Adaptive Behavior
Clinical Adaptive Test/Clinical Linguistic Auditory Milestone Scale*	Capute and Accardo (1996)	Birth–36 months	Language, Problem Solving, and Visual-Motor Skills.
Clinical Evaluation of Language Fundamentals Preschool	Wiig, Secord, and Semel (2020, 2004, 1992)	3–6 years, 11 months	Language Skills

(Continued)

Assessment Name	Author(s) (Year of Publication)	Age Range	Developmental Domains or Areas Assessed
Denver Developmental Screening Test	Frankenburg, Dodds, Archer, and Bresnick (1990) Frankenburg, Fandel, Sciarillo, and Burgess (1981) Frankenburg, Goldstein, and Camp (1971) Frankenburg and Dodds (1967)	Birth–6 years	Gross Motor, Language, Fine Motor-Adaptive, Personal-Social, and Behavior.
Detroit Tests of Learning Aptitude – Primary*	Hammill and Bryant (2005, 1991)	3–9 years	Cognitive, Language, Attention, and Motor Abilities
Developmental Activities Screening Inventory*	Fewell and Langley (1984)	Birth–5 years	Perceptual, Motor, and Cognitive Skills
Developmental Assessment for Individuals with Severe Disabilities*	Dykes and Mruzek (2012)	6 months–adulthood	Sensory-Motor, Language, Social-Emotional, Activities, and Academics
Developmental Assessment of Young Children*	Voress, Maddoc, and Hammill (2012)	Birth–5 years	Cognitive, Communication, Social-Emotional Development, Physical Development, and Adaptive Behavior
Developmental Indicators for the Assessment of Learning	Mardell and Goldenberg (2011) Mardell-Czudnowski and Goldenberg (1998, 1990, 1983)	2 years, 6 months–5 years, 11 months	Visual, Motor, Quantitative Concepts, Language, Self-Help, Personal Information, and Social-Emotional Skills

Developmental Programming for Infants and Young Children*	Schafer and Moersch (1981)	0–36 months	Visual-Fine Motor Development
Developmental Profile*	Alpern (2020) Alpern, Boll, and Shearer (2007, 1986)	Birth–21 years, 11 months DP-II – Birth–9 years, 5 months	Physical, Adaptive Behavior, Social-Emotional, Cognitive, and Communication
Developmenal Test of Visual Motor Integration* (3rd rev.)	Beery (1989)	2–15 years	Visual-Motor
Devereux Early Childhood Assessment–Clinical Form	LeBuffe and Naglieri (2002, 1999)	2–5 years, 11 months	Initiative, Self-Control, and Attachment
Differential Ability Scales	Elliott (2007, 1990)	2 years, 6 months–17 years, 11 months	Cognitive Abilities
Dynamic Indicators of Basic Early Literacy Education*	Good and Kaminski (2002)	Grades K–3	Initial Sound Fluency, Letter Naming Fluency, Phoneme Segmentation Fluency, Nonsense Word Fluency, Oral Reading Fluency, Oral Retelling Fluency, Word Use Fluency
Early Childhood Inventory*	Gadow and Sprafkin (2014, 2010, 2000)	3–5 years	Emotional and Behavior Disorders
Early Coping Inventory	Zeitlin, Williamson, and Szczepanski (1988)	4–36 months	Sensorimotor Organization, Reactive Behaviors, Self-Initiated Behaviors

(Continued)

Assessment Name	Author(s) (Year of Publication)	Age Range	Developmental Domains or Areas Assessed
Early Functional Communication Profile	Jensen (2012)	2–10 years	Joint Attention, Social Interaction, Communicative Intent, Social Interaction
Early Screening Inventory Early Screening Inventory–Kindergarten (ESI-K) Early Screening Inventory–Preschool (ESI-P) Early Screening Inventory–Revised (ESI-R)	Meisels and Marsden (2019) Meisels, Marsden, Wiske, and Henderson (1997)	ESI-P: 3–4 years, 5 months ESI-K: 4 years, 6 months–5 years, 11 months ESI-R: 3–6 years; Preschool version 3–4½ years	Visual Motor/Adaptive, Language and Cognition, and Gross Motor Skills.
Early Screening Project	Walker, Seversen, and Feil (1995)	3–5 years	Social-Emotional
Early Screening Profiles	Harrison, A. Kaufman, N. Kaufman, Bruininks, Rynders, Ilmer, Sparrow, and Cicchetti (1990)	2–6 years, 11 months	Cognitive/Language Profile, Motor Profile, Self-Help/Social Profile, Articulation Survey, Home Survey and Health History Survey, and Behavior Survey
Expressive One-Word Picture Vocabulary Test*	Gardner (1990)	2 years, 11 months–11 years, 11 months	Vocabulary, Auditory Processing, and Auditory Visual-Verbal Association

Expressive Vocabulary Test*	Williams (2007)	2 years, 6 months–90+ years	Vocabulary Acquisition
Evaluating Acquired Skills in Communication*	Marcott (2009)	3 months–6 years	Prelinguistic Skills, Semantics, Syntax, Morphology, Pragmatics
Eyberg Child Behavior Inventory and the Sutter-Eyberg Student Behavior Inventory	Eyberg and Pincus (1999)	2–16 years	Conduct
First STEP: Screening Test for Evaluating Preschoolers	Miller (1993)	2 years, 9 months–6 years, 2 months	Cognition, Communication, Motor, Social-Emotional, Adaptive Behavior
Fluharty Preschool Speech and Language Screening Test*	Fluharty (2000)	3–6 years, 11 months	Articulation and Language (Receptive, Expressive, and Composite)
Functional Emotional Assessment Scale	Greenspan, DeGangi, and Wieder (2001)	7 months–48 months	Emotional Functioning
Gesell Developmental Schedules	Knobloch, Stevens, and Malone (1980) Gesell and Amatruda (1941) Gesell (1925b)	Revised: 1 week–36 months Original: 4–60 months	Adaptive, Motor (Gross & Fine), Language, and Personal-Social
Gesell School Readiness Test	Ilg and Ames (1972)	2 years, 6 months–6 years, 11 months	Adaptive and Language Development

(Continued)

Assessment Name	Author(s) (Year of Publication)	Age Range	Developmental Domains or Areas Assessed
Gilliam Asperger's Disorder Scale	Gilliam (2001)	3–22 years	Social Interaction, Restricted Patterns, Cognitive Patterns, and Pragmatic Skills.
Gilliam Autism Rating Scale*	Gilliam (2005)	3–22 years	Stereotyped Behaviors, Communication, and Social Interaction
Goldman-Fristoe Test of Articulation*	Goldman and Fristoe (2000)	2–21 years	Consonant Phonemes
Greenspan Social-Emotional Growth Chart	Greenspan (2004)	Birth–42 months	Social -Emotional
Griffiths Developmental Scale*	Griffiths (1967)	1–60 months	Locomotor, Hearing and Speech, Eye and Hand Coordination, Performance, Practical Reasoning, and Personal-Social
Hawaii Early Learning Profiles, Strands Preschool Version	Vort Corporation (1999)	3–6 years	Attachment, Separation, Autonomy
Hiskey-Nebraska Test of Learning Aptitude	Hiskey (1966)	3–16 years, 6 months	Visual Attention, Memory, Classification, Spatial Reasoning, and Eye-Hand Coordination
Howes Peer Play Scale	Howes and Matheson (1992)	Toddler–59 months	Parallel Play, Parallel Aware Play, Simple Social Play, Complementary and Reciprocal Play, and Complex Social Pretend Play
Infant Development Inventory	Ireton (2006, 1994)	Birth–18 months	Cognitive, Language Motor, Social-Emotional Skills, and Adaptive functioning

Infant Psychological Development Scale	Uzgiris and Hunt (1975)	2 weeks–2 years	Object Permanence, Use of Objects as Means, Learning and Foresight, Development of Schemata, Development of an Understanding of Causality, Conception of Objects in Space, Vocal Imitation, and Gestural Imitation
Infant-Toddler and Family Instrument	Apfel and Provence (2001)	6–36 months	Motor (Gross & Fine) Social-Emotional, Language, Coping, and Self-Help
Infant-Toddler Developmental Assessment*	Provence, Erikson, Vater, Palmeri, Pruett, and Rosinia (2016)	Birth–36 months	Motor (Gross & Fine), Relationship to Inanimate Objects/Cognition, Language/Communication, Self-Help/Adaptive, Relationship to Persons, Emotions and Feeling States, and Coping Behavior
Infant-Toddler Social and Emotional Assessment; Brief Infant-Toddler Social and Emotional Assessment	Carter and Briggs-Gowan (2004); Briggs-Gowan and Carter (1998)	12–36 months	Social-Emotional
Infant-Toddler Symptom Checklist	DeGangi, Poisson, Sickel, and Wiener (1995)	7–30 months	Self-Regulation, Attention, Sleep, Eating/Feeding, Dressing, Bathing and Touch, Movement, Listening and Language, Looking and Sight, and Attachment/Emotional Functioning

(Continued)

Assessment Name	Author(s) (Year of Publication)	Age Range	Developmental Domains or Areas Assessed
Iowa Tests of Basic Skills*	Hoover, Hieronymous, Frisbie, and Dunba (1996)	Grades K–8	Cognitive and Language Development
Kaufman Assessment Battery for Children	Kaufman and Kaufman (2018, 2004, 1983)	3–18 years	Cognitive Abilities
Kaufman Speech Praxis Test for Children*	Kaufman (1995)	24–72 months	Speech and Language
Kaufman Survey of Early Academic and Language Skills	Kaufman and Kaufman (1993)	3–6 years, 11 months	Language Skills, Pre-Academic Skills, and Articulation
Kent Inventory of Developmental Skills*	Reuter, Katoff, and Gruber (2000)	Birth–15 months or up to age 6 when severe developmental disabilities are present	Cognitive, Motor, Communication, Self-Help, and Social Skills
Khan-Lewis Phonological Analysis*	Lewis and Khan (2002)	2–21 years, 11 months	Reduction Processes, Place and Manner Processes, and Voicing Processes
Learning Accomplishment Profile-Diagnostic Standardized Assessment	Nehring, A., Nehring, E. Bruni, and Randolph (1992)	30–72 months	Fine Motor Manipulation, Fine Motor Writing, Cognitive Matching, Cognitive Counting, Language Naming, Language Comprehension, Gross Motor Body Movement, and Gross Motor Object Movement

Leiter International Performance Scale*	Roid and Miller (2013, 1997)	2– 20 years, 11 months	Reasoning, Visualization, Memory, and Attention
MacArthur Story Stem Battery	Emde, Wolf, and Oppenheim (2003)	3–7 years	Attachment, Response to Authority, Response to Family Conflict, Response to Getting Caught Doing a Transgression, and Separation Anxiety
McCarthy Scales of Children's Abilities	McCarthy (1972)	2 years, 6 months–8 years, 6 months	Cognitive and Motor Behaviors
Meadow/Kendall Social-Emotional Assessment Inventories for Deaf and Hearing-Impaired Students Preschool Form	Meadow (1983)	3–6 years, 11 months	Communication
Mental Health Screening Tool	California Institute for Mental Health (2000)	Birth–5 years	Social-Emotional
Merrill-Palmer–Revised Scales of Development*	Roid and Sampers (2004)	1 month–6 years, 6 months	Cognitive, Language, Motor (Fine & Gross), Social-Emotional, Self-Help, and Adaptive Skills
Metropolitan Readiness Test*	Nurss and McGaurvan (1995)	Pre-K–Grade 1	Basic and Advanced Language and Mathematics Skills
Milani-Comparetti Neurodevelopmental Screening Examination*	Milani-Comparetti and Gidono (1967)	Birth–24 months	Neuromotor Function
Miller Assessment for Preschoolers*	Miller (1988)	2 years, 9 months–5 years, 8 months	Motor, Language, and Cognition
Modified Checklist for Autism in Toddlers*	Robbins, Fein, Barton, and Green (1999)	16–30 months	Proto-declarative Pointing, Gaze Monitoring, and Pretend Play

(Continued)

Assessment Name	Author(s) (Year of Publication)	Age Range	Developmental Domains or Areas Assessed
Mullen Scales of Early Learning: AGS Edition	Mullen (1995)	Birth–68 months	Gross Motor (birth to 33 months only), Fine Motor, Visual Reception, Receptive Language, and Expressive Language
NEPSY	Korkman, Kirk, and Kemp (2007, 1998)	3–16 years, 11 months	Executive Functioning/Attention, Language, Memory/Learning, Sensorimotor Functioning, Visuospatial Processing, and Social Perception
Northwestern Syntax Screening Test*	Lee (1971)	3–7 years, 11 months	Identify Language Deficiencies
Oral and Written Language Scales*	Carrow-Woolfolk (2011)	3–21 years, 11 months	Lexical/Semantics, Syntax, Pragmatics, Supralinguistics
Ostrov Early Childhood Play Project Observation System	Ostrov (2005)	36 months–6 years	Aggressive Behavior and Play Behavior
Parent Interview for Autism*	Stone and Hogan (1993)	Preschool level and below	Communication, Language, Social Relating, Affective Responses, Sensory, Motor, Play, and Behavior Skills, and Need for Sameness
Parents' Evaluations of Developmental Status*	Glascoe (2012)	Birth–8 years	Language, Motor, Self-Help, Early Academic Skills, and Behavior and Social-Emotional/ Mental Health
Peabody Developmental Motor Scales*	Folio and Fewell (2000)	Birth–5 years	Reflexes, Stationary, Locomotion, Object Manipulation, Grasping, and Visual-Motor Integration

Peabody Picture Vocabulary Test*	Dunn (2018)	2 years, 6 months–90+ years	Receptive and Expressive Vocabulary Acquisition
Penn Interactive Peer Play Scale	Fantuzzo, Coolahan, Mendez, McDermott, and Sutton-Smith (1998)	Preschool Children	Play Interaction, Play Disruption, and Play Disconnection
Personality Inventory for Children*	Wirt, Lachar, Klinedinst, Seat, and Broen (1977)	3–16 years	Social-Emotional Adjustment
Pervasive Developmental Disorders Screening Test*	Siegel (2004)	12–48 months	Behavior Development
Photo Articulation Test*	Pendergast (1969)	3–12 years	Speech Analysis
Photo Articulation Test	Lippke, Dickey, Selmar, and Soder (1997)	3–8 years, 11 months	Speech Analysis
Preschool and Kindergarten Behavior Scales	Merrell (2003, 1994)	3–6 years	Social Skills and Problem Behavior (Externalizing & Internalizing)
Preschool Behavior Checklist	McGuire and Richman (1988)	2–5 years, 11 months	Behavior and Emotional Difficulties
Preschool Behavior Questionnaire	Behar and Stringfield (1974)	3–6 years	Emotional Problems
Preschool Child Observation Record*	HighScope Educational Research Foundation (2003)	2½-6 years	Initiative, Social Relations, Creative Representation, Movement and Music, Language and Literacy, and Mathematics and Science

(Continued)

Assessment Name	Author(s) (Year of Publication)	Age Range	Developmental Domains or Areas Assessed
Preschool Developmental Inventory *	Ireton (1988)	3–5 years, 5 months	Language, Motor Self-Help, Personal, and Social
Preschool Language Assessment Instrument*	Blank, Rose, and Berlin (2003)	3–5 years, 11 months	Matching, Analysis, Reordering, Reasoning, Receptive Mode, and Expressive Mode
Preschool Language Scale *	Zimmerman, Stelner, and Pond (2011)	Birth–7 years, 11 months	Total Language, Auditory Comprehension, Expressive Communication
Pre-Literacy Skills Screening	Crumrine and Lonegan (1999)	3–5 years, 11 months	Letter Knowledge and Phonological Awareness
Primary Test of Nonverbal Intelligence	Ehrler and McGhee (2008)	3–9 years, 11 months	Cognitive Skills
Psychoeducational Profile: TEACCH Individualized Psychoeducational Assessment for Children with Autism Spectrum Disorders *	Schopler, Lansing, Reichler, and Marcus (2005)	2–7 years, 6 months, or children functioning within this age range	Education Planning and ASD Diagnosis
Receptive One-Word Picture Vocabulary Test*	Gardner (1985)	2–11 years, 11 months	Receptive and Expressive Vocabulary Skills
Receptive Expressive Emergent Language Test*	Bzoch, League, and Brown (2020, 2003) Bzoch and League (1991)	Birth–3 years	Receptive and Expressive Language

Reynell Developmental Language Scales *	Reynell and Gruber (1990)	1–6 years	Expressive Language and Verbal Comprehension
Reynell-Zinkin Scales*	Reynell and Zinkin (1979)	Birth–4 years	Social Adaptation, Sensorimotor, Exploration of Environment, Response to Sound/Verbal Comprehension, Expressive Language and Nonverbal Communication
Scales of Independent Behavior	Bruininks, Woodcock, Weatherman, and Hill (1996, 1984)	Birth–80+ years	Motor, Social/Communication, Personal Independence, and Community
Screening Tool for Autism in Two-Year-Olds	Stone, Coonrod, and Ousley (2000)	24–35 months	Play, Imitation, Directing Attention, and (not scored) Response to Requests
Sensory Processing Measure Preschool*	Parham and Ecker (2010)	2–5 years	Social Participation, Vision, Hearing, Touch, Body Awareness, Balance and Motion, Planning and Ideas, and Total Sensory Systems
Sequenced Inventory of Communication Development	Hedrick, Prather, and Tobin (1984, 1975)	4–48 months	Communication Skills (Receptive and Expressive)
Smith–Johnson Nonverbal Performance Scale	Smith and Johnson (1977)	2–4 years	Cognitive Skills
Social Communication Questionnaire*	Rutter, Bailey, and Lord (2003)	4 months–0 years; minimum mental age of 2 months–0 years	Social Development and Play, Communication, and Repetitive and Restrictive Behavior

(Continued)

Assessment Name	Author(s) (Year of Publication)	Age Range	Developmental Domains or Areas Assessed
Social Competence and Behavior Evaluation Preschool*	LaFreniere and Dumas (1995)	30–76 months	Social Skills
Social Responsiveness Scale	Constantino and Gruber (2012)	2 years, 6 months–18 years	Social (Awareness, Cognition, Communication, Motivation), Restricted Interests and Repetitive Behavior
Social Skills Improvement System Rating Scales	Gresham and Elliot (2008)	3–18 years	Communication, Engagement, Bullying, and Autism Spectrum
Social Skills Rating System	Gresham and Elliot (1990)	3–18 years	Social Skills, Problem Behavior (Externalizing & Internalizing), Hyperactivity, and Academic Competence
Stanford-Binet Intelligence Scale(s)	Roid (2005) Thorndike, Hagen, and Sattler (1986) Terman and Merrill (1973, 1960, 1937) Terman (1916)	2–90 years 2–24 years 1 year, 6 months – 18 years 3–14 years	Cognitive Abilities
Strengths and Difficulties Questionnaire	Goodman (1997)	3–16 years	Emotional Symptoms, Conduct Problems, Hyperactivity/Inattention, Peer Relationship Problems, and Prosocial Behavior
Structured Photographic Expressive Language Test*	Werner and Kresheck (1983)	3–5 years, 11 months	Diagnose Language Impairment
Stuttering Severity Instrument*	Riley and Bakker (2009)	2–10 years and older	Speech Development

Symbolic Play Scale	Westby (2000, 1991)	8 months–5 years (and older children with learning problems)	Decontextualization, Thematic Content, Organization, Self-Other Relations, and Language
Symbolic Play Test*	Lowe and Costello (1988)	12–36 months	Cognitive and Expressive Language
Temperament and Atypical Behavior Scale	Neisworth, Bagnato, Salvia, and Hunt (1999)	11–71 months	Atypical Self-Regulatory Behavior
Test for Auditory Comprehension of Language*	Carrow-Woolfolk (1985)	3–10 years	Receptive Spoken Vocabulary, Grammar, and Syntax
Test Observation Form	McConaughy and Achenbach (2004)	2–18 years	Behavior, Affect, and Test-Taking Style During Testing Sessions
Test of Early Communication and Emerging Language	Huer and Miller (2011)	2 weeks–24 months or older if the child has moderate to severe language delays	Receptive and Expressive Language
Test of Early Language Development*	Hresko, Reid, and Hammill (2018, 1999, 1991)	3–7 years, 11 months 2–7 years, 11 months	Language

(Continued)

Assessment Name	Author(s) (Year of Publication)	Age Range	Developmental Domains or Areas Assessed
Test of Early Mathematics Ability*	Ginsburg and Baroody (2003)	3–8 years, 11 months	Numbering Skills, Number-Comparison Facility, Numeral Literacy, Mastery of Number Facts, Calculation Skills, and Understanding of Concepts
Test of Early Reading Ability–Deaf or Hard of Hearing	Reid, Hresko, Hammill, and Wiltshire (1991)	3–13 years, 11 months	Early Reading
Test of Early Reading Ability*	Reid, Hresko, Hammill, and Wiltshire(2001)	3 years, 6 months–8 years, 6 months	Alphabet, Conventions, and Meaning
Test of Gross Motor Development*	Ulrich (2000)	3 years–10 years, 11 months	Gross Motor Skill Development
Test of Irregular Word Reading Efficiency*	Reynolds and Kamphaus (2007b)	3–94 years	Reading Comprehension
Test of Visual-Motor Skills	Gardner (1995)	2–13 years	Visual-Motor Integration
Test of Visual-Motor Skills	Martin (2010)	3–90 years	Visual Perception, Motor Planning, and/or Execution
The Ounce Scale	Meisels, Marsden, Dombro, Weston, and Jewkes (2003)	Birth–3½ years	Personal Connections, Feelings About Self, Relationships with Other Children, Understanding and Communication, Exploration and Problem Solving, and Movement and Coordination

The Temperament Assessment Battery for Children	Martin (1988)	3–7 years	Activity, Adaptability, Approach/Withdrawal, Emotional Intensity, Distractibility, and Persistence
Token Test for Children*	McGhee, Ehrler, and DiSimoni (2007)	3–12 years, 11 months	Receptive Language
Transdisciplinary Play-Based Assessment*	Linder (2008)	Infancy–6 years	Cognitive Abilities, Social-Emotional Functioning, Communication and Language Skills, and Sensory-Motor Development
Verbal Behavior Milestones Assessment and Placement Program*	Sundberg (2014)	Birth–48 months	Language and Social Skills
Vineland Adaptive Behavior Scales	Sparrow, Balla, and Cicchetti (2005, 1984) Sparrow, Cicchetti, and Saulnier (2016)	Birth–19 years	Communication, Daily Living Skills, Socialization, and Motor Skills
Vineland Social–Emotional Early Childhood Scales	Sparrow, Balla, and Cicchetti (1998)	Birth–72 months	Social and Emotional Functioning
Wechsler Preschool and Primary Scale of Intelligence (WPPSI)	Wechsler (2012, 2002, 1989, 1967)	WPPSI I-III: 2 years, 6 months–7 years, 3 months WPPSI-IV: 2 years, 6 months–7 years, 7 months	Cognitive Ability

(Continued)

Assessment Name	Author(s) (Year of Publication)	Age Range	Developmental Domains or Areas Assessed
Woodcock-Johnson	Schrank, McGrew, and Mather (2014) Woodcock, McGrew, and Mather (2001) Woodcock and Johnson (1989, 1977)	2–90 years 3–80 years (1977)	Academic Achievement, Oral Language, Scholastic Aptitude, and Overall Cognitive Skills
Work Sampling System*	Meisels, Jablon, Dichtelmiller, Dorfman, and Marsden (2001)	Grades Pre-K – 6	Art and Fine Motor, Movement and Gross Motor, Concept and Number, Language and Literacy, and Personal and Social Development

Note: Although many assessments and screening assessments have been revised one or more times, we did not write "revised" or "2nd edition," for example, for ease of reading unless required for clarity * = There are multiple editions of this assessment, but space limitations precluded listing all of them except for some of the most popular assessments (e.g., WPPSI).

NOTES

1 The Centers for Disease Control and Prevention consider infants to be between 0 and 12 months, toddlers to be between 12 and 36 months, and preschoolers between 36 and 60 months. Retrieved from: https://www.cdc.gov/ncbddd/childdevelopment/positiveparenting/index.html.

2 Retrieved from: https://www.acf.hhs.gov/ohs/about/history-head-start and https://eclkc.ohs.acf.hhs.gov/about-us/article/head-start-timeline.

3 Sources for this section include the following: https://www.pearsonassessments.com/professional-assessments/products/authors/bayley-nancy.html; https://psychology.jrank.org/pages/65/Nancy-Bayley.html; http://psychology.iresearchnet.com/developmental-psychology/history-of-developmental-psychology/nancy-bayley; https://psychology.jrank.org/pages/65/Nancy-Bayley.html.

4 "An unpublished 1958 version of the BSID covered the first 15 months of life and was employed in a research program sponsored by the National Institute of Neurological Diseases and Blindness" (Whatley, 1987, p. 38).

Two

HOW TO ADMINISTER THE BAYLEY–4

Vincent C. Alfonso, Joseph R. Engler, and Andrea D. Turner
Gonzaga University and Pearson Assessments

The *Bayley Scales of Infant and Toddler Development–Fourth Edition* (Bayley–4; Bayley & Aylward, 2019a) is a standardized, norm-referenced assessment that requires practitioners to follow the administration procedures outlined in the Bayley–4 Administration Manual (Bayley & Aylward, 2019b). When administering the Bayley–4, as with any assessment, practitioners must be sure to know as much as possible about the examinee, the referral question(s), and the goals of assessment (Alfonso et al., 2020; Black & Matula, 2000). As discussed throughout this chapter, there are many considerations for administration of the Bayley–4, all of which require practitioners to have a thorough understanding of the challenges in assessing infants and toddlers (e.g., mood variability, shorter attention span, limited language skills). These considerations include building rapport with infants and toddlers and their caregivers, experiencing assessments with infants and toddlers, and an understanding of typical infant and toddler development (Bayley & Aylward, 2019b).

PREPARATION FOR DEVELOPMENTAL ASSESSMENT

Practitioner Preparation

Practitioners can never be too prepared for assessing infants and toddlers. It is imperative that practitioners become familiar with the Bayley–4 standard administration procedures, test items, and materials (e.g., Record Form, manipulatives). This typically requires hours of studying the manuals and practicing the test items and materials. The most qualified practitioners should not only study the manuals, test items, and materials extensively, but should also seek training opportunities with professional colleagues, practice test administrations with typically developing young children, and receive supervision from qualified professionals during initial administrations of the Bayley–4 to infants and toddlers in a clinical or research setting. In addition, practitioners should be aware of ethical considerations when assessing young children such as test security (see Rapid Reference 2.1).

≡ *Rapid Reference 2.1*

Ethical Considerations When Assessing Young Children

Test users have an obligation to protect test security and follow guidelines for appropriate test use (American Educational Research Association et al., 2014). The following is a partial list of the guidelines for practitioners to follow when using the Bayley–4.

- Practitioners must follow their professional ethical guidelines regarding test use and security and during testing administration and interactions with the caregiver and child.
- Per the Bayley–4 Administration Manual, "the Bayley–4 should only be administered by practitioners with graduate-level or professional training and experience in the administration and interpretation of standardized clinical instruments" (Bayley & Aylward, 2019b, p. 7).
- Bayley–4 administration and scoring of responses can be completed by a trained technician or research assistant under supervision; however, graduate-level or professional training in assessment is required of the person who will be interpreting the test results.
- Practitioners should refrain from testing children whose demographic, cultural, educational, clinical, or medical histories differ greatly from the children with whom the practitioner has testing experience and/or training. Practitioners are encouraged to seek supervision and/or consultation for cases that are outside of their area of expertise if there is not an option for another practitioner to conduct testing for the child (e.g., in underserved areas where another professional may be many miles away or cost-prohibitive).
- Practitioners are responsible for ensuring that test materials are kept secure and are not shared with people other than qualified professionals. Caregivers of the child being assessed have the right to test results and may be given copies of summaries or diagnostic reports that include information about test results; however, copyrighted test materials (e.g., item content, protocols) should not be shared, as this compromises the validity of the Bayley–4.

(Continued)

- If the Bayley–4 is involved in litigation, review of the test should be limited (as permitted by law) to those who are legally or ethically bound to protect test security.
- Information about the Bayley–4 should not be shared with unqualified professionals in any form. Bayley–4 users must exercise caution even when providing professional training, whether live, audio, or video, to safeguard test information as much as possible.
- It is prohibited for materials to be presented in a way that unqualified professionals or the general public may purchase or view partial or complete portions of the test. Pictures, slide shows, videos, or any other representation of Bayley–4 content on personal or educational Internet websites, social media video sharing platforms, and auction sites is prohibited.
- NCS Pearson, Inc. owns the copyright to all Bayley–4 test items, norms, and other testing materials and must approve in writing the copying or reproduction of any test materials.

The above user responsibilities, copyright restrictions, and test security issues are delineated in the Bayley–4 Administration Manual (Bayley & Aylward, 2019b) and/or are stated or consistent within the guidelines detailed in the *Standards for Educational and Psychological Testing* (Standards; American Educational Research Association et al., 2014). This is not an exhaustive list of the guidelines practitioners are obligated to follow for testing, and practitioners should be familiar with the *Standards* prior to Bayley–4 use.

Rapid Reference 2.2 lists several practitioner preparation tips that may be useful prior to a testing session. Furthermore, a good understanding of typical infant and toddler development and behavior is also necessary to prepare fully for Bayley–4 administration.

≡ *Rapid Reference 2.2*

Practitioner Preparation Tips

Before the testing session, practitioners must take care to prepare themselves for the test administration. The practitioner may benefit from awareness of the following tips.

- Anything that may affect the practitioner's mood state should be attended to before the testing session, as patience and calmness are required for testing infants and toddlers. Practitioners should take care to:
  - have an appropriate amount of sleep for optimal functioning,
  - take any prescribed medications as directed,

(Continued)

- attend to other needs such as eating and hydration,
- be aware of their own negative mood states, as a young child will be less likely to cooperate and may even begin to show irritation or shut down completely if they feel pressured, rushed, or pick up on negative cues from the practitioner, which compromises the testing results,
- take a break to engage in deep breathing or other brief self-care activity if feeling restless or hurried or having a bad day.
- As many items may require sitting on the floor, moving from the floor to a seated position, and demonstrating gross motor items, comfortable clothing that allows for bending, stooping, and crawling around on the floor is recommended.
- Appropriate footwear should be considered, as practitioners should be comfortable, but also because crawling on the floor can scuff the toes of shoes over time.
- Practitioners should consider removing or hiding jewelry items that could be easily grabbed or distracting to the child, and in some instances could cause injury to the practitioner or child.
- Practitioners should also be aware of the possibility that young children may grab at eyewear.

Test Material Preparation

Before each test administration, the practitioner should ensure that all test materials are accounted for and inspected so that nothing poses a safety risk to the young child, such as loose or broken manipulatives. The Bayley–4 test materials and the testing environment (e.g., small table, mats) must be thoroughly cleaned and sanitized after each administration as recommended by the Centers for Disease Control and Prevention (CDC; cdc.gov). Finally, food pellets used during the test administration should be replaced after each session (Bayley & Aylward, 2019b). Following these recommendations sets the stage for a safe and efficient test administration.

Testing Environment Preparation

For reliable and valid assessment results, the practitioner must establish and maintain an environment conducive to a positive experience. The testing room should be quiet, comfortable, and well-lit (Black & Matula, 2000). In addition, loud noises and potentially distracting visual stimuli (e.g., bright lights, toys, bright wall coverings or pictures, or unusual furniture or equipment) should be avoided to prevent distracting the child. The testing area must be large enough to accommodate the child's gross motor skills, such as crawling, walking, running, and jumping (Bayley & Aylward, 2019b; Black & Matula, 2000). Rapid Reference 2.3 lists materials that need to be provided by the practitioner.

≋ *Rapid Reference 2.3*

Materials Provided by the Practitioner

- Blue tape to secure stepping path
- Facial tissue
- Food pellets (Cheerios® or other ½ inch diameter snack that will not stick to the child's hands, is caregiver-approved, and to which the child has no allergies or sensitivities)
- Object to hide practitioner's entire head (e.g., large clipboard, binder, notepad, blanket)
- Several sheets of 8.5 × 11 inch blank white paper
- Standard stairs (three steps that are 6½ inches high and 10 inches deep, with a width of at least 24 inches; stairs with a handrail or next to a wall are preferred to provide support to the child as needed)
- Stopwatch

Source: Bayley and Aylward (2019b)

Bayley–4 administration typically includes the child, the caregiver, and the practitioner. No more than three adults (including the practitioner) should be present during the assessment and the presence of other children should be avoided, if possible (Bayley & Aylward, 2019b). The presence of a caregiver is important for keeping the child comfortable and calm and for meeting the child's needs as they arise during testing (e.g., providing a snack when hungry, changing a diaper, consoling when upset). In addition, the presence of the caregiver is invaluable for obtaining valid assessment results via Caregiver Questions that give information about the child's typical behavior when needed throughout the administration and to assist the practitioner with administering items (Bayley & Aylward, 2019b, 2019c).

Appropriate seating is needed for the child, caregiver, and practitioner. A small table and at least two chairs should be in the testing room for administration of items requiring a flat surface. The table and chairs should be comfortable and at an appropriate height for most young children. The seating arrangement should be conducive to efficient test administration and minimize the need for locating materials. The practitioner typically sits across from the child, but may need to sit behind or to the side of the child for items that require the practitioner be out of the child's line of sight. The seating arrangement is flexible such that any arrangement is acceptable if it is conducive to the child completing items and does not present a distraction or compromise focus (Bayley & Aylward, 2019b). Practitioners should review the Materials Setup or Examiner/Caregiver Position sections in the Bayley–4 Administration Manual for illustrations regarding the optimal position of the practitioner or caregiver in relation to the child (Bayley & Aylward, 2019b).

Infant or Toddler and Caregiver Preparation

The infant or toddler should be accompanied to the assessment by a caregiver who knows the child well. The practitioner should explain to the caregiver what to expect during testing, emphasizing that a variety of different tasks will be presented, including some that will be easy for the child and others that will be hard. The practitioner should ask the caregiver to refrain from rephrasing the instructions, giving additional help to the child, or prompting or intervening in other ways unless otherwise instructed. Reassuring the caregiver that the practitioner will make it clear when to intervene assists in building rapport and may help the caregiver feel more relaxed about the testing session (Bayley & Aylward, 2019b).

Caregivers should prepare themselves and the child for testing (e.g., adequate sleep the night before). The practitioner and caregiver should find a testing time that best suits the child's needs, such as when the child is typically alert and content, and avoiding regular feeding and nap times that may lead the child to be uncooperative or irritable during test administration. If the child or caregiver is sick, the testing session should be rescheduled. In order for caregivers to prepare best for test administration, they should be given reasonable expectations for how long the assessment will take, with extra time added on to the average administration time for the child's age to account for any delays in getting started, breaks to meet the child's or caregiver's needs, or to account for a child who may take longer than average to complete the test. Such preparation may include ensuring that caregivers have food or drink if the child becomes hungry or thirsty and that there are supplies (e.g., diapers, wet wipes) available for children who are not yet toilet trained. Taking the necessary time to prepare the infant or toddler and caregiver ensures that rapport is established among all parties and increases the validity of the test results (Aylward 2020a; Bayley & Aylward, 2019b; Black & Matula, 2000). Rapid Reference 2.4 provides examples of how to establish rapport with young children and caregivers. Rapid Reference 2.5 provides helpful tips for a valid Bayley–4 assessment.

≡ *Rapid Reference 2.4*

Tips for Establishing Rapport with Young Children and Caregivers

Tips for Rapport with Young Children

Building rapport with the infant or toddler eases the anxiety of the child and caregiver and sets the stage for a positive assessment that will yield valid testing results (Bayley & Aylward, 2019b). Some tips are now given for establishing and maintaining rapport with a young child.

- The practitioner should work to maintain an easy, calm, and soothing manner with the child, including using a soothing and encouraging voice and making frequent eye contact (Aylward, 2020a).
- A playful approach to the item presentation may encourage engagement from the child (Bayley & Aylward, 2019b).
- Anxious or shy children can sometimes be wary of people who express too much excitement and movement until they become more familiar with their environment. It is best to introduce yourself to the caregiver and infant and take some time to observe the infant's behavior and mood before determining the best way to approach the child (Aylward, 2020a; Bayley & Aylward, 2019b).
- Including the caregiver in the assessment process and using the Caregiver Questions decreases anxiety for the child (and caregiver) and decreases the likelihood of inhibited responding in a child because of the presence of a "stranger" (e.g., the practitioner) or as a consequence of being in unfamiliar surroundings (Aylward, 2020a; Bayley & Aylward, 2019b).
- It is appropriate to ask questions about the child's interests or day, even if the child has yet to build the appropriate vocabulary to respond. Infants and toddlers have a rich mental life and may understand what is being said or enjoy the way in which it was said and respond positively.
- Warm smiles, encouraging words, and sometimes clapping and expressing excitement at the attempt or completion of a task are often positive ways to build rapport with children. It is important for the practitioner to provide general encouragement for effort and cooperation and not only for correct responses.
- It is important for the practitioner to ensure the child does not feel rushed with responses. There is a balance between having the assessment conducted quickly and rushing the child to respond, thereby missing the chance to see the infant demonstrate the skill being assessed.
- There may be times it is unclear if the child's response is purposeful, and the item should be readministered, when not prohibited by the instructions, to give the child the chance to demonstrate the skill (Bayley & Aylward, 2019b).

(Continued)

Tips for Rapport with Caregivers

Taking the time to build rapport with the caregiver is essential for facilitating a positive assessment experience for the child, caregiver, and practitioner. Attempts to establish rapport and good communication are important to help the caregiver understand the purpose of accurate reporting for the assessment (Bayley & Aylward, 2019b). Some tips are now given for establishing and maintaining rapport with the caregiver.

- The stage is set for building rapport with the caregiver from the moment the caregiver is contacted for scheduling an appointment. It is important to try to make the experience of scheduling the appointment and providing an orientation to what is expected during the assessment as pleasant and collaborative as possible.
- The practitioner should provide the caregiver with information about the check-in procedures, testing environment, and what to expect during the testing session prior to the testing appointment.
- Caregivers benefit from warm smiles and words of encouragement from the practitioner.
- The caregiver is more likely to feel comfortable when the practitioner exudes an attitude of respect for the caregiver's knowledge of and relationship with the child.
- Including the caregiver in the assessment process and using the Caregiver Questions decreases anxiety for the caregiver and child (Aylward, 2020a; Bayley & Aylward, 2019b, 2019c).
- The practitioner may continue to build rapport with the caregiver by briefly explaining what the practitioner is doing with the child and why as the test administration progresses.
- Occasionally, a caregiver may be surprised that the child demonstrated a new skill within the testing session. This is an opportunity for the practitioner to join with the caregiver and child in the joy of discovering something new and celebrating the developmental milestone. This also provides an opportunity to encourage positive interactions and developmentally appropriate play between the caregiver and child and to assist the caregiver in learning about emerging skills expected for the child.

≡ Rapid Reference 2.5

Helpful Tips for a Valid Bayley–4 Assessment

- Follow standard administration procedures with provided materials from the Bayley–4 kit in addition to required materials provided by the practitioner. The practitioner should identify the potential range of items to be administered, and relevant materials should be out of view (e.g., set to the side, under a table, and/or under a blanket) of the examinee until the respective item is presented.

(Continued)

- Ensure all items needed for the assessment are accounted for, sanitized, have no broken pieces or parts, and are readily available during the assessment.
- Ensure that appropriate seating is available, there is sufficient room to carry out all assessment activities, and a mat or blankets are available for items administered on the floor.
- The testing environment should be at a comfortable temperature and as free from visual and auditory distractors as possible.
- The testing appointment should be scheduled at a time that does not interfere with the child's routines, such as eating or napping, and the child should be rescheduled if sick.
- Testing in a room where medical procedures are performed could be potentially distressing for children, particularly for children who have experienced medical trauma or have frequent medical visits.
- Avoid having additional people besides the practitioner, child, and caregiver(s) in the testing room, with no more than three adults and no other children, if possible, to decrease distractions.

Sources: Aylward (2020a); Bayley and Aylward (2019b); Black and Matula (2000)

ADMINISTRATION FORMATS

There are three administration and scoring options for the Bayley–4: paper administration and scoring, paper administration with digital scoring and reporting, and digital administration, scoring, and reporting. Each of these is described briefly in the next sections.

Paper Administration Format

Paper administration of the Bayley–4 Cognitive, Receptive Communication, Expressive Communication, Fine Motor, and Gross Motor subtests is described in Chapters 3 and 4 of the Administration Manual (Bayley & Aylward, 2019b). The paper Record Form is used to record the child's responses and calculate raw scores for these subtests and the scales they comprise (see Chapter 3, for detailed information on scoring). A paper Stimulus Book and Response Booklet are used for some items, depending on the child's age. The paper Social-Emotional and Adaptive Behavior Questionnaire is completed by the caregiver, with directions for the caregiver printed on the questionnaire. Administration and scoring instructions for the Social-Emotional and Adaptive Behavior Scales are located in Chapter 5 of the Administration Manual. Practitioners have the option of entering responses obtained during paper administration into Pearson's Q-global®

platform, which is a secure online testing platform. Scores are then calculated digitally, which decreases scoring errors, and a report may be generated based on the scores.

Digital Administration Format

Digital administration of the Bayley–4 on Q-global is designed for use on mobile devices, laptops, and PCs. Standardized administration of the Bayley–4 items is the same as with paper administration; however, instead of the practitioner using a separate printed Administration Manual and Record Form, these are combined on a single tablet, laptop, or PC screen for easier accessibility during testing (Bayley & Aylward, 2019b). Instructions and items are presented on screen, and all administration and scoring is fully automated. Digital administration on Q-global facilitates correct administration of age-appropriate items, guides the practitioner through administration and scoring of trials and items, and provides resources to support test administration and scoring of the Cognitive, Receptive Communication, Expressive Communication, Fine Motor, and Gross Motor subtests (Bayley & Aylward, 2019b). The practitioner may save time during administration because the digital administration navigates to the next appropriate trial or item, as compared with the practitioner having to reference the Administration Manual or Record Form or try to rely on memory for that information. The items are administered based on the standardized administration rules and allow for administration based on groupings of related and series items.

In addition, the Social–Emotional and Adaptive Behavior Scales can be administered via Q-global. The instructions and items are presented on screen and the entire administration and scoring are fully automated. These assessments can be sent to the caregiver via email per Remote On-Screen Assessment (ROSA) on Q-global, for which the respondent (typically the caregiver) must have a working email and access to a computer, tablet, or other mobile device with internet connectivity. It is recommended the caregiver (and practitioner) complete these items at a time that may be more convenient than

---

CAUTION 2.1

Practitioners may believe the digital format of the Bayley–4 on Q-global is fully automated, including the tasks required for the child to complete. This is a misconception as the child and caregiver interact with materials in the same way as with paper administration, including use of the manipulatives, stimulus book, and response booklet as appropriate for the child's age (see Materials List in Figure 2.1). The practitioner is still required to provide the materials listed in Rapid Reference 2.3.

during the testing session (e.g., when the caregiver is home). An advantage of the digital administration is that it eliminates the possibility of missing data and ensures that all scores are derived (Bayley & Aylward, 2019b). See Chapter 8: Digital Administration, for more information on assessment procedures using Q-global.

ADMINISTRATION TIME

The time to administer the performance-based subtests of the Cognitive, Language, and Motor Scales of the Bayley–4 depends on several factors, including practitioner, environmental, caregiver, and child factors. Practitioner factors include familiarity with the Bayley–4 administration procedures and items, experience with testing infants and toddlers, how materials are organized and the assessment is planned, and whether features designed to increase test administration efficiency are used (Bayley & Aylward, 2019b). Environmental factors may include the weather, the time of day (e.g., whether the session is scheduled close to or during an anticipated event in the child's day such as eating, a nap, or transition between home and external caregiver/school), external noises that may be distracting, availability of required equipment, the time it takes to set up based on the environment, and the proximity of required items (e.g., stairs) to the testing room.

Caregiver behaviors, including cooperativeness, mood, responsiveness to the child, and the time it takes them to provide answers may also affect testing time. Child factors affecting testing time may include biological needs that require attention (e.g., diaper changes, toileting, feeding, napping), the child's temperament, the child's mood state, how much sleep the child had the night before, if the child is hungry or tired, age, level of functioning, the amount of time the child takes to consider and complete items, and comfort and cooperation with the practitioner. Every effort should be made to administer all items during one testing session. However, if the child is showing signs of fatigue or is upset, allow as many breaks as necessary (Bayley & Aylward, 2019b). If the testing session cannot be resumed, a second testing session should be scheduled as soon as possible (Bayley & Aylward, 2019b).

The testing time for the Bayley–4 is approximately 35 minutes for children ages 1–12 months; 63 minutes for children ages 13–24 months; and 68 minutes for children ages 25–42 months (Bayley & Aylward, 2019b). Table 2.1 reports the testing time for the Cognitive, Language, and Motor Scales subtests for the normative sample. Average times were also calculated according to the Special Groups included in the Bayley–4 validity studies and are listed in Table 2.2. These testing times are based on administration of all item trials and all

Caregiver Questions appropriate for the child's age. When features designed for administration efficiency are used, practitioners may experience a shorter administration time than listed. For example, practitioners are not required to record the response for all trials or use all Caregiver Questions during administration, and administering related items together may decrease testing time (Bayley & Aylward, 2019b). In addition, the efficiencies of navigation, recording, and scoring with the digital administration may make the testing time shorter.

The average administration time for completing the Social–Emotional and Adaptive Behavior Questionnaire is 20–35 minutes. The Social–Emotional subtest typically takes the respondent 10 minutes to complete. The completion time for the Adaptive Behavior subtest is dependent on the child's age and level of functioning and typically takes 10–25 minutes (Bayley & Aylward, 2019b).

Table 2.1   Time Required (in Minutes) to Complete the Bayley–4, by Various Percentages of the Normative Sample

Age in months	50%	75%	90%	95%
1–12	35	50	73	86
13–24	63	84	103	111
25–42	68	88	102	108

Note: From Bayley Scales of Infant and Toddler Development, Fourth Edition (Bayley™–4). Copyright © 2019 NCS Pearson, Inc. Reproduced with permission. All rights reserved.

Table 2.2   Average Time (in Minutes) to Complete the Bayley–4, by Special Group

Special group (ages 1–42 months)	Average time in minutes
Autism Spectrum Disorder (ASD)	71
Developmental Delay (DD)	53
Down Syndrome (DS)	69
Language Delay (LD)	67
Moderate/Late Premature (MLP)	63
Motor Impairment (MI)	56
Prenatal Drug/Alcohol Exposure (PDAE)	55
Specific Language Impairment (SLI)	62
Very/Extremely Premature (VEP)	57

Note: From Bayley Scales of Infant and Toddler Development, Fourth Edition (Bayley™–4). Copyright © 2019 NCS Pearson, Inc. Reproduced with permission. All rights reserved.

TEST MATERIALS

Manipulatives

The Bayley–4 materials were created with considerations for child development, features that are interesting and appealing to children, and safety. Children should be supervised at all times when interacting with Bayley–4 materials to ensure safety, as young children often mouth objects and may engage with materials in a way that is unexpected to adults (Bayley & Aylward, 2019b). Figure 2.1 shows

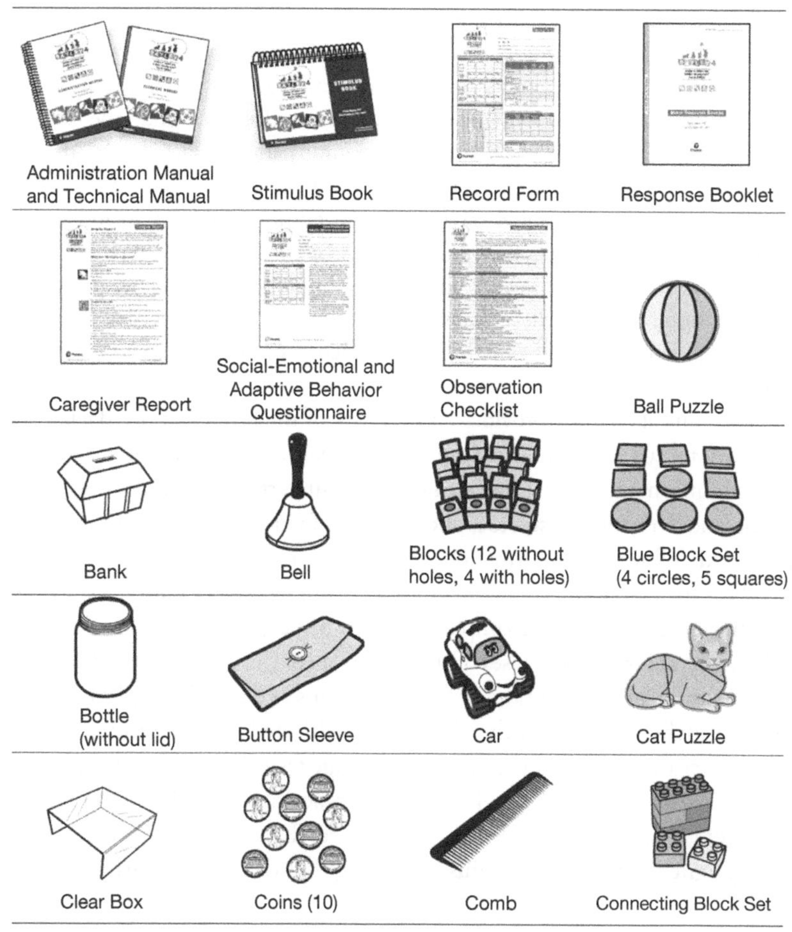

Figure 2.1   Bayley–4 Test Kit Materials.
Note: From Bayley Scales of Infant and Toddler Development, Fourth Edition (Bayley™–4). Copyright © 2019 NCS Pearson, Inc. Reproduced with permission. All rights reserved.

illustrations of some test materials included in the Bayley–4 test kit. Appendix D of the Administration Manual (Bayley & Aylward, 2019b) provides a list of materials needed for each subtest. The practitioner is required to provide additional materials for test administration, as noted earlier in Rapid Reference 2.3.

Manuals and Stimulus Book

There are two manuals that accompany the Bayley–4: the Administration Manual (Bayley & Aylward, 2019b) and the Technical Manual (Bayley & Aylward, 2019c). The Administration Manual provides an overview of the test content and general information, including start points, reverse rules, discontinue rules, and detailed information needed to administer and score the Cognitive, Language, and Motor Scales. Additionally, instructions for how to complete the Social–Emotional and Adaptive Behavior Questionnaire, the Caregiver Report, and the Behavior Observation Inventory are included. Finally, information regarding the recording and scoring procedures on the Record Form and on Q-global is provided (note that detailed information for digital navigation and administration is included in the separate *Bayley–4 Digital Administration User's Guide* [Bayley & Aylward, 2019d] that is included in the Resource Library on Q-global). The appendices in the Administration Manual include the norms and conversion tables needed for accurate scoring, supplemental tables, and Bayley–4 accommodations and modifications (Bayley & Aylward, 2019b).

The Technical Manual provides an overview of the history of the Bayley Scales from 1969 to 2019. In addition, the revision goals of the Bayley–4 are listed and discussed. Information about the research procedures, standardization, norms development, and derivation of scores is also included. Evidence of reliability and validity is presented, followed by information regarding interpretation of results. Finally, the appendices include information regarding developmental risk indicators, inclusion and exclusion criteria for the sample, and a list of people and sites involved in the development and research phases of the Bayley–4 (Bayley & Aylward, 2019c).

The Stimulus Book contains certain test items and should be placed approximately 6 inches away from the child and positioned with the front cover facing the practitioner so that the appropriate page faces the child. Administration instructions for items are provided on the practitioner's side of the Stimulus Book. Items may be administered using the easel feature to keep the Stimulus Book upright or with the Stimulus Book lying flat (Bayley & Aylward, 2019b).

Record Form/Q-global, Response Booklet, and Observation Checklist

The paper Record Form and the Bayley–4 on Q-global are designed to make navigation through the test administration and scoring as simple and easy as possible. They provide opportunities for recording and scoring the child's responses or Caregiver Questions and include information on start points, reverse and discontinue rules, and time limits. The paper Record Form included in the Bayley–4 includes the items for the Cognitive, Language, and Motor Scales (Bayley & Aylward, 2019b). In addition, separate paper Record Forms for the Cognitive, Language, and Motor Scales are available for purchase. These may be appropriate for use if the referral question is targeted to one specific area, or if the scales of the Bayley–4 will be administered by more than one professional (e.g., Developmental Pediatrician, Psychologist, Speech–Language Pathologist, Occupational Therapist, Physical Therapist). When two different professionals are administering the Cognitive and Receptive Communication subtests, coordination is needed to avoid repetition of the shared items from those subtests. More information about recording responses on the paper Record Form and on Q-global is provided later in this chapter.

The Behavior Observation Inventory (BOI) is found on the back page of the Record Form. The BOI is completed with the caregiver immediately after administering the Bayley–4 Cognitive, Language, and Motor Scales. The purpose of the BOI is to rate whether or not a child's performance is typical. The practitioner responds to each statement by placing a checkmark in the column that describes how often the behavior was observed during testing. For caregiver ratings, the description of each behavior is read aloud to the caregiver to rate the degree to which each statement is typical of the child's behavior (Bayley & Aylward, 2019b). The ratings are: (1) Not at all typical: Never or Rarely; (2) Somewhat typical: Some of the time; and (3) Typical: Most of the time. The practitioner and caregiver ratings can be compared and used for qualitative information in combination with scores and analysis from the Bayley–4 that may be useful in intervention planning (Bayley & Aylward, 2019c; see also Chapter 4). The digital version of the BOI is available to download in the Q-global Resource Library. The Response Booklet is used for completing several items on the Fine Motor subtest. The Response Booklet should be positioned such that only the item being administered can be seen and in a way that is most conducive to the child completing the task (Bayley & Aylward, 2019b).

The Observation Checklist may be used to identify and help score items that are based on incidental observation. Incidental observation is important to the administration of the Bayley–4, as the practitioner should score as many items by incidental observation as possible. This includes spontaneous behaviors during interactions with the caregiver (Bayley & Aylward, 2019b). Practitioners must be familiar with the Bayley–4 items to prevent missing incidental observations upon greeting the child and caregiver and setting them up to begin the testing session, between administration of items, or when the child and caregiver are taking a

Item	2-point scoring criteria	Observed
COGNITIVE		
1. Calms When Picked Up	Consistently calms within 30 seconds when picked up and remains calm.	☐
2. Looks at Object	Looks continuously at object for 7 to 10 seconds.	☐
5. Recognizes Caregiver	Expression immediately changes to indicate caregiver recognition on at least 1 occasion.	☐
6. Reaction to Caregiver	Displays a reaction that is clearly anticipatory.	☐
12. Responds to Surroundings	Quiets, looks around, and displays interest in surroundings.	☐
13. Explores Object	Attends to the sight, sound, or feel of rattle by touching, shaking, or engaging in other playful activity.	☐
14. Brings to Mouth	Consistently carries objects to mouth.	☐
15. Inspects Own Hands	Clear and sustained inspection of hand(s).	☐
17. Reaches/Obtains Objects	Persistently reaches for and obtains object.	☐
19. Bangs Object	Intentional and frequent banging of object.	☐

Figure 2.2 Observation Checklist Excerpt.
Note: From Bayley Scales of Infant and Toddler Development, Fourth Edition (Bayley™–4). Copyright © 2019 NCS Pearson, Inc. Reproduced with permission. All rights reserved.

break. The Bayley–4 Administration Manual (Bayley & Aylward, 2019b) includes instructions for eliciting behaviors if they are not observed incidentally. To prevent disruption of the interaction when first greeting the child and caregiver, or in other situations when stopping to record data may be awkward, the practitioner using Q-global administration may want to note inconspicuously observations on the Observation Checklist and record data in Q-global later (Bayley & Aylward, 2019b). Figure 2.2 shows part of the Observation Checklist. See Chapter 3 for more information on scoring of items based on incidental observations.

Social–Emotional and Adaptive Behavior Questionnaire and Caregiver Report

The Social-Emotional and Adaptive Behavior Questionnaire includes items completed by a designated respondent, typically the caregiver, to describe the social–emotional and adaptive behavior functioning of the child. The practitioner must make sure the caregiver is willing and motivated to complete the questionnaire accurately and objectively (e.g., refraining from reporting the child's best performance instead of what is typical; Bayley & Aylward, 2019b).

The Social–Emotional Scale is adapted from the *Greenspan Social–Emotional Growth Chart: A Screening Questionnaire for Infants and Young Children* (Greenspan, 2004) and is comprised of the Social–Emotional subtest (Bayley &

Aylward, 2019b). Major social and emotional developmental milestones are assessed that should be met by certain ages. Skills measured include self-regulation, interest in surroundings, communication of needs, engagement with others and establishment of relationships, using emotions in a manner that is interactive and purposeful, and solving problems using emotional signals or gestures (Bayley & Aylward, 2019b).

The Adaptive Behavior Scale is based on the *Vineland Adaptive Behavior Scales* (3rd ed.), *Comprehensive Parent/Caregiver Form* (Vineland–3; Sparrow et al., 2016) and includes an overall Adaptive Behavior standard score, as well as scores in three domains: Communication, Daily Living Skills, and Socialization. The Communication domain includes the Receptive and Expressive subdomains, the Daily Living Skills domain includes the Personal subdomain, and the Socialization domain includes the Interpersonal Relationships and Play and Leisure subdomains. The Adaptive Behavior Scale assesses the child's everyday behaviors and functioning. The emphasis is on what the child actually and typically does, not on what the child could potentially do or the child's best performance (Bayley & Aylward, 2019b; Sparrow et al., 2016).

The Caregiver Report is a tool the practitioner uses to summarize the child's performance on the Bayley–4 for the caregiver (Bayley & Aylward, 2019b). It begins with a general description of the Bayley–4. Next, the Cognitive, Language, and Motor Scales are described by summarizing the skills assessed for infants, toddlers, and preschoolers for each scale. The Social–Emotional and Adaptive Behavior Scales are also briefly summarized.A section is then included for the practitioner to transfer subtest and subdomain scaled scores from the Record Form and Social–Emotional and Adaptive Behavior Questionnaire to the Subtest/Subdomain Score Profile. The following page on the Caregiver Report begins the *Activities for You and Your Child* section that suggests age-appropriate activities in which the caregiver can engage the child to foster positive development. Finally, the comments section at the end of the form is used to add recommendations or observations that help the caregiver understand the child's performance. Digital administration on Q-global automatically generates a Caregiver Report after an assessment is submitted (Bayley & Aylward, 2019d).

TYPES OF ITEMS ON THE BAYLEY–4

The Cognitive, Language, and Motor Scales are completed based on interaction with the child and the caregiver. In assessing these areas of development, the Bayley–4 incorporates administration of structured items to measure the child's ability to learn and adapt to novel situations. In addition, the Social–Emotional and Adaptive Behavior Questionnaire includes items presented to the caregiver (or other designated respondent if the parent or caregiver is not participating in the assessment) related to the behaviors the child engages in or the caregiver has observed related to social–emotional and adaptive functioning (Bayley & Aylward, 2019b). Furthermore, direct observation is used to determine the accomplishment of developmental milestones and important behaviors for the child's age. The caregiver is directly involved in the assessment to assist with administration of items and to collect historical information important for scoring of behaviors that cannot be directly observed in the testing session (Bayley & Aylward, 2019b). Rapid Reference 2.6 describes the types of items used for the Bayley–4 assessment. It is important to note that the Cognitive and Expressive Communication subtests share six items, which only need to be administered once, as explained in Don't Forget 2.1.

≡ Rapid Reference 2.6

Types of Items on the Bayley–4

The Bayley–4 includes several types of structured items, including demonstration and sample items, multiple trial items, series items, and related items. Items that describe behaviors that may be demonstrated by children are also part of the Social–Emotional and Adaptive Behavior Questionnaire (Bayley & Aylward, 2019b).

Demonstration and Sample Items

- Demonstration items are included that allow the practitioner or caregiver to show the child how to complete the item and allow the practitioner to observe how the child reacts to a novel task.
- Sample items give the child an opportunity to practice completing the task before being scored on performance and provide the opportunity for the practitioner to see how a child may process information and apply learning from the practitioner's instructions, demonstration, or corrective feedback.
- The practitioner must be careful to follow standardized instructions regarding the number of times information can be presented, repeated, and the amount and type of assistance given.
- Providing more help or feedback than is allowed within the standardized instructions is not considered a standardized administration, and therefore the score would not be valid or reportable for that item or scale.

(Continued)

Multiple Trial Items

- Some Bayley–4 items require administration of multiple trials, which include recording and scoring of each trial response.
- The score for a multiple trial item is typically determined by the number of correct trial responses.
- On Q-global, item scores are suggested based on the selected responses for the trials, and the item scoring criteria should be reviewed to verify correct scoring before advancing to the next item.

Series Items

- Series Items require the same item instructions, but different levels of performance for scoring. Series items are indicated in the Administration Manual (Bayley & Aylward, 2019b).
- Series items are indicated on the Record Form in a lightly shaded oval area to the left of the item number with an "S," and the items within the series listed under the S. The number of the item the practitioner is administering is underlined within the shaded area.
- On Q-global, series items are configured into a single administration, and all of the items in the series are automatically scored.

Related Items

- Related items require the use of the same test materials or similar activities but have different administration instructions.
- Related items are indicated in the Administration Manual (Bayley & Aylward, 2019b) in a table at the end of the administration instructions for each related item.
- Related items are indicated on the Record Form as a list of items labeled with an "R" to the left of the item number. The number of the item the practitioner is administering is underlined within the rectangular shaded box.
- If an item is part of a series and a related item, the "S" list is to the left of the "R" list by the item number.
- Administering related items together may be helpful to maintain the flow of a test administration by keeping a child's attention on a particular object or book for quick administration of multiple items instead of presenting and removing the same materials several times throughout the test administration.
- Items deemed to be developmentally inappropriate per the practitioner's clinical judgment and/or items that would occur past the discontinue point should not be administered despite being in the related item group (Bayley & Aylward, 2019b).
- Bayley–4 on Q-global allows for administration of related items in serial order according to the item grouping.

(Continued)

- Related item groups are not comprehensive and may be modified or created based on practitioner preference, personal administration style, clinical judgment, and presentation and response style of the child.

Items on the Social–Emotional and Adaptive Behavior Scales

- For the Social–Emotional subtest and the Adaptive Behavior subdomains, the items are worded as statements that describe a behavior the child may exhibit or a behavior the caregiver may easily elicit from the child.
- The caregiver provides a rating for each statement based on the number of choices for each scale (e.g., six possible ratings for the Social–Emotional subtest and three possible ratings for the Adaptive Behavior subdomains).

Source: Bayley and Aylward (2019b)

DON'T FORGET 2.1

There are six items that are the same on the Cognitive and Receptive Communication subtests. Whether administered first on the Cognitive or Receptive Communication subtest, the item is scored the same and should be administered only one time.

Items with Caregiver Questions

An important new feature of the Bayley–4 is the addition of items with Caregiver Questions, which are included on 51 items. These items assist with scoring by obtaining information about the child's typical behavior across settings, not just within the contrived setting of a one-time testing session. In addition, Caregiver Questions help to decrease the testing time and avoid administration of items that are more likely to be refused by the child. For example, children are more likely to refuse some language and motor items, as well as items that the child may already be self-aware are difficult (Aylward, 2020a; Bayley & Aylward, 2019b, 2019c). Furthermore, use of Caregiver Questions helps avoid missing test data (Bayley & Aylward, 2019b, 2019c).

The majority of Caregiver Questions are associated with structured test items. For example, Item 13 of the Expressive Communication subtest is a structured item that includes a Caregiver Question (Bayley & Aylward, 2019b). The practitioner can then score the item according to the caregiver response. The instructions indicate that the item score may be based on incidental observations of the child, the caregiver's interaction with the child, or the practitioner's interaction with the child (Bayley & Aylward, 2019b). Scoring criteria for responses (e.g., often, not often, not at all) are included in the Administration Manual (Bayley & Aylward, 2019b). The Bayley–4 includes a small number of items scored based solely on the response to a Caregiver Question. This is a change from the *Bayley Scales of Infant and Toddler Development–Third Edition* (Bayley, 2006) and replaces the administration of complicated items that required several manipulatives and the artificial construction of play scenarios, which did not always elicit the desired response from the child (Bayley & Aylward, 2019b).

The Caregiver Questions are not intended to improve scores. Instead, they are to be used when a child's response is unclear, the child is uninterested or refusing to complete an item, or it seems the behavior is more likely to occur in familiar surroundings (NCS Pearson, Inc., 2021a). If the practitioner notices that there are frequent discrepancies between the observed behavior during the testing session and the Caregiver Question responses, the validity of the Caregiver Question scores may be in question, and the practitioner must use clinical judgment in interpretation of these scores (Bayley & Aylward, 2019b; NCS Pearson, Inc., 2021a).

BAYLEY–4 ADMINISTRATION GUIDELINES

The standardized administration procedures in the Bayley–4 Administration Manual (Bayley & Aylward, 2019b) must be followed when administering items on the Cognitive, Language, and Motor Scales and for the completion of the Social–Emotional and Adaptive Behavior Questionnaire. Following these procedures ensures that a child's scores can be compared appropriately to the normative sample. Changes to instructions, including wording or presentation of items, is considered deviation from standard instructions and decreases the reliability and validity of the test results; however, following standardized procedures does not equate to having a rigid presentation of items and interactions with the child and caregiver. The practitioner must be sensitive to the needs of the child being assessed and, as mentioned earlier in this chapter, foster a supportive environment that will be more conducive to a positive testing experience for the child and caregiver (Bayley & Aylward, 2019b).

Recording Information on Record Forms

Prior to test administration, the practitioner should complete the demographic information on the front of the paper Record Forms and the Social–Emotional and Adaptive Behavior Questionnaire. Similarly, the demographic information should be provided in Q-global when using the digital administration.

Calculating Test Age

Accurate calculation of the child's test age is essential to identify the start point for subtest administration. On the Record Form and Social–Emotional and Adaptive Behavior Questionnaire, the Calculation of Child's Age table can be used to help calculate the test age. The year, month, and day of the testing date are entered in the first row. If testing must be completed on more than one day, the first testing date is used (Bayley & Aylward, 2019b).

The child's date of birth is recorded in the second row. The test age is then calculated in the third row by subtracting the birth date from the test date. For test age calculations, all months are entered as 30 days. The last row of the table requires conversion of years, months, and days into months and years, with the number of years multiplied by 12 and added to the number of months. Days are not rounded upward to the nearest month (e.g., 21 months, 18 days is not rounded to 22 months). Figure 2.3 shows the Calculation of Child's Age table. The test age is automatically calculated in Q-global when the test date and date of birth are entered (Bayley & Aylward, 2019d).

Because of the assumption that all months have 30 days, these calculation procedures may not provide the exact age of the child. Typically, this does not affect the start point; however, for children nearing the transition between two ages, a practitioner may want to recalculate the child's age more precisely using a calendar or digital age calculator to verify the manual age calculation (Bayley & Aylward, 2019b). Pearson offers a web-based age calculator on its website that requires entry of the test date and birth date to calculate the chronological test age. This can be found at https://images.pearsonclinical.com/images/agecalculator/agecalculator.htm

<table>
<tr><td colspan="5" align="center">Calculation of Child's Age</td></tr>
<tr><td></td><td align="center">Year</td><td align="center">Month</td><td></td><td align="center">Day</td></tr>
<tr><td>Test date</td><td>2019</td><td>5̶ 6</td><td></td><td>32̶ 2</td></tr>
<tr><td>Birth date</td><td>2017</td><td>1</td><td></td><td>15</td></tr>
<tr><td>Test age</td><td>2</td><td>4</td><td></td><td>17</td></tr>
<tr><td rowspan="2">Test age in months and days</td><td align="center">Years x 12</td><td align="center">Months</td><td align="center">Total months</td><td align="center">Days</td></tr>
<tr><td align="center">24 +</td><td align="center">4 =</td><td align="center">28</td><td align="center">17</td></tr>
</table>

Figure 2.3   Calculation of Child's Age.

Note: From Bayley Scales of Infant and Toddler Development, Fourth Edition (Bayley™–4). Copyright © 2019 NCS Pearson, Inc. Reproduced with permission. All rights reserved.

Adjustment for Prematurity				
	Year	Month		Day
Test date	2019	8		6
Expected birth date	2019	1		2
Adjusted test age	0	7		4
	Years x 12	Months	Total months	Days
Adjusted test age in months and days	0 +	7 =	7	4

Figure 2.4   Test Age: Adjusted for Prematurity.
Note: From Bayley Scales of Infant and Toddler Development, Fourth Edition (Bayley™–4). Copyright © 2019 NCS Pearson, Inc. Reproduced with permission. All rights reserved.

(NCS Pearson, Inc, 2021b) or by entering *Pearson chronological age calculator* in the search bar of any web browser.

Beginning Below Chronological Age. The Bayley–4 Administration Manual (Bayley & Aylward, 2019b) recommends adjustment of the test age for prematurity up to 24 months of age for children born at 36 weeks gestation or less. For children born more than 16 weeks premature, the practitioner may consider correction up to 3 years (Aylward, 2020a, 2020b). The Adjustment for Prematurity table on the Record Form can be used to determine the adjusted test age. The test date and expected birth date are recorded, and the expected birth date is subtracted from the test date. The adjusted age is the start point for the child. If the adjusted test age is less than 16 days, the Bayley–4 may still be administered to collect qualitative data, but normative data are not available (Bayley & Aylward, 2019b). Figure 2.4 shows the Adjusted for Prematurity table. The Bayley–4 on Q-global automatically calculates the child's adjusted test age and determines the appropriate start points when the child's actual birth and expected birth dates are entered.

Guidelines for Administering the Cognitive, Language, and Motor Scales

Order of Subtest Administration

The five performance-based subtests of the Bayley–4 are typically administered in the order presented on the Record Form: Cognitive, Receptive Communication, Expressive Communication, Fine Motor, and Gross Motor and this order should be followed as much as possible; however, the test was standardized using a flexible approach, such that administration based on infant behaviors and responses is acceptable as long as items are presented in a standardized way (Bayley & Aylward, 2019b). For example, a child may be having a difficult time settling down, so starting with the Gross Motor subtest tasks may help the child settle down, gain trust with the practitioner, and self-regulate.

Determining Starting Point, Reverse Rule, and Discontinue Rule

For each subtest, the practitioner must determine the starting point and administer items from that point, following reverse rules if applicable, until the discontinue rule is met or all subtest items are administered. The Bayley–4 normative data were calculated for ages 1 month through 42 months. The age range is divided into 17 categories, which are displayed in the Start Points table on the cover page of the Record Form. To identify the start point, the practitioner locates the letter in the Start Point column that corresponds with the child's test age or adjusted test age in months and days. For example, a child whose test age is 21 months, 14 days would start with the item for each subtest that is associated with Start Point L. The start point letter is useful for identifying where to begin each subtest and is found within an arrow on the left side of the corresponding item number on the Record Form and in the Administration Manual (Bayley & Aylward, 2019b). Start points are automatically identified and navigated to with Q-global administration.

The reverse rule for the Bayley–4 is the same for all five subtests. If the child does not obtain a perfect score of 2 (i.e., a score of 1 or 0) on the first three items administered, the practitioner must go back to the previous start point and administer the items in forward sequence. This rule is applied until the child obtains a perfect score of 2 on the first three items at any start point, or until Item 1 is administered. Once three perfect scores are obtained, the items are administered in forward sequence until the discontinue rule is met or all subtest items are administered.

The discontinue rule is also the same for all five subtests. Administration on a subtest stops when the child has obtained a score of 0 on five consecutive items (i.e., the ceiling) or when all subtest items are administered. Previously administered items with a score of 0 that were used to apply the reverse rule count toward the discontinue rule. If for any reason items were administered above the ceiling and received a score of 1 or 2, those scores should be considered a score of 0 for raw score calculation purposes.

Basal and Ceiling Rules and Timing

The basal for each subtest is the first three consecutive scores of 2 at any given start point. If the child achieves a basal at their age-appropriate start point, the items are administered in forward sequence until the discontinue rule is met (Bayley & Aylward, 2019b). For example, a child who begins at Start Point P on the Expressive Communication subtest obtaining a score of 2 on Items 21, 22, and 23 has established a basal and the practitioner continues administration in forward sequence until the discontinue rule is met or all items in the subtest are administered.

A basal may be established at a lower start point if the reversal rule is applied at the age-appropriate start point. For example, a child with a test age of 28 months, 10 days has a Start Point of N on the Fine Motor subtest (i.e., Item 18). The child obtains a score of 0 on Item 18. The practitioner must then reverse to the previous Start Point J-L at Item 13 because of the imperfect score on Item 18. The child obtains a perfect score of 2 on Items 13 and 14, but a score of 1 on Item 15. The practitioner must then reverse again to the previous start point F-I at Item 9. The child successfully completes Items 9, 10, and 11 with a perfect score, and these three scores of 2 in a row establish the basal. The practitioner then continues administration at Item 12 in a forward sequence until the discontinue rule is met. The previously administered items are not re-administered, but they are considered in calculating the discontinue rule when applicable (Bayley & Aylward, 2019b).

Multiple Basals. The Bayley–4 start points were chosen to accommodate most children with some degree of delay in development. If developmental delay is suspected for a particular subtest, the practitioner may reverse one start point prior to the age-appropriate start point, and reverse further as needed. If the child is administered items before the age-appropriate start point and a "second" basal is established at the age-appropriate start point, a perfect score is assigned to all items before the second (i.e., highest) basal even if the child did not obtain a perfect score on those items (Bayley & Aylward, 2019b).

For example, a child with a calculated test age of 14 months, 2 days has a Start Point of J. On the Cognitive subtest, this child would start at Item 27. However, based on the caregiver report, the child is not yet grasping objects well so the practitioner decides to begin administration at Start Point I to accommodate the possible delay in development. The child establishes a basal with a perfect score on Items 19, 20, and 21 and the practitioner continues administration in a forward sequence. Once the age-appropriate Start Point J is reached, the child surprises the caregiver and the practitioner by obtaining a perfect score on Items 27, 28, and 29. Thus, two basals have been established. In this situation, the highest basal at the original start point is used, and all items below Item 27 are scored as 2 regardless of the obtained score (Bayley & Aylward, 2019b).

A distinct advantage to the digital administration of the Bayley–4 is the automatic navigation to appropriate start points for the child's test age (or adjusted age if premature), and the practitioner has the ability to navigate to a lower start point if desired. The navigation to items based on the basal and ceiling rules is automatic, and no items are repeated if they have been previously administered. Once the basal and ceiling are established, the scores below the established basal are automatically scored as 2, and any items administered above the ceiling are scored as 0.

When exact timing is required for items, the timer is listed in the materials section for that item on the Record Form. Timing for the Bayley–4 uses whole numbers, and the time is not rounded up to the next second. For example, a display of 4.31 seconds on a stopwatch is recorded as 4 seconds and 125.98 is recorded as 125 seconds. When a timer is not listed and the item mentions completion of a task within a specific amount of time, the practitioner may use a less precise way of tracking the rate of passing time, such as counting silently, if needed. For example, Item 16 on the Cognitive subtest requires the practitioner to observe the child interacting with a manipulative for 5 seconds or less. To maintain rapport and prevent frustration, the child may be allowed to finish a task when nearing completion even if the time limit has been exceeded. Item scores should reflect the child's performance within the indicated time limit (Bayley & Aylward, 2019b). Administration on Q-global includes a timer for recording completion time, eliminating the need for an additional timer and potentially reducing timing errors.

Item Administration

Once the practitioner has identified the appropriate start point for a child, the item is administered according to the instructions in the Administration Manual for that item and subsequent test items. The test items within each subtest are presented in developmental sequence for each subtest, which facilitates the child's experience of success at the beginning of each subtest (Bayley & Aylward, 2019b). Administration of items for each subtest is conducted in a forward sequence unless the reverse rule is applied. There is flexibility in administration of the items, including administration of series and related items together to increase testing efficiency, and when the child is engaged with the materials and removal of those materials would interfere with the flow of the administration. Flexibility in administration of subtests and items was built into the Bayley–4 to optimize the child's performance while adhering to standardized procedures (Bayley & Aylward, 2019b). Practitioners must score as they go in order to determine whether a basal and ceiling have been established and to avoid administering more items than necessary (Bayley & Aylward, 2019b).

The item descriptions in the Administration Manual follow the same format throughout every performance-based subtest. Each item description includes the item number, item title, materials, and position of the child when presenting the item. The item administration instructions follow, which provide the practitioner with the information regarding what to do, including instructions in black font. Verbatim instructions or questions are indicated with bold font. Scoring criteria are also listed.

The Record Form is used to reference item sequence and groupings and to determine what is needed for each trial and item, as well as to record item responses. The Record Form should be readily accessible, and it is recommended that a clipboard be used to hold the Record Form and provide a hard writing surface (Bayley & Aylward, 2019b). On the Record Form, the practitioner can quickly reference the item number and item title, and the materials needed to present the item.

Starting Positions. Each item on the Cognitive, Language, and Motor Scales specifies the starting position for the child. The positioning of the child is important to the standardized administration and scoring of the items listing a specific starting position. When the position is listed as *Not Specified*, the practitioner should use clinical judgment regarding the optimal position for the item based on the child's age, especially when the item is part of a series. Rapid Reference 2.7 provides a list and explanation of the recommended starting positions. See pages 24–26 in Chapter 3 of the Bayley–4 Administration Manual (Bayley & Aylward, 2019b) for illustrations and a further explanation of the starting positions.

≡ *Rapid Reference 2.7*

Recommended Starting Positions for Performance-Based Item Administration

Level Supine	• Child is lying on back with head and trunk fully supported and slightly elevated
Elevated Supine	• Child is on back with head and trunk fully supported and slightly elevated • May include an infant carrier/seat, on a wedge, or with other positioning equipment to elevate/recline to approximately 15° to 25° upright
Prone	• Child is on stomach
Cradled	• Child is on back, held snugly with the caregiver's arm and trunk • Child's body is mostly perpendicular to caregiver's trunk, with child's head supported near caregiver's elbow and caregiver's other hand providing support to child's back, bottom, and legs • Child may be mostly flat or elevated in the caregiver's arms

(Continued)

Supported at Shoulder	• Child is picked up by caregiver and placed in a vertical position at caregiver's shoulder • Child is held facing the caregiver with head resting on caregiver's shoulder • One of caregiver's forearms is supporting the child's lower body while the other is supporting the back, if needed
Supported Sitting	• Child is supported in an upright position, facing forward, typically in a caregiver's lap • Practitioner is usually seated at the table directly across from child, unless otherwise specified, and presents materials on table in front of child • Child may be supported in an infant carrier/seat, or other positioning equipment with head and trunk fully supported, and equipment elevated to near-upright position of approximately 60° to 70°
Seated	• Child is seated at testing table or chair tray • Chair may be toddler chair, highchair, booster seat, or other chair or seat that provides correct height for child to fit appropriately at table surface • Child may also sit in caregiver's lap at table's surface • Child must show good sitting stability or be provided with external positioning assistance (e.g., foam positioning pads or towel rolls) typically used by child • Best if child's feet are supported, but this is not required • Practitioner is usually seated at the table directly across from the child, unless otherwise specified, and presents materials on table in front of child
Social Sitting	• Any mutually agreeable sitting arrangement that facilitates attention to the task • Child and caregiver are sitting casually on the floor or in chairs that may not be the same size • May be side by side or facing each other • May be with or without a table surface • Common arrangement is both facing forward with child in caregiver's lap
Floor Sitting	• Child sits on floor • Firm and stable surface that is cushioned or padded • Child may sit with legs bent or straight, or in a variation of those
Upright	• Child lifted to vertical position with feet on exam surface • Caregiver (or practitioner) hands placed under the child's armpits and fingers spread around child's trunk for support
Standing	• Child stands alone or with support per item directions

Source: Bayley and Aylward (2019b)

Guidelines for Administering the Social–Emotional and Adaptive Behavior Questionnaire

To assess the child's social–emotional development and adaptive behavior, the Bayley–4 uses information provided by the child's primary caregiver on the Bayley–4 Social–Emotional and Adaptive Behavior Questionnaire. The questionnaire is divided into the Social–Emotional Scale and the Adaptive Behavior Scale (Bayley & Aylward, 2019b). The questionnaire may be administered using paper forms, paper forms with digital scoring and reporting on Q-global, and digital administration, scoring, and reporting, including ROSA on Q-global. A reliable respondent must be selected to complete the Social–Emotional and Adaptive Behavior Questionnaire, and information regarding selecting a respondent is included in Rapid Reference 2.8.

CAUTION 2.2

If it is not possible to locate a respondent who knows the child well, the results of the Social–Emotional and Adaptive Behavior Questionnaire should be interpreted with caution. The scores may not accurately reflect the child's true functioning; however, the scores may provide some item-level information helpful to the overall developmental or clinical conceptualization that informs the determination for further evaluation (Bayley & Aylward, 2019b).

≡ Rapid Reference 2.8

Selecting the Respondent to Complete the Social–Emotional and Adaptive Behavior Questionnaire

Before administering the Social–Emotional and Adaptive Behavior Questionnaire, the first task for the practitioner is to select the individual who will provide the responses for the questionnaire.

- The primary caregiver is typically the best respondent because they spend the most time with the child and should have the most extensive knowledge about the child's functioning in a variety of areas.
- The primary caregiver is usually a parent, but could be a relative such as a grandparent, aunt, uncle, or a non-relative such as a foster parent or caregiver in a residential care facility.
- To ensure a valid assessment, the respondent must:
  - be very knowledgeable about the child's everyday activities and behaviors,
  - have frequent and extended contact with the child,
  - live in the same home as the child.

Source: Bayley and Aylward (2019b)

Determining Starting Points and Discontinue Rules on the Social–Emotional and Adaptive Behavior Questionnaire

Regardless of the child's age, the respondent starts with Item 1 on the Social–Emotional subtest and at Item 1 on each subdomain of the Adaptive Behavior Scale. For the Social–Emotional subtest, the respondent is instructed to stop at the age-appropriate stop point listed at the bottom of sets of items on the questionnaire. For example, if the child is 2 months old, the respondent stops at *Stop here if your child is 0–3 months old* on the questionnaire; however, if the child was premature, the adjusted age in months is used to calculate the stop point, and the practitioner may highlight and point out the appropriate stop point to the respondent if using a paper form (Bayley & Aylward, 2019b).

For the Adaptive Behavior Scale, the practitioner should notify the respondent that each section needs to be completed, answering every question until circling 0 (i.e., Never) five times in a row for that subdomain. The respondent then moves to the next subdomain until all subdomains have been completed (Bayley & Aylward, 2019b). Discontinue rules for adaptive behavior subdomains can be confusing for respondents so the practitioner must be sure the respondent understands when to stop.

Item Administration of the Social–Emotional and Adaptive Behavior Questionnaire

The practitioner instructs the respondent to read and respond to all items within the required item sets and to rate the extent to which the child performs the behaviors or the adaptive skills, when needed. The instructions for the parent or caregiver are on the front page of the questionnaire. It is important for the respondent to recognize that the questionnaire consists of two parts: Social–Emotional and Adaptive Behavior. The instructions describe what is being assessed and informs the respondent that the child is not expected to demonstrate all skills on the form. The practitioner should make sure the respondent understands that there are different rating systems for the Social–Emotional Scale and Adaptive Behavior Scale (Bayley & Aylward, 2019b). In addition, it is prudent for the practitioner to check the responses once the Social–Emotional and Adaptive Behavior questionnaire is submitted by the respondent. There may be items that require further clarification, or follow-up may be needed if more than 15% of items are marked as *Can't Tell* or *Estimated* on the Social–Emotional and Adaptive Behavior Scales, respectively (Bayley & Aylward, 2019b). Chapter 3 contains more information about *Can't Tell* and *Estimated Items*.

If the respondent has difficulty completing certain items, the practitioner may want to follow up regarding the reasons why, as this could indicate more reasons for further evaluation or serve to reassure the practitioner that the child is progressing as expected. Language and/or cultural differences may be reasons that a respondent has difficulty completing the questionnaire (Bayley & Aylward, 2019b). The questionnaire is written at approximately a fifth-grade reading level to help ensure that the respondent has the ability to read the form; however, the items may be read to the respondent if the respondent is unable to read or expresses anxiety about the assessment process. Steps for reading these items to respondents are found on page 270 in Bayley and Aylward (2019b).

The respondent should select and circle one rating for each item. The sample ratings on pages 2 and 5 of the questionnaire shows the respondent how to circle the behavior frequency, and the practitioner should point out these samples to ensure the respondent understands the expectations (Bayley & Aylward, 2019b). The Social–Emotional Scale is on pages 2–4 of the questionnaire. When introducing the Social–Emotional Scale to the respondent, it is helpful for the practitioner to review the ratings to ensure the respondent knows what they mean (Bayley & Aylward, 2019b). On the Social–Emotional Scale, one of the following six ratings is selected for each item to best describe how often a particular behavior is observed: 0 (Can't tell), 1 (None of the time), 2 (Some of the time), 3 (Half of the time), 4 (Most of the time), or 5 (All of the time). Respondents circle 0 *Can't Tell* if unsure whether the child has or has not displayed the behavior or does not know the child well enough to respond with confidence. Figure 2.5 shows the ratings for the Social–Emotional Scale as they appear on the questionnaire.

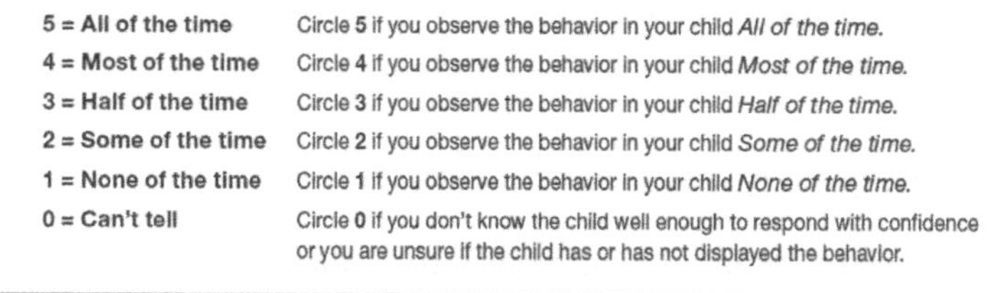

Figure 2.5   Social–Emotional Scale Item Ratings.
Note: From Bayley Scales of Infant and Toddler Development, Fourth Edition (Bayley™–4). Copyright © 2019 NCS Pearson, Inc. Reproduced with permission. All rights reserved.

Adaptive Behavior Scale

Scoring

2 = Usually or often	Circle 2 if your child *usually* or *often* performs the behavior without help or reminders. (Or if he/she has outgrown the behavior.)
1 = Sometimes	Circle 1 if your child *sometimes* performs the behavior without help or reminders.
0 = Never	Circle 0 if your child *never* performs the behavior or never performs it without help or reminders.
	Some reasons why you might circle a score of 0 are:
	▓ Your child has not learned the behavior.
	▓ Your child is not physically able to perform the behavior.
	▓ Your child is not expected or allowed to perform the behavior because of his/her age.
	▓ Your child can perform the behavior but chooses not to.

Figure 2.6 Adaptive Behavior Scale Frequency Based Item Ratings.
Note: From Bayley Scales of Infant and Toddler Development, Fourth Edition (Bayley™–4). Copyright © 2019 NCS Pearson, Inc. Reproduced with permission. All rights reserved.

The Adaptive Behavior Scale is found on pages 5–12 of the questionnaire. When introducing the Adaptive Behavior Scale to the respondent, the practitioner should point out that this part of the questionnaire includes multiple subdomains and to remind the respondent of the differences in the stop point and rating system (Bayley & Aylward, 2019b). For the Adaptive Behavior Scale, a behavior frequency rating scale is used: 2 (Usually or often), 1 (Sometimes), and 0 (Never). The reasons a respondent may rate a child's behavior as 0 *Never* include the fact that the child has not yet learned the behavior, the child is not physically able to perform the behavior, the child may not be expected or allowed to perform the behavior due to age, or the child may be able to perform the behavior but chooses not to. Figure 2.6 shows the ratings for the Adaptive Behavior Scale as they appear on the questionnaire. Respondents are encouraged to make a best guess if they are unsure about the frequency of an item, and the Estimated box should be checked (Bayley & Aylward, 2019b).

ASSESSING CHILDREN WITH DISABILITIES

Practitioners may need to adjust assessment procedures to decrease the impact of a disability or condition on test performance. This is especially true for a child diagnosed with an impairment in vision, hearing, or neuromotor functioning (Aylward, 2020a). The Bayley–4 provides an opportunity to observe and record how a child interacts with people and presented materials in a "structured, yet playful" way that facilitates gathering meaningful clinical information from the assessment (Bayley & Aylward, 2019b, p. 323). When assessing a child with a disability (whether previously diagnosed or suspected), the goal of the Bayley–4 assessment remains the same as with typically developing children—to measure the child's development and abilities as accurately as possible while maintaining the validity of the test results (Aylward, 2020a). Appropriate adaptations to the testing environment, positioning of the child, presentation of materials, types of materials used, time limits, response formats, and provision of corrective feedback can assist with analyzing a child's strengths and needs, which may be helpful with intervention planning and determination of eligibility for access to relevant support programs (Bayley & Aylward, 2019b). Caution must be exercised when applying norm-referenced scores to a child with a physical, neurological, or sensory impairment (Bayley & Aylward, 2019b).

> ## DON'T FORGET 2.2
>
> "Each child with a disability is unique and there is no specific accommodation that is appropriate for all children." (Aylward, 2020a, p. 85)

When assessing children with disabilities, it becomes even more important for practitioners to have familiarity and understanding of the Bayley–4 items and test procedures (Bayley & Aylward, 2019b), as well as typical child development and the ways that a neurodevelopmental, neuromotor, sensory, or physical disability may affect development and behavior (Aylward, 2020a). This includes an understanding of the possible accommodations and modifications that may be needed in order to provide a valid and clinically useful assessment for the child. The testing strategy should be individualized to the child's needs, as every child with an impairment or disability is unique and there is no one testing strategy to employ (Aylward, 2020a; Bayley & Aylward, 2019b). A balance must be struck between giving the child the chance to interact with the testing materials in the standardized way and the practitioner's knowledge of the child's impairment and appropriate accommodations and modifications to address potential needs. To obtain quantitative and qualitative information, a strategy described by Aylward (2020a) includes starting with the standardized administration and adjusting the administration incrementally if the child is unable to complete an item. Providing cues, prompts, and adjustments to feedback and reinforcement of the child's response (e.g., frequent praise, fist bumps, high fives, clapping) may be other helpful strategies (Aylward, 2020a; Bayley & Aylward, 2019b). Rapid Reference 2.9 lists several features and accommodations of the Bayley–4 that facilitate its use with children who have a disability. General approaches to assessing infants and toddlers with disabilities are outlined in Appendix A of the Bayley–4 Administration Manual (Bayley & Aylward, 2019b) and Chapter 9 of *Bayley–4 Clinical Use and Interpretation* (Aylward, 2020a).

≡ *Rapid Reference 2.9*

Bayley–4 Features and Accommodations That Facilitate Use with Children with Disabilities

The Bayley–4 includes many features and accommodations that make it appropriate for use for assessment of children with disabilities including:

- Simplification of directions
- Decreased language load for non-language concepts
- Less scripting of directions
- Utilization of parent report on many items
- Scoring per incidental observation on many items
- Several accommodations consistent with state assessment standards embedded throughout:
  - Individual testing
  - Use of adaptive equipment for positioning
  - Testing with the child facing the practitioner
  - Allowing a variety of individualized response types
- Use of gesturing and encouragement (e.g., praise, applause, fist bumps, high fives) included in instructions for flexible item administration
- Polytomous scoring approach (discussed more in Chapter 3) to measure approximation of skills in addition to mastery
- Graded levels of support for item administration (see Appendix C in the Administration Manual [Bayley & Aylward, 2019b] for examples)

Sources: Aylward (2020a) and Bayley and Aylward (2019b)

Appendix C of the Bayley–4 Administration Manual (Bayley & Aylward, 2019b) includes the accommodations that can be used for children with physical or sensory impairments and guidelines for determining whether an accommodation would significantly alter standardized administration to the point that validity of the scores would be in question (Aylward, 2020a). Accommodations are adaptations to the way test content is presented or the way the child is allowed to respond; the integrity of the construct(s) being measured is preserved in order to maintain standardized administration (Aylward, 2020a; Bayley & Aylward, 2019b). Rapid Reference 2.10 lists accommodations to the Bayley–4 that can be made for children with visual, hearing, and motor impairments. Accommodations are useful when it is difficult to determine whether a child with a disability has the capacity to demonstrate a skill or behavior. Accommodations may be considered a fairer assessment of a child's ability on a particular construct by allowing the chance for the child to demonstrate

≡ *Rapid Reference 2.10*

Bayley–4 Accommodation Features on the Cognitive, Language, and Motor Scales for Children with a Visual, Hearing, or Motor Impairment

For all children with a disability, scheduling assessments at optimal times to lessen fatigue, taking frequent breaks, and maintaining shortened testing sessions may be necessary accommodations to gain the best perspective on the child's abilities (Bayley & Aylward, 2019b). The following accommodations are also recommended for visual, hearing, and motor impairments.

<u>Vision Impairment</u>
- Positioning manipulatives and stimuli where the child can best see them, including:
  - Moving stimuli closer to the child
  - Moving stimuli to one side of their visual field
  - Placing stimuli flat on a table surface
  - Placing items upright or slanted on an easel
- Using glasses, magnifying aids, or assistive equipment for vision enhancement
- Decreasing glare and adjusting lighting
- Extra time for visual scanning of material
- Shorter testing sessions to prevent fatigue from attending to visual stimuli
- Enhancing contrast of the table surface to see test materials better
- Enhancing contrast of picture stimulus with a high-contrast frame
- Assistance with motor tasks affected by visual impairment, including:
  - Child holding and manipulating items
  - Placing items into the child's hands
  - Using manual guiding for identification of response choices

<u>Hearing Impairment</u>
- Use of amplification system (e.g., hearing aid, auditory trainer, or cochlear implant)
- Minimizing ambient noise (e.g., blowers, fans, air conditioners, radios, televisions)
- Minimizing noise with use of noise-absorbing accessories (e.g., rugs, curtains, acoustic panels)
- Facing the child for all communication methods and remaining within a few feet of the child
- Taking time to understand the child's communication strengths because understanding a child's idiosyncratic use of language improves the longer the practitioner is around the child
- Using a variety of ways to communicate encouragement (e.g., demonstrative gestures, smiles, praise, and touch such as fist bumps, high fives, and pats on the back if acceptable to the child and caregiver)

(Continued)

<u>Motor Impairment</u>
- Positioning (based on parent or motor therapist suggestions) that promotes optimal physical control for the child to point, verbalize, or manipulate materials
- Positioning of materials for optimal participation in tasks
  - Presenting materials very close to a child with limited reaching ability
  - Moving an item closer
  - Stabilizing a body part
  - Stabilizing materials with non-slip material or suction cups
- Considering alternative components of responding that indicate awareness of concepts (e.g., eye gaze, facial expression, posture changes, activity level changes)

Modifications to the Bayley–4 testing procedures for children with visual, hearing, and motor impairments, which modify the tasks in a manner that precludes use of norm-referenced scoring, are also listed in Appendix C of the Bayley–4 Administration Manual (Bayley & Aylward, 2019b).
Sources: Aylward (2020a) and Bayley and Aylward (2019b)

DON'T FORGET 2.3

There may be times when a practitioner wants to use the Bayley–4 to assess a child whose chronological age falls outside the test age range. For example, a child who is 6 years old who does not yet exhibit the ability to complete age-appropriate items may be given the Bayley–4 to assess performance on tasks that are more consistent with the child's actual ability level. For such cases, developmental age equivalents may be used to describe the child's performance. Standard scores cannot be derived. There are limitations to using developmental age equivalents, which are discussed in Chapter 4.

a skill or behavior without the score being dictated by the constraints of the disability (Aylward, 2020a; Bayley & Aylward, 2019a).

Modifications are changes to the content of the test such that test item administration can no longer be considered standardized (Aylward, 2020a; Bayley & Aylward, 2019b). Modifications may be appropriate for a child with a significant disability, and the data obtained in that situation may be used qualitatively to evaluate strengths, needs, and emerging skills, as well as to inform intervention planning; however, the data obtained based on modifications cannot be used to compare a child's performance to the normative sample (Aylward, 2020a; Bayley & Aylward, 2019b). Clinical judgment is required for determining the appropriate use of accommodations and modifications on a case-by-case basis.

The Bayley–4 Technical Manual (Bayley & Aylward, 2019c) includes lists of items and behaviors that may assist practitioners with clinical decision making. Appendix A contains a list of items that may be considered developmental risk indicators or "red flags," including movement and muscle tone indicators and autism spectrum disorder indicators, for development that may be helpful in interpretation of the results if a pattern of items from the list is established. It is important not to take any one item or behavior out of context as a developmental risk indicator. Rather, "clusters of abnormalities…are much more reliable in prediction of later dysfunction than are isolated signs. The predictive power of abnormal findings and the amount of concern increase corresponding to an increase in the number of these findings. The *functional significance* of an abnormal finding is critical" (Aylward, 2020a, p. 98).

It is also important to note that a child with a disability may perform a behavior differently than a child without a disability (Bayley & Aylward, 2019b). For example, a child may use sign language or an electronic communication aid to express themselves. Credit is given to a child who successfully demonstrates the target behavior, even if performed in an alternative way. In addition, the wording of items should be considered carefully when crediting performance. For example, when evaluating expressive communication, many of the items use the word, "says," and credit may be given if the child is able to answer correctly using sign language or an electronic communication aid. A child may also be credited as "hearing" an item if the child responded to sign language rather than verbalizations (Bayley & Aylward, 2019b). This information regarding crediting a child's ability to perform a behavior via alternative means should be explained to the respondent completing the Social–Emotional and Adaptive Behavior Questionnaire prior to administration (Bayley & Aylward, 2019b).

MANAGING UNUSUAL OR PROBLEM BEHAVIORS DURING TESTING

An infant or toddler may engage in behaviors during testing that make administration of items challenging. There can be a wide variety of reasons for this behavior, some of which are typical and should be expected by any user of the Bayley–4. Refusal to complete items, refusal to give up manipulatives and move to the next task, temper tantrums, falling asleep, toileting accidents, and crying will likely all be encountered at one time or another by a practitioner who tests infants and toddlers. In some cases, a young child may be referred for a developmental assessment due to challenging behaviors that are out of the typical expectations for their age. These challenging behaviors (e.g., throwing objects, biting, screaming, spitting) may be associated with delayed development, trauma history, or a neurological or developmental disability. In all cases, the practitioner must remain calm and have a plan for how to manage such difficult circumstances.

As was emphasized earlier in this chapter, good practitioner preparation sets the stage for a positive testing session regardless of the child's problem behaviors. When a practitioner is prepared, more time can be spent attending to the child's behavior and needs and less time with attempting the correct administration of the items. Testing efficiencies built into the Bayley–4, such as administering series and related items together, refraining from repetition of trials once a perfect score is obtained, and using Caregiver Questions when applicable, should be understood and used by the practitioner as much as is appropriate for the child being tested (Bayley & Aylward, 2019b). In addition, many challenges during testing can be avoided by appropriate timing of the assessment (e.g., avoiding feeding and nap times). However, there are times that scheduling cannot account for the child's schedule, and the best a practitioner can do is maintain a positive demeanor and administer the items as efficiently as possible while attempting to accommodate the child's needs. It is also important for the practitioner to manage frustration levels in these situations and to continue to engage the child positively with a calm and playful approach.

If a child is not responding and starting to act inappropriately with a given item, the practitioner may try to transition the child to a more engaging, fun task. If possible, the practitioner should try to remove any objects or stimuli within the testing environment that may be the focus of negative behavior and try to move quickly to the next task, paying as little attention to the problem behavior as possible and encouraging more positive interactions (Black & Matula, 2000). Typically, the behavior on which the practitioner focuses attention will increase, whether positive or negative (Bailey, 2015). If a child continues to refuse responses, is struggling with attending to a task, and/or is fussing, yelling, or crying, it is best to take a break. Although it is important to try to complete testing in one session, it may not be possible if the practitioner is not successful in re-engaging the child in the testing session.

There are times when a child may perseverate on a certain manipulative item or picture. This may be more likely for a child who demonstrates behaviors consistent with an autism spectrum disorder diagnosis. If this becomes a problem for continued administration of the test, try to finish this item set quickly, and then take a break to refocus the child's attention. While the child is taking the break, the practitioner can remove the item that was leading to the perseveration. After returning from break, the child may look for the preferred item and quickly transitioning the child to an engaging task will give a chance for the testing to continue. If the child references the item(s) he or she was fond of, the practitioner can make a validating statement such as, "That [toy, picture, object] is fun, and this [toy, picture, object] is fun, too." The practitioner can then engage in using or playing with the object in a playful way, and encourage the child to do the same, to capture the child's attention and interest. The practitioner may also find success in using the preferred object as reinforcement for completion of the tasks, but this will only work if the child is willing to give up the object.

TELEPRACTICE AND THE BAYLEY–4

The COVID-19 global pandemic introduced challenges for testing that had not been encountered before. Suddenly, the ability to conduct in-person testing became restricted and/or introduced testing conditions that compromised standardization. This is especially true for assessing infants and toddlers, as remote assessment of cognitive, language, and motor skills through practitioner interaction with young children is not feasible. Rapid Reference 2.11 summarizes guidance provided by Pearson for professionals considering telepractice use of the Bayley–4.

≡ Rapid Reference 2.11

Telepractice Administration of the Bayley–4

Pearson, Inc. has provided a guidance document that urges postponement of testing using the Bayley–4 if at all possible, as standard administration of the Bayley–4 cannot be conducted via telepractice administration. However, if an assessment cannot be postponed and is necessary for the benefit of the child, the guidance document on the Pearson, Inc. website https://www.pearsonassessments.com/professional-assessments/digital-solutions/telepractice/telepractice-and-the-Bayley–4.html) provides considerations regarding how practitioners may be able to obtain qualitative data that may inform recommendations for intervention in conjunction with other measures of development and functioning. The Bayley–4 Q-global digital assets needed for telepractice administration are available for purchase from Pearson.

The telepractice guidance document on the Pearson website includes a thorough description of considerations and methods for using the Bayley–4 for telepractice. This document should be read and understood before any attempt by a practitioner to use the Bayley–4 in a telepractice format. Below is a brief summary for practitioners considering telepractice administration of the Bayley–4.

Practitioner Responsibilities
- Follow best practice recommendations and ethical codes.
- Follow telepractice regulations and all legal requirements.

(Continued)

- Develop competence with assessment via telepractice through consultation, collaboration, and ongoing professional development.
- Use clinical judgment to determine whether assessment via telepractice is appropriate.
- Document all considerations, procedures, and conclusions, especially regarding how administration differed from standardized procedures and the conditions under which telepractice was deemed necessary.

Administration Methods via Telepractice

- Social–Emotional & Adaptive Behavior Scale questionnaire completed by parents or caregivers:
  - Using Q-global for ROSA, which does not require video contact.
  - Using Q-global for On-Screen Administration (OSA) via videoconferencing.
- The Cognitive, Language, and Motor subtests **CANNOT** be administered in a standardized format via telepractice. Cognitive, Language, and Motor Scales are administered by a qualified professional through observation and direct interaction with the child.
- Some qualitative information regarding cognitive, language, and motor skills may be available through observation and Caregiver Questions.

Considerations If Using Telepractice

- Review Appendix A of the *Bayley–4 Technical Manual*.
- Review Chapters 8, 9, and 10 of *Bayley–4 Clinical Use and Interpretation* (Aylward, 2020a).
- This approach does not allow for calculation of scores for cognitive, language, and motor skills. However, practitioners can use observations and information from the caregiver to inform their clinical opinion, according to Part C of the IDEIA (Individuals with Disabilities Education Improvement Act of 2004).
- The Item Presentation Summary in the Q-global resource library provides details of items for which information can be obtained through observation and Caregiver Questions.

The practitioner is encouraged to review the general information on the Pearson telepractice overview web page, as well as the five factors listed in the Telepractice and Bayley–4 guidance document, to consider when planning for telepractice administration, which are too extensive to describe here. These factors include the telepractice environment and equipment, assessment procedures and materials, examinee considerations, examiner considerations, and other considerations.

At the time of publication for this book, telepractice guidance posted on the Pearson Clinical Assessments website was intended for use only during the COVID-19 global pandemic. Use of the Bayley–4 via telepractice may not be permitted by Pearson, Inc. for other uses. Practitioners must check the Pearson Clinical website for guidance on how to use the Bayley–4 materials in a non-standardized way. If this guidance no longer exists on the website, it must be assumed that telepractice administration is no longer an acceptable way of collecting qualitative

(Continued)

developmental information about a child using the Bayley–4. Practitioners should contact Pearson, Inc. customer support with further questions regarding telepractice administration.
Source: NCS Pearson, Inc. (2020). *Administering the Bayley Scales of Infant and Toddler Development* (4th ed.) *via Telepractice.* https://www.pearsonassessments. com/professional-assessments/digital-solutions/telepractice/telepractice-and-the-Bayley–4.html.

TEST YOURSELF

1. **Professional-level training and familiarity with the Bayley–4 administration procedures and items are necessary because:**
   a) Testing infants and toddlers presents considerations and challenges unique to the age range
   b) The practitioner must be able to move quickly and smoothly between items to keep the child's interest, attention, and cooperation
   c) The practitioner may need to make accommodations for a child who has an impairment
   d) All of the above
2. **The scores from the Bayley–4 are sufficient evidence to diagnose a developmental disability.**
   True or False
3. **What are the three options for Bayley–4 administration and scoring?**
4. **The basal and discontinue criteria for the Cognitive, Language, and Motor subtests are:**
   a) 3 consecutive scores of 2 at an age start point; 5 consecutive scores of 0
   b) 5 consecutive scores of 2 at an age start point; 5 consecutive scores of 0
   c) 3 consecutive scores of 2 at an age start point, 3 consecutive scores of 0
   d) different for each subtest
5. **The child's caregiver is minimally involved in the Bayley–4 assessment because the practitioner is a highly trained expert and is able to elicit responses from the child better than the caregiver.**
   True or False
6. **Digital administration of the Bayley–4 includes:**
   a) The child interacting with stimuli presented on an electronic device
   b) The practitioner accessing item administration information and recording responses on an electronic device

    c) A game-like interactive experience for the child on a tablet

    d) A computer workstation so the child can complete the assessment

7. **The Adaptive Behavior Scale uses items from the Vineland-3.**
True or False

8. **The terms "accommodation" and "modification" should not be used interchangeably when discussing adaptations made to Bayley–4 items because they refer to different levels of adaptation.**
True or False

9. **All Bayley–4 items can be scored by a caregiver report.**
True or False

10. **List the five scales of the Bayley–4.**

Answers: 1. (d); 2. False; 3. Paper administration and scoring, paper administration with digital scoring and reporting, and digital administration, scoring, and reporting; 4. (a); 5. False; 6. (b); 7. True; 8. True; 9. False; 10. Cognitive, Language, Motor, Social–Emotional, and Adaptive Behavior.

REFERENCES

Alfonso, V. C., Engler, J. R., & Lepore, J. C. C. (2020). Assessing and evaluating young children: Developmental domains and methods. In V. C. Alfonso & G. J. DuPaul (Eds.), *Healthy development in young children: Evidence-based interventions for early education* (pp. 13–44). American Psychological Association. Retrieved from https://doi.org/10.1037/0000197-002.

American Educational Research Association, American Psychological Association, & National Council on Measurement in Education (2014). *Standards for educational and psychological testing.* American Educational Research Association.

Aylward, G. P. (2020a). *Bayley–4 clinical use and interpretation.* Academic Press.

Aylward, G. P. (2020b). Is it correct to correct for prematurity? Theoretic analysis of the Bayley–4 normative data. *Journal of Developmental & Behavioral Pediatrics, 41*, 128–133.

Bailey, B. A. (2015). *Conscious discipline: Building resilient classrooms.* Loving Guidance.

Bayley, N. (2006). *Bayley Scales of Infant and Toddler Development* (3rd ed.). *Administration manual.* Pearson.

Bayley, N., & Aylward, G. P. (2019a). *Bayley Scales of Infant and Toddler Development* (4th ed.). Pearson.

Bayley, N., & Aylward, G. P. (2019b). *Bayley Scales of Infant and Toddler Development* (4th ed.). *Administration manual.* Pearson.

Bayley, N., & Aylward, G. P. (2019c). *Bayley Scales of Infant and Toddler Development* (4th ed.). *Technical manual.* Pearson.

Bayley, N., & Aylward, G. P. (2019d). *Bayley Scales of Infant and Toddler Development* (4th ed.). *Digital administration user's guide.* Pearson.

Black, M. M., & Matula, K. (2000). *Essentials of Bayley Scales of Infant Development–II assessment.* John Wiley & Sons.

Greenspan, S. I. (2004). *Greenspan Social-Emotional Growth Chart: A Screening Questionnaire for Infants and Young Children [Measurement Instrument].* Harcourt Assessment.

Individuals With Disabilities Education Improvement Act of 2004, Pub. L., No. 108–446, 118 Stat, 2647.

NCS Pearson, Inc. (2020). *Administering the Bayley Scales of Infant and Toddler Development (4th ed.) via telepractice.* https://www.pearsonassessments.com/ professional-assessments/digital-solutions/telepractice/telepractice-and-the-Bayley–4.html.

NCS Pearson, Inc. (2021a, February 13). *Bayley Scales of Infant and Toddler Development* (4th ed). Retrieved from Pearson Assessments: https://www. pearsonassessments.com/store/usassessments/en/Store/Professional-Assessments/Cogniton-%26-Neuro/Bayley-Scales-of-Infant-and-Toddler-Development-%7C-Fourth-Edition/p/1000001996.html?tab=faq.

NCS Pearson, Inc. (2021b, February 13). *Chronological Age Calculator.* Retrieved from Pearson Clinical: https://images.pearsonclinical.com/images/ ageCalculator/ageCalculator.htm.

Sparrow, S. S., Cicchetti, D. V., & Saulnier, C. A. (2016). *Vineland Adaptive Behavior Scales* (3rd ed.). Pearson.

Three

HOW TO SCORE THE BAYLEY–4

Vincent C. Alfonso, Joseph R. Engler, and Andrea D. Turner
Gonzaga University and Pearson Assessments

The *Bayley Scales of Infant and Toddler Development–Fourth Edition* (Bayley–4; Bayley & Aylward, 2019a) offers a variety of scores to understand better a young child's current developmental functioning across cognitive, language, motor, social-emotional, and adaptive behavior areas. Therefore, this chapter begins by providing an overview of scores available across Bayley–4 scales, subtests, domains, and subdomains. Then, we discuss general scoring procedures that may be helpful when administering the Bayley–4. Next, we discuss how to convert raw scores to scaled or standard scores as a way of comparing any child's performance to the normative population (which is discussed in detail in Chapter 4). In addition, we describe how to calculate, and where to find, confidence intervals, developmental age equivalents, growth scale values (GSVs), and percent delays for reporting purposes. We conclude with a brief discussion on how to score the Bayley–4 using Q-global®.

SCORES AVAILABLE FOR THE BAYLEY–4

There are several scores available for the Bayley–4; namely, scaled scores, standard scores, and percentile ranks. A summary of scores available across the Cognitive, Language, Motor, Social–Emotional, and Adaptive Behavior Scales is found in Table 3.1. It is important to note that certain scores cannot be derived for certain scales, subtests, domains, or subdomains. For example, age equivalents and GSVs are not available for the Motor Scale. Nevertheless, the Bayley–4 provides multiple ways of calculating and reporting scores that are valuable to a practitioner.

Essentials of Bayley™–4 Assessment, First Edition. Vincent C. Alfonso, Joseph R. Engler and Andrea D. Turner.
© 2022 John Wiley & Sons, Inc. Published 2022 by John Wiley & Sons, Inc.

Table 3.1 Bayley–4 Score Types

domain subdomain	Scaled score	Standard score	Percentile rank	Confidence interval	Age equivalent	Growth scale value
Cognitive (COG)		✓	✓	✓		
Cognitive (CG)	✓				✓	✓
Language (LANG)		✓	✓	✓		
Receptive Communication (RC)	✓				✓	✓
Expressive Communication (EC)	✓				✓	✓
Motor (MOT)		✓	✓	✓		
Fine Motor (FM)	✓				✓	✓
Gross Motor (GM)	✓				✓	✓
Social-Emotional (SOEM)		✓	✓	✓		
Social-Emotional (SE)	✓					

Scale domain subdomain	Scaled score	Standard score	Percentile rank	Confidence interval	Age equivalent	Growth scale value
Adaptive Behavior (ADBE)		✓	✓	✓		
Communication (COM)		✓	✓	✓		
Receptive (REC)	✓				✓	✓
Expressive (EXP)	✓				✓	✓
Daily Living Skills (DLS)		✓	✓	✓		
Personal (PER)	✓				✓	✓

(Continued)

Table 3.1 (Continued)

domain subdomain	Scaled score	Standard score	Percentile rank	Confidence interval	Age equivalent	Growth scale value
Socialization (SOC)		✓	✓	✓		
Interpersonal Relationship (IPR)	✓				✓	✓
Play and Leisure (PLA)	✓				✓	✓

Note: From Bayley Scales of Infant and Toddler Development, Fourth Edition (Bayley™–4). Copyright © 2019 NCS Pearson, Inc. Reproduced with permission. All rights reserved.

A brief overview is given of the types of scores available for the Bayley–4, as well as confidence intervals, developmental age equivalents, GSVs, and percent delays.

SCALED SCORES, STANDARD SCORES, AND PERCENTILE RANKS

A scaled score is a conversion of a raw score to a standardized scale and represents a child's performance on a subtest or subdomain relative to peers (Bayley & Aylward, 2019c). For the Bayley–4, scaled scores range from 1 to 19, with a mean of 10 and a standard deviation (SD) of 3. Based on this metric, a score of 7 is equivalent to 1 SD below the mean. Conversely, a score of 13 is equivalent to 1 SD above the mean (Bayley & Aylward, 2019b). Scaled scores can be calculated for all Bayley–4 subtests and for the Adaptive Behavior subdomains, which allow for comparison of a child's performance to the normative sample. Standard scores, which are similar to scaled scores, are derived from the sum of subtest and subdomain scaled scores. The standard scores on the Bayley–4 have a mean of 100 and an SD of 15. For example, standard scores of 85 and 115 are equivalent to 1 SD below and above the mean, respectively. For the Cognitive, Language, Motor, and Social–Emotional Scales, the standard scores range from 45 to 155. For the Adaptive Behavior Scale, standard scores range from 40 to 160.

Percentile ranks are derived for scaled and standard scores. Percentile ranks have a mean and median of 50, with a range from 1 to 99. A percentile rank indicates

Table 3.2   Relation of Standard and Scaled Scores to Standard Deviations from the Mean, Percentile Rank, and Descriptive Classification

Scaled score	Standard score	SDs from mean	Percentile rank	Descriptive classification
–	160	+4	>99.9	Extremely high
–	155	+3 2/3	>99.9	Extremely high
–	150	+3 1/3	>99.9	Extremely high
19	145	+3	99.9	Extremely high
18	140	+2 2/3	99.6	Extremely high
17	135	+2 1/3	99.0	Extremely high
16	130	+2	98.0	Extremely high
15	125	+1 2/3	95.0	Very high
14	120	+1 1/3	91.0	Very high
13	115	+1	84.0	High average
12	110	+2/3	75.0	High average
11	105	+1/3	63.0	Average
10	100	0	50.0	Average
9	95	–1/3	37.0	Average
8	90	–2/3	25.0	Average
7	85	–1	16.0	Low average
6	80	–1 1/3	9.0	Low average
5	75	–1 2/3	5.0	Very low
4	70	–2	2.0	Very low
3	65	–2 1/3	1.0	Extremely low
2	60	–2 2/3	0.4	Extremely low
1	55	–3	0.1	Extremely low
–	50	–3 1/3	<0.1	Extremely low
–	45	–3 2/3	<0.1	Extremely low
–	40	–4	<0.1	Extremely low

the child's relative standing to other children in the same age group of the normative sample. Specifically, percentile ranks indicate the percentage of same-aged children in the standardization sample who performed equal to or below the score for the child being tested (Bayley & Aylward, 2019b). Table 3.2 is a reproduction of Table 5.1 in the Technical Manual and shows the

CAUTION 3.1

Caution is warranted when using percentile ranks to compare across scales within the Bayley–4 or to scores on other measures. They are also not an accurate way to make comparisons of testing results at different developmental stages for the child.

relation between Bayley–4 scaled scores, standard scores, SDs from the mean, percentile ranks, and descriptive classifications (Bayley & Aylward, 2019c). Readers are also encouraged to see Chapter 4, for interpretive and reporting guidelines for scaled scores, standard scores, and percentile ranks.

CONFIDENCE INTERVALS, DEVELOPMENTAL AGE EQUIVALENTS, GROWTH SCALE VALUES, AND PERCENT DELAYS

In addition to scaled scores, standard scores, and percentile ranks, practitioners can also obtain confidence intervals, developmental age equivalents, GSVs, and percent delays on the Bayley–4. An in-depth discussion is precluded from this chapter due to space limitations and each of the aforementioned is described in Chapter 4. Thus, only a brief overview is provided here. A confidence interval describes a band of scores around an obtained score within which the child's true score is likely to fall (Sattler, 2018). Confidence intervals for the Bayley–4 are calculated at the 90% or 95% confidence level. The practitioner has the option of choosing which confidence interval is most appropriate.

Developmental age equivalents estimate the chronological age (in months) at which a typically developing child would obtain the same total raw score or demonstrate the skills observed for the child being assessed. Developmental age equivalents are derived by calculating the average raw scores obtained on a test by children at different ages (Sattler, 2018). Chapter 5 of the Technical Manual provides more information regarding the steps that were followed to derive the age equivalents for the Bayley–4 (Bayley & Aylward, 2019c). Developmental age equivalents involve a fair amount of controversy, however, and should be used only when they can be easily understood and interpreted by practitioners and caregivers alike. Rapid Reference 4.3 in Chapter 4, highlights some of the limitations of developmental age equivalents. On the Bayley–4, developmental age equivalents are available for the Cognitive, Receptive Communication, Expressive Communication, Fine Motor, and Gross Motor subtests and the Adaptive Behavior Scale subdomains.

GSVs are used to follow the young child's developmental growth over time (e.g., between two administrations of the Bayley–4 that occurred at different ages) for each performance-based subtest and the Adaptive Behavior Scale subdomains. They are not available for the Social–Emotional subtest. The GSVs are derived from the total raw score and have a mean of 500 and an SD of 25. The GSVs provide a way to document an individual child's progress or improvement over time independent of comparisons to same-age peers. They are not used for comparison between subtests or subdomains. Due to measurement error when comparing GSVs from one testing session to another, it is important to determine the statistical significance of a change in GSVs (Bayley & Aylward, 2019b).

> **DON'T FORGET 3.1**
>
> The GSVs provide a way to document an individual child's progress or improvement over time independent of comparisons to same-age peers. They are not used for comparison between subtests or subdomains.

Percent delay is derived from age equivalents. The percent delay is usually calculated by dividing the developmental age of a child by the child's chronological age, multiplying that value by 100, then subtracting that percentage from 100%. For example, a child who is 19 months old with an age equivalent of 12 months would be considered to have a 37% delay or be functioning at 63% of the child's expected developmental ability. Percent delay is frequently used for determining eligibility for early intervention services (Individuals with Disabilities Education Improvement Act, 2004, Part C) and may differ by state, with qualifications of services for a 20%, 30%, or 40% delay (Bayley & Aylward, 2019b).

GENERAL SCORING PROCEDURES

There are several general scoring procedures that practitioners should be made aware. They include polytomous scoring, quantitatively and qualitatively-based scoring, incidental observations, multiple responses and self-corrections, and scoring caregiver responses. Further, each of these general scoring procedures is likely to be encountered during a typical Bayley–4 administration and, thus, should be thoroughly understood prior to administering the instrument. Although these will be discussed in this chapter, readers are encouraged to see Bayley and Aylward (2019b) for more information.

The Bayley–4 includes new polytomous scoring for the Cognitive, Language, and Motor Scales, which assigns a score of 2, 1, or 0 for observed behaviors and/

or caregiver responses to individual items. This represents a change from dichotomous scoring of previous versions of the Bayley Scales, which gave either full or no credit by assigning a score of 1 or 0, respectively. Polytomous scoring has an advantage over the dichotomous scoring approach for young children who are demonstrating emerging skills within a particular item or area. In addition, polytomous scoring provides a clear direction for discerning the extent to which a young child has developed a skill. Polytomous scoring applies a score of 2 for mastery level skills, which indicates that the child can successfully demonstrate the skill most of the time. A score of 1 is assigned to emerging skills, which indicates the child inconsistently demonstrates the skill, or the skill is present to some degree, yet mastery of the skill is expected to develop eventually. A score of 0 is assigned to skills that are not present, indicating the absence of the skill or ability being measured, and may indicate a delay or deficit. Table 3.3 summarizes polytomous scoring and provides an approach to polytomous scoring.

The Social–Emotional and Adaptive Behavior Scales utilize a different scoring procedure from the Cognitive, Language, and Motor Scales, as well as from each other. This can be attributed to the Social–Emotional

DON'T FORGET 3.2

The Bayley–4 includes new polytomous scoring for the Cognitive, Language, and Motor Scales, which assigns a score of 2, 1, or 0 for observed behaviors and/or caregiver responses to individual items. This represents a change from dichotomous scoring of previous versions of the Bayley Scales, which gave either full or no credit by assigning a score of 1 or 0, respectively.

Table 3.3   Bayley–4 Scoring Approach Summary

Skill level	Score	Description
Mastery	2 points	This score reflects successful mastery of a task or skill. Consider a 2-point score to reflect proficiency that occurs consistently or almost all of the time.
Emerging	1 point	This score reflects an emerging skill or performance on a task that does not suggest mastery but is present to some degree. The skill is inconsistent or present only some of the time but is anticipated to eventually develop into mastery.
Not present	0 points	This score reflects when a skill is not yet present. The absence of the skill or ability may be either a delay or a deficit.

Note: From Bayley Scales of Infant and Toddler Development, Fourth Edition (Bayley™–4). Copyright © 2019 NCS Pearson, Inc. Reproduced with permission. All rights reserved.

and Adaptive Behavior Scales relying on ratings from the caregiver as compared to direct observation and/or caregiver responses. The Social–Emotional Scale utilizes a six-point Likert scale for scoring purposes, which requires the caregiver to assign one of the following ratings to each item: 0 (can't tell), 1 (none of the time), 2 (some of the time), 3 (half of the time), 4 (most of the time), or 5 (all of the time). A score of 0 is assigned if the caregiver is unsure if the child has displayed the behavior or if the caregiver does not know the child well enough to answer with confidence. In such cases, the practitioner may want to follow up with questions to clarify 0-point responses. On the Adaptive Behavior Scale, a three-point scale is used based on a frequency of observed behavior. The caregiver assigns one of the following ratings for each item: 0 (never), 1 (sometimes), and 2 (usually or often). A score of 0 is assigned when the child has not yet learned the behavior, is not physically able to perform the behavior, is not expected or allowed to perform the behavior due to age, or chooses not to perform the behavior despite being able.

Quantitative observation is used for scoring many of the Bayley–4 items. Quantitative observation refers to the number of trials with a correct response and is used on timed items and/or items that require a certain number of manipulatives to be placed (e.g., Pegboard, Pink Board, or Blue Board Series). It is imperative that a practitioner follows the quantitative scoring criteria and refrains from overriding a score based on clinical judgment or observation (i.e., qualitative scoring) at all times. In addition to quantitatively-based scoring, the Bayley–4 has several items that require clinical judgment because they are scored based on qualitative observation and, therefore, require qualitatively-based scoring. The polytomous scoring approach for each item helps guide the practitioner in the decision-making process regarding how to score an item based on qualitative data. As described above, the child's performance is scored in terms of proficiency in a skill area or if the skill is not fully developed or is absent. A review of page 31 in Bayley and Aylward (2019b) provides detailed information on quantitatively and qualitatively-based scoring.

Incidental observations are indispensable to the administration of the Bayley–4, as it allows a practitioner to score as many items by incidental observation as possible. The Observation Checklist may be used to identify and score items based solely on observation. These behaviors include verbal behaviors and interactions with the caregiver that occur spontaneously. It is recommended that a practitioner be familiar with the Bayley–4 items to prevent missing incidental observation opportunities upon greeting the young child and caregiver and prior to the testing session, between administration of items, or when the child and caregiver take a break. A practitioner who is not fully familiar with the Bayley–4 items may miss this opportunity to record an incidental observation of the child engaging in joint attention with the caregiver.

Although Q-global includes efficient navigation to test items that can be scored by observation, it may disrupt the natural flow of the interaction with the child and caregiver in some situations, such as upon first greeting them, to record incidental observations on the practitioner's device in that moment. This is another example of the importance of practitioner familiarity with the items that can be scored by incidental observation, as it may be more conducive to the flow of the testing session to note observations unobtrusively on the Observation Checklist and record the scores in Q-global later (Bayley & Aylward, 2019b).

There are times when a young child may provide more than one response to an item. If the child self-corrects with a response after the initial response, appropriate credit is given. If the practitioner can discern that a later response is intended to replace a previous one, the intended response is scored. On timed items, the best response given within the time limit is scored. In addition, verbal prompts may be needed at times to help clarify a response from the child. For example, a child may point to more than one response on the Stimulus Book. The practitioner should then say, "Point to just one picture." If the child points to only one picture, that response is scored. If multiple pictures are chosen again, the response is scored as incorrect. A correct and incorrect response from the child can be given to the same item. If it is not clear which is the intended response, the practitioner can ask something like, "Which one is it?" or "Which one did you mean?" to elicit the intended response and score that response.

For items that can be responded to by the caregiver (e.g., Caregiver Questions), the practitioner may ask the caregiver how often the child demonstrates the behavior when attempting it, or when given the opportunity. The item is scored as 2 points (i.e., mastery) if the child demonstrates the behavior *almost every time* or *often*. The item is scored 1 point (i.e., emerging) if the behavior is performed *some of the time* or *not often*. The item is scored 0 points (i.e., not present) if the behavior is performed *none of the time* or *not at all*. Table 3.4 provides more thorough explanations for scoring Caregiver Questions.

There is no limit on how many Caregiver Questions may be asked in place of structured item scores. However, caregiver responses should only be used if the caregiver is someone who has frequent and extended contact with the child. If discrepancies are noted between the observed performance of the child during the

CAUTION 3.2

Caregiver Questions should only be used in place of structured item scores if the individual responding has frequent and extended contact with the child. Otherwise, the validity of the scores may be questionable.

Table 3.4 Caregiver Question Scoring Summary

Caregiver response	Score	Description
Almost every time or Often	2 points	Use this score when the caregiver indicates that the child is consistently able to perform a task when he or she tries, that the child responds the same way almost every time, or that the child is able to perform a task at least 75% of the time when given the opportunity.
Some of the time or Not often	1 point	Use this score when the caregiver indicates that the child performs a task inconsistently or intermittently when given the opportunity; that the child responds as expected only some of the time; or that the child is able to perform a task, but not at least 75% of the time when given the opportunity.
None of the time or Not at all	0 points	Use this score when the caregiver indicates that a skill or behavior is not yet present in any form, that the child attempts the behavior but is never successful, or that the child is not able to perform a task when given the opportunity.

Note: From Bayley Scales of Infant and Toddler Development, Fourth Edition (Bayley™–4). Copyright © 2019 NCS Pearson, Inc. Reproduced with permission. All rights reserved.

testing session and the caregiver responses, the scores based on the Caregiver Questions are considered potentially invalid.

SCORING RESPONSES ON THE PAPER RECORD FORM

Scoring the paper Record Form includes several steps that culminate in the completion of the Summary section on the front page of the Record Form. The steps include calculating total raw scores for each subtest and subdomain, transferring raw scores to the Summary section, converting the raw scores to scaled scores and standard scores, and then calculating confidence intervals, age equivalents, and GSVs. As a result, a practitioner has all of the information necessary to interpret the results of the test. There are slight variations in scoring the Cognitive, Language, and Motor Scales as compared to the Social–Emotional and Adaptive Behavior Scales so each is discussed separately.

Calculating Total Raw Scores for the Cognitive, Language, and Motor Subtests

On the Record Form, pages 3–47 include a box at the bottom to record the sum of the scores for all items on each page (e.g., page 3 total, page 4 total, etc.). For administering a subtest, total raw scores are calculated for each subtest. It is important to remember that once a basal is established (i.e., three consecutive perfect scores at an appropriate start point), all items below the basal are scored as 2, unless the basal starts at Item 1. Items between the basal and ceiling (i.e., five consecutive scores of 0) are scored according to the child's performance or the response given to a Caregiver Question. If any items were administered after the ceiling, they are scored as 0 regardless of the child's performance or the caregiver's response. The practitioner assigns a page total on each page and then sums the page totals to calculate the total raw score provided on the last page of each subtest. A separate box is included for clarity. This occurs for all Cognitive, Language, and Motor subtests. The total raw score for each subtest is then transferred to the first page of the Record Form in the raw score column for the corresponding subtest. It is important that the practitioner pays close attention to the calculation and transfer of raw scores on the Record Form, and double checks this information for accuracy. Rapid Reference 3.1 lists some common scoring errors made by practitioners when calculating total raw scores.

To illustrate calculating a total raw score, please consider the following example for August. August is an 8-month, 20-day-old child who begins with Item 12 (Start Point H) on the Cognitive subtest. This item is at the bottom of page 4, and August obtains a raw score of 2 on that item. Because a basal is yet to be established, the

≡ Rapid Reference 3.1

Common Errors in Calculating Subtest Raw Scores

- Not including raw scores for items below the basal (scored 2 points) that were not administered in the total raw score
- Not adding the points from all boxes at the bottom of the Record Form within a particular subtest
- Transferring total raw scores incorrectly from inside the Record Form to the front page of the Record Form
- Miscalculating the total raw score sum
- Including points earned after the discontinue criterion was met
- Not double checking totals and the data transferred to the Record Form

Adapted from Flanagan, D. P., & Alfonso, V. C. (2017). *Essentials of WISC-V assessment.* John Wiley & Sons, Inc.

practitioner leaves the box at the bottom of page 4 temporarily blank. On the next page, August obtains a raw score of 2 for items 13–19. As a result, a raw score of 14 is entered in the page 5 total box. The basal is established and the practitioner moves to page 6 of the Record Form, on which August obtains a raw score of 1 on items 20 and 21 and a raw score of 0 for the remaining five items on the page. The ceiling is established and the subtest is discontinued, with a total raw score of 2 entered in the page 6 total box. The practitioner goes back and enters a total of 10 (i.e., 2 points for the 5 items) in the page 3 total box and a total of 14 (i.e., 2 points for the 7 items) in the page 4 total box because full credit is given to items below the basal. Next, the scores in the page total boxes are added resulting in a Cognitive total raw score of 40 (10 + 14 + 14 + 2) on page 16 of the Record Form. The Cognitive total raw score is recorded and transferred to the Cognitive raw score box on the first page of the Record Form in the Total Raw Score to Scaled Score Conversion table of the Summary. This process is followed for the remaining subtests.

Converting Total Raw Scores to Scaled Scores for the Cognitive, Language, and Motor Subtests

Once total raw scores are calculated and transferred to the raw score column on the front page of the Record Form, the practitioner converts the raw scores to scaled scores. The Record Form refers to Table A.1 of the Administration Manual to assist in this process (Bayley & Aylward, 2019b). The test age or adjusted test age of the child determines which portion of Table A.1 is used. The practitioner finds the quadrant with the age range that corresponds with the child's test age or adjusted test age to use. Next, the practitioner locates the subtest abbreviation (see Chapter 1, for subtest abbreviations), and looks under that abbreviation, where all available subtest raw scores are found, and finds the raw score (or range of raw scores) that matches the young child's performance. Directly to the left or right of the raw score is the corresponding scaled score value within the shaded bands on either side of the quadrant. Once identified, the scaled score is recorded and transferred to the front page of the Record Form in the scaled score column for the corresponding subtest. The practitioner must continue to pay close attention and double check the accuracy when obtaining the scaled scores from Table A.1 and transferring the scores to the Record Form. Rapid Reference 3.2 lists the common scoring errors made by practitioners when obtaining scaled scores.

To continue the example above with August, the practitioner looks in Table A.1 and locates the ages 8:16–9:15 quadrant found on page 290 in the Administration Manual (Bayley & Aylward, 2019b). A Cognitive raw score of 40 is found in the range of 39–41 and corresponds to a scaled score of 5. This value is entered in the scaled score column for the Cognitive subtest. This process is followed for the remaining performance-based subtests.

Rapid Reference 3.2

Frequent Errors in Obtaining Scaled Scores

- Using a score conversion table that references the wrong age group
- Referencing a score conversion table for the wrong subtest
- Misreading across the rows of the score conversion tables
- Transferring scaled scores incorrectly from the conversion table to the Record Form
- Mistakenly confusing total raw scores with scaled or standard scores when they are within the same range
- Neglecting to double check the accuracy of calculations and the data obtained from relevant tables

Adapted from Flanagan, D. P., & Alfonso, V. C. (2017). *Essentials of WISC-V assessment.* John Wiley & Sons, Inc.

Reporting Age Equivalents

The next column to complete on the Record Form is age equivalents. The age equivalent column is associated with Table B.1 in the Administration Manual (Bayley & Aylward, 2019b). To obtain the age equivalent, the practitioner looks under the appropriate subtest abbreviation, similar to calculating scaled scores, and finds the obtained raw score (or range of raw scores) that matches the young child's performance. The practitioner then looks to the shaded area directly to the right or the left of the raw score to find the age equivalent in the corresponding row. Once identified, the age equivalent is recorded and transferred to the first page of the Record Form. Continuing with the example of August, a raw score of 40 on the Cognitive subtest corresponds with an age equivalent of 6:00 (i.e., 6 months, 0 days). This value is entered in the age equivalent column for the Cognitive subtest. This process is repeated for each of the performance subtests.

Reporting GSVs

The last column to complete on the Summary section is the GSV. Table B.2 in Appendix B of the Administration Manual is used to obtain this score. Finding the GSV is different from finding the previously mentioned scores in that the practitioner must first look in the shaded region labeled 'Raw score.' When the practitioner locates the raw score that matches the young child's performance, the practitioner should look directly to the right under the appropriate subtest abbreviation. That value is the GSV for the young child. The value is then recorded and transferred to the GSV column on page 1 of the Record Form. For August, the GSV corresponding with a total raw score of 40 on the Cognitive subtest is 483. This process is then repeated for each of the performance subtests and Adaptive Behavior subdomains.

Calculating Standard Scores, Percentile Ranks, and Confidence Intervals for the Cognitive, Language, and Motor Subtests

Before the practitioner can obtain standard scores, the sum of scaled scores must be calculated. The scaled score column in the Summary section on page 1 of the Record Form includes cells that are labeled with 1, 2, and 3 in the lower right corner. The numbers correspond to the same numbers in the Sum of Scaled Scores to Standard Score Conversion table directly below the Summary section. The Cognitive scaled score is transferred to the box labeled with a 1. To calculate the sum of scaled scores for the Language Scale, the practitioner adds the Receptive Communication scaled score and the Expressive Communication scaled score. That score is then recorded and transferred to the box labeled with a 2 in the table. The same process is repeated for the Fine Motor and Gross Motor subtests to obtain the sum of scaled scores for the Motor Scale (i.e., box 3). The values entered in boxes 1, 2, and 3 should match for both conversion tables.

Next, the practitioner uses Table A.4 in Appendix A of the Administration Manual (Bayley & Aylward, 2019b) to obtain the standard score, percentile rank, and confidence interval for each scale. The efficient part about obtaining these scores is that all are found in one table, which should decrease the likelihood of making an error. The practitioner should first find the scale abbreviation located toward the top of the table. Then, the practitioner should go down the respective column to find the sum of scaled scores value that matches the sum of scaled scores described above. When found, the practitioner should look directly to the left into the shaded region titled "Standard score." That score is recorded and transferred to the front page of the Record Form. Located directly to the right of the standard score is the percentile rank (labeled as PR). This score is also recorded and transferred to the Record Form. The confidence intervals are located at the bottom of the table and are listed as a single digit under the corresponding scale column. To calculate the confidence interval, the practitioner first decides what level of confidence interval is desired (e.g., 90% or 95%; see Chapter 4, for more details on how to decide the level of confidence interval) and that value is recorded at the top of the confidence interval column of the Record Form. Then the corresponding value is subtracted from and added to the standard score and recorded on the Record Form.

To extend the example with August, the Cognitive subtest scaled score obtained by the child is 5, which corresponds to a standard score of 75 and a percentile rank of 5. The 95% confidence interval is chosen and written in the confidence interval column on the Record Form. The 95% confidence level for the Cognitive Scale is ±7, so the confidence interval range would be recorded on the Record Form as 68–82 in the confidence interval column.

SOCIAL–EMOTIONAL AND ADAPTIVE BEHAVIOR SCORING AND ANALYSIS

Once the respondent completes the Social–Emotional and Adaptive Behavior Questionnaire, the practitioner must review the items to determine if every age-appropriate item includes a rating. If an item was not rated, the practitioner should follow up with the respondent to obtain a rating. This is particularly important for the Social–Emotional Scale, as all items within an age band are necessary to calculate the total raw score and to obtain the norm-referenced scores. In addition, the number of *Can't Tell* and *Estimated* items should be noted to determine if further follow-up with the respondent is needed to clarify responses or to find an individual more suitable for completing the question-naire. More information on *Can't Tell* and *Estimated* items is now provided.

Social–Emotional Subtest/Scale

On the Social–Emotional Questionnaire, the first step in calculating the total raw score is to sum all of the responses for items 1–8 to obtain the Sensory Processing total raw score. Once summed, the practitioner records that score in the box at the bottom of page 2 of the Social–Emotional and Adaptive Behavior Questionnaire. The Sensory Processing score helps to examine potential difficulties in the child's sensory processing capacities (e.g., sensitivity to colors, sounds, touch, or movement). Next, items 1–35 are summed for the Social–Emotional total raw score, and that score is recorded in the box at the end of page 4.

> **DON'T FORGET 3.3**
>
> The Sensory Processing score of the Social–Emotional Scale helps to examine potential difficulties in the child's sensory processing capaci-ties (e.g., sensitivity to colors, sounds, touch, or movement).

At the bottom of page 4, there is a box for calculating the percentage of *Can't Tell* items. This is completed by taking the number of times the respondent circled 0 and entering that number in box A, and entering the total number of items administered in box B. The value in box A is divided by the value in box B and multiplied by 100 to obtain the percentage of items responded to as *Can't Tell*. If more than 15% of the items are responded to as *Can't Tell*, the practitioner should follow up with the respondent to determine if the respondent knows the child well enough to complete the questionnaire. A new respondent may be used to complete the questionnaire if the original respondent was not familiar with the child to complete the questionnaire. Scores should be interpreted with caution if an alternative respondent is not available.

The Summary section on page 13 of the Social–Emotional and Adaptive Behavior Questionnaire provides a way to record and derive scaled scores, standard scores, and percentile ranks for the Social–Emotional Subtest/Scale. These scores are recorded and derived similarly to the Cognitive, Language, and Motor subtests but using a different table. After recording and transferring the Social–Emotional raw score to the Summary section, Table A.2 in Appendix A of the Administration Manual (Bayley & Aylward, 2019b) is used to find the corresponding scaled score. On Table A.2, the child's age range is located across the top row with all the possible raw scores below. The practitioner finds the child's age range and then locates the obtained raw score below. When the raw score is found, the practitioner looks directly to the shaded areas on the left or right to find the appropriate scaled score. The scaled score is recorded and transferred to the Summary section. The scaled score is then used to look up the standard score, percentile rank, and confidence interval in Table A.4 using the same procedure described for finding these scores for the Cognitive, Language, and Motor Scales. These scores are then transferred to their corresponding columns in the Summary section. In addition, the raw score and scaled score for the Social–Emotional Subtest are transferred to the Social–Emotional and Adaptive Behavior Raw and Scaled Scores table at the bottom of the first page of the Record Form. Age equivalents are available for the Social–Emotional Subtest, but are not included in the appendices of the Bayley–4 Administration or Technical Manual. These scores are available within the Pearson Q-global Resource Library or can be requested from Pearson customer support if the practitioner does not have access to Q-global (NCS Pearson, Inc., 2021).

The supplemental analysis on page 13 of the Summary section is the next table to be completed. The Sensory Processing raw score calculated earlier is transferred to the raw score column in the Supplemental Analysis table. Table B.6 in Appendix B of the Administration Manual (Bayley & Aylward, 2019b) is used to find the Sensory Processing cut score. The practitioner finds the child's age (use adjusted age if premature) and corresponding Sensory Processing raw score underneath the appropriate "possible challenges," "emerging mastery," or "full mastery" column. Once located, the practitioner checks the box for the category that reflects the Sensory Processing raw score on the Supplemental Analysis table. In the highest stage mastered column, practitioners identify the highest stage in which the respondent circled a score of 4 or 5 for all items within that stage. The number of that stage is recorded under the appropriate section.

Plotting the child's highest stage mastered can be completed on the Social–Emotional Growth Chart at the bottom of page 13. The stages for emotional development are listed on the vertical axis, while age bands are marked on the horizontal axis. A 45° line indicates the age range at which mastery of each stage for emotional development is expected. The practitioner plots the intersection of the line corresponding to the highest mastered designation and the line indicating the child's age range. Figure 3.1 shows an example of a completed Social–Emotional Growth Chart for a child whose adjusted age is 12 months. The responses on the Social–Emotional subtest included some 2s and 3s within Stage 1, and so the child's highest stage mastered designation was 1. This is plotted in Figure 3.1 with a black X. The stage for emotional development at which the child is expected to be functioning for their age is plotted along the line and

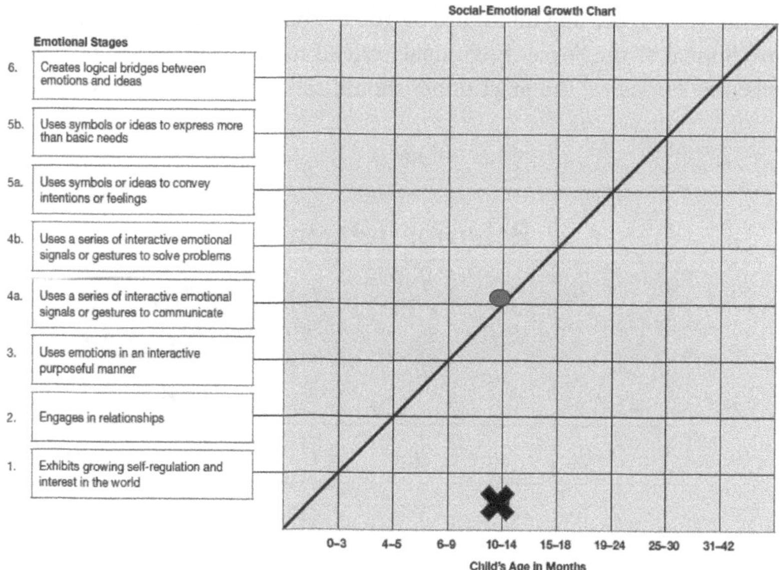

Figure 3.1   Example of Completed Social–Emotional Growth Chart.
Note: From Bayley Scales of Infant and Toddler Development, Fourth Edition (Bayley™–4). Copyright © 2019 NCS Pearson, Inc. Reproduced with permission. All rights reserved.

indicated with a dot. The plotting of these values indicates that the child's emotional development is delayed, as functioning is at Stage 1: Exhibits growing self-regulation and interest in the world, but the child is expected to be functioning at Stage 4a: Uses a series of interactive emotional signals or gestures to communicate.

Adaptive Behavior Scale

The Adaptive Behavior Scale includes five subdomains that are scored separately and are also used to calculate the Adaptive Behavior standard score. These scores are recorded and derived in much the same way as with the scales for the Cognitive, Language, and Motor subtests but use different tables. To calculate the subdomain total raw scores, the practitioner totals the responses for each of the subdomains: Receptive (23 items), Expressive (28 items), Personal (30 items), Interpersonal Relationships (20 items), and Play and Leisure (19 items). A total raw score box is located at the bottom of each of the subdomains for recording the total.

In addition, at the end of each subdomain is a table for calculating the number of *Estimated* items. The number of times the respondent checked the *Estimated* box for an item (see Figure 3.2) is entered in the A box, and the number of items administered is entered in the B box. The value in the A box is then divided by the value in the B box and multiplied by 100 to obtain the percentage of *Estimated* items. Similar to the Social–Emotional Scale, if more than 15% of the items are checked as *Estimated*, the practitioner should follow up with the respondent to

Behavior frequency			
Usually or often	Sometimes	Never	Estimated
②	1	0	☒
2	1	0	☐
2	1	0	☐

Figure 3.2   Example of Checked Estimated Item.
Note: From Bayley Scales of Infant and Toddler Development, Fourth Edition (Bayley™–4). Copyright © 2019 NCS Pearson, Inc. Reproduced with permission. All rights reserved.

RECEPTIVE (Items 1–23)
Total Raw Score (max. = 46): **16**

Total Estimated items	**2** A
Total administered items	**15** B
(A ÷ B) x 100 =	**13** % estimated

Figure 3.3   Calculating Percentage of Estimated Items.
Note: From Bayley Scales of Infant and Toddler Development, Fourth Edition (Bayley™–4). Copyright © 2019 NCS Pearson, Inc. Reproduced with permission. All rights reserved.

determine if the respondent knows the child well enough to complete the questionnaire. A new respondent may be used to complete the questionnaire if the original respondent was not adequately familiar with the child to report on their behavior. Scores should be interpreted with caution if an alternative respondent is not available.

Figure 3.3 provides an example for calculating the percentage of *Estimated* items for the Receptive subdomain. This example shows that the respondent checked the *Estimated* box twice and completed 15 items. Thus, 13% of the items for the Receptive subdomain were *Estimated* items. This is an acceptable number of *Estimated* items for a subdomain, indicating that the respondent was likely to be sufficiently familiar with the young child to complete the questionnaire.

Once total raw scores have been entered into the boxes at the end of each subdomain, these scores can be transferred to the Total Raw Score to Scaled Score Conversion table in the Summary section on page 14. Each total raw score is entered into the raw score column for the corresponding subdomain. Next, raw scores can be converted to scaled scores by looking at Table A.3 in Appendix A of the Administration Manual (Bayley & Aylward, 2019b). The practitioner chooses the quadrant that corresponds to the chronological age (or adjusted age if using) of the child. The subdomain abbreviations (see Chapter 1 for all subdomain abbreviations) are listed at the top of the corresponding columns. To obtain each subdomain scaled score, the practitioner finds the obtained raw score underneath the appropriate subdomain column and then looks directly to the left or right of the raw score to find the appropriate scaled score in the shaded region. This score is then recorded and transferred to the scaled score column of the Adaptive Behavior Scale Summary section. For example, an 8-month-old child with a raw score of 10 on the Receptive subdomain obtains a scaled score of 9.

Next, age equivalents are derived for each subdomain. The raw score of each subdomain is used to obtain the corresponding age equivalents found in Table B.7 in Appendix B of the Administration Manual (Bayley & Aylward, 2019b). With this table, the practitioner locates the total raw score (or range of raw scores) that correspond to the obtained raw score for each subdomain. The practitioner finds the obtained raw score listed below the respective subdomain abbreviation, and looks directly to the left or the right to find the age equivalent (in months) in the shaded region. For example, a Receptive subdomain raw score of 10 corresponds to an age equivalent of 5:15 (e.g., 5 months, 15 days). The age equivalent is recorded and transferred to the age equivalent column for each subdomain in the Summary section.

The last column in the Adaptive Behavior Scale Summary section is for the GSVs. The table used for converting a raw score to the GSV is Table B.8 in Appendix B of the Administration Manual (Bayley & Aylward, 2019b). In this table, the practitioner finds the raw score obtained on each respective subdomain in the far left or right columns (i.e., shaded areas) and then looks across the row to locate the GSV. This is completed separately for each subdomain. For example, if a child obtained a raw score of 10 on the Receptive subdomain, the GSV is 478. Each GSV is located and recorded in the appropriate column for the respective subdomain on the Summary page.

The practitioner can now complete the Sum of Scaled Scores to Standard Score Conversion table on the Summary page. First, the practitioner should calculate the sum of scaled scores in the Total Raw Score to Scaled Score Conversion table. The practitioner sums the Receptive and Expressive scaled scores to obtain the sum of scaled scores for the Communication domain. The sum of scaled scores is recorded in the box with the 1 in the bottom right corner. The Interpersonal Relationships and Play and Leisure subdomains are totaled, and the sum is entered in the box with a 3 for the Socialization domain. Finally, the three sums of scaled scores boxes (i.e., boxes labeled 1–3) are summed and entered into the box with a 4 for the Adaptive Behavior score. Each of these scores is transferred to the corresponding numbered boxes in the sum of scaled scores column of the Sum of Scaled Scores to Standard Score Conversion table.

Next, the standard scores, percentile ranks, and confidence intervals for the Communication, Daily Living Skills, and Socialization domains and the Adaptive Behavior Scale are obtained. Table A.5 in the Administration Manual (Bayley & Aylward, 2019b) is used to find these scores. The practitioner locates the sum of scaled scores obtained for each domain underneath the appropriate domain abbreviation. Once the sum of scaled scores is found, the practitioner should look directly to the left to find the appropriate standard score in the shaded region. The percentile rank is found in the column directly to the right of the standard score column (labeled PR). The values used to determine the confidence interval at the 90% and 95% confidence level are found at the bottom right corner of the table. The procedure for calculating the confidence interval is similar to that described in the *Calculating Standard Scores, Percentile Ranks, and Confidence Intervals for the Cognitive, Language, and Motor subtests* section in this chapter. The standard score, percentile rank, and confidence interval are recorded for the Communication, Daily Living Skills, and Socialization domains and the Adaptive Behavior Scale. To the right of the Summary section on the same page, there are graphs for plotting subdomain and standard scores. In addition, page 15 of the Social–Emotional and Adaptive Behavior Questionnaire includes a section for supplemental and GSV analysis. The procedures for completing the score plots and the supplemental and GSV analysis are described in the following sections.

Plotting the Profiles of the Scaled Scores and Standard Scores

On the Record Form, page 2 includes graphs on which to plot scores. Plotting scores provides a visual depiction of the range of scores and their relation to one another, which can assist in interpretating and reporting of scores. First, the Subtest/Subdomain Score Profile is found at the upper left side of the page and provides a way to plot each subtest or subdomain scaled score calculated for the Bayley–4 to view in one profile. The abbreviations for each subtest or subdomain are at the top of the profile, and the range of scaled scores from 1 to 19 are listed on either side of the graph. For each subtest and subdomain, scaled scores are transferred to the box under the appropriate subtest or subdomain abbreviation. These scores are taken from the Summary sections of the Record Form and the Social–Emotional and Adaptive Behavior Questionnaire. The raw and scaled scores from the Social–Emotional and Adaptive Behavior Questionnaire should be transferred to the bottom of page 2 for easier reference when plotting scaled scores. The practitioner places an X or other desired mark on the dot that corresponds to the obtained scaled score for each subtest or subdomain. A line is drawn between each mark.

Next, the Standard Score Profile is completed. This graph is located on the upper right side of page 2 on the Record Form. The abbreviations for each of the Bayley–4 scales are listed at the top of the table. The practitioner transfers the standard score values from the first page of the Record Form and from the respective Summary sections of the Social–Emotional and Adaptive Behavior Questionnaire. The range of standard scores is listed on both sides of the profile, with the highest value at the top. Similar to the Subtest/Subdomain Score Profile, the practitioner places an X or other mark (e.g., a dot) on the line that corresponds to the standard score obtained for each of the scales and draws a line between each mark.

Similar profile analysis is available for the Adaptive Behavior Scale on the right side of page 14 of the Social–Emotional and Adaptive Behavior Questionnaire. For the Subdomain Score Profile, the practitioner transfers from the Summary table the scaled scores from each of the subdomains under the respective subdomain abbreviation. The obtained scaled score is then plotted by putting an X or other mark on the dot for each subdomain, and a line is drawn between each mark. Next, the Standard Score Profile is completed. The standard score values for the Communication, Daily Living Skills, and Socialization domains and the Adaptive Behavior Scale are transferred from the Sum of Scaled Scores to Standard Score Conversion table on the bottom left of page 14 to their respective columns in the Standard Score Profile. These values are then plotted by putting an X or other mark on the line that corresponds to the standard score for each scale, with a line drawn between each mark.

Supplemental Analysis for the Cognitive, Motor, Language, and Adaptive Behavior Scales

The Supplemental Analysis section on page 2 of the Record Form provides a way to calculate comparisons between scores that indicate if a child performed significantly higher or lower in one developmental area than another. The first discrepancy comparison calculates the difference between the scaled scores for the Language subtests and the Motor subtests. Scores for the Receptive and Expressive Communication subtests are transferred to the Score 1 and Score 2 columns labeled with RC and EC, respectively. The same transfer of scores takes place to the Score 1 and Score 2 columns labeled with the abbreviations for the Fine Motor and Gross Motor subtests (i.e., FM and GM). The difference is then calculated for these sets of scores. Table B.3 in Appendix B of the Administration Manual (Bayley & Aylward, 2019b) provides the critical value by which the absolute value of the difference is compared to determine if the difference is statistically significant. The critical value is found in one of the significance level columns (e.g., .05 or .10) for the respective scaled score comparison (see Chapter 4 for more on deciding the significance level to use). That value is then entered into the critical value column, while the significance level desired is checked at the top of the significance level column. When the absolute value of the calculated difference between the scaled scores is larger than the critical value, the difference is statistically significant. The practitioner then circles Y or N for each scaled score comparison to signify if the difference is significant.

Whether the scaled score comparison difference is statistically significant or not, the base rate is recorded in the final column. The base rate, which is also found in Table B.3, conveys the percent of children in the normative sample who obtained the same or greater difference in scaled scores. In Table B.3, difference values are listed that correspond to various base rate percentages. The practitioner looks across the row for the given comparison to determine the base rate for the respective scaled score difference. For example, if a child whose Receptive Communication scaled score is 4 points higher than the Expressive Communication scaled score, the difference is statistically significant at the .05 and .10 levels. The corresponding base rate for that difference is ≤5% (e.g., 5% of the children in the normative sample had the same or larger difference between the Receptive Communication and Expressive Communication scaled scores). If the difference between scores is not shown on the row for the comparison in the relevant table, the practitioner starts at the last base rate column (e.g., ≤2) and reads across the row to the left to locate the difference that is less than that obtained by the child. For example, if the difference between the RC and EC scaled scores is 6, the corresponding base rate is <2%. Practitioners should be attentive to which scaled score is greater since base rates may differ.

A similar procedure is used to calculate differences between the Cognitive and Language, Cognitive and Motor, and Language and Motor standard scores. Table B.4 in Appendix B of the Administration Manual (Bayley & Aylward, 2019b) is used to determine the critical values and base rates for these standard discrepancy comparisons. In addition, the Adaptive Behavior Scale includes a Supplemental Analysis section found on page 15 of the Social–Emotional and Adaptive Behavior Questionnaire. Similar procedures may be followed for determining scaled score discrepancies between the Receptive and Expressive subdomains and the Interpersonal Relationships and Play and Leisure subdomains, and for determining the standard score discrepancies between the Communication and Daily Living Skill, Communication and Socialization, and Daily Living Skills and Socialization domains. The critical values and base rates for the subdomain discrepancies are found in Table B.9, while the critical values and base rates for the domain discrepancies are found in Table B.10.

Growth Scale Value Analysis for the Cognitive, Motor, Language, and Adaptive Behavior Scales

The Bayley–4 provides a way to measure the growth of a child's performance over repeated assessments; namely, GSVs. This measure is available for the Cognitive, Receptive Communication, Expressive Communication, Fine Motor, and Gross Motor subtests. GSVs can also be evaluated on the Adaptive Behavior Scale for the Receptive, Expressive, Personal, Interpersonal Relationships, and Play and Leisure subdomains.

For the Cognitive, Language, and Motor subtests, page 2 of the Record Form includes a table labeled Growth Scale Value Analysis, on which the administration dates and raw score, scaled score, and GSVs are recorded in the respective columns for the first administration and the second administration of the subtests. The practitioner subtracts the GSV on the first test administration from the second test administration. The difference is then recorded in the difference column in the row corresponding to the second administration. Table B.5 in Appendix B of the Administration Manual (Bayley & Aylward, 2019b) includes critical values by which to compare the difference between administrations to determine if the difference is statistically significant. The practitioner circles Y if the absolute value of the difference is equal to or larger than the critical value or N if it is less than the critical value. The procedure is similar for the Growth Value Analysis on the Adaptive Behavior Scale. Table B.11 is used to reference the critical values needed to determine if a GSV difference between the first and second administration is statistically significant.

> **CAUTION 3.3**
>
> Practitioners must ensure there is an accurate transfer of scaled and standard scores when completing score profiles, supplemental analysis, and GSV analysis. A mistake could lead to inaccurate interpretation and reporting of scores. All score transfers should be double checked and verified for accuracy. An advantage of administration and/or scoring on Q-global is that all scores are calculated automatically after being entered by the practitioner or as a result of using a mobile device to administer the test, thereby greatly decreasing the possibility of scoring mistakes.

SCORING RESPONSES ON Q-GLOBAL

The Q-global platform provides two options for administration and scoring of the Bayley–4. Practitioners may use the paper Record Form to record responses and observations and enter the raw scores and relevant information into Q-global once the test administration is completed. Alternatively, the practitioner may use a mobile electronic device to record responses and observations directly in Q-global during administration of the Bayley–4. For both options, all scores and discrepancy comparisons are automatically calculated once the assessment is submitted. Digital administration has distinct advantages for scoring, including increasing the accuracy of application of administration and scoring rules. In addition, the practitioner does not have to look up each score in various tables in the manual appendices, which saves time and decreases the likelihood of scoring errors. Furthermore, completion of the Social-Emotional and Adaptive Behavior Questionnaire can be completed by Remote On-Screen Administration (ROSA) by the child's caregiver, either on an electronic device in the test setting or at their convenience by opening a link sent through email, completing the questionnaire, and submitting the questionnaire when finished. That data are then automatically scored in Q-global. Chapter 8 provides an in-depth description of the digital scoring features of the Bayley–4.

> **DON'T FORGET 3.4**
>
> When using Q-global to enter scores or for digital administration of the Bayley–4, all scores and discrepancy comparisons are automatically calculated once the assessment is submitted.

TEST YOURSELF

1. **Bayley–4 scaled scores have a mean of 10 and a standard deviation of 3.** True or False

2. **There are no limitations to consider when using percentile ranks to describe a child's performance on the Bayley–4.** True or False

3. **Percent delay...**
   a) Is often used for determination of eligibility for early intervention services
   b) Criteria for eligibility of services varies by state
   c) Is derived from age equivalents
   d) All of the above

4. **The Bayley–4 scoring approach...**
   a) Is the same as the Bayley-III
   b) Is now polytomous (e.g., 2, 1, 0)
   c) Requires determining if a child passes or fails an item
   d) All of the above

5. **Items administered below the basal are awarded full credit regardless of performance on those items unless the basal starts at Item 1.** True or False

6. **Growth Scale Values (GSVs)…**
    a) Are used to track a child's developmental progress between two Bayley–4 administrations
    b) Measure how much a child has grown since the last office visit
    c) Compare a child's growth in an area to their same-aged peers
    d) Should never be reported
7. **Supplemental analysis and GSV analysis are only available for the Cognitive, Language, and Motor scales.** True or False
8. **For Caregiver Questions:**
    a) Care should be taken not to administer too many
    b) The respondent can be anyone who knows the child
    c) The responses are used in combination with the child's performance to calculate an average score for the item
    d) There is no limit to how many Caregiver Questions may be asked in place of structured item scores
9. **To consider the Adaptive Behavior Scale valid, less than 25% of the items can be estimated.** True or False
10. **Manual entry of data from a paper Record Form into Q-global or digital administration on an electronic device using Q-global derives all scores and discrepancy comparisons automatically.** True or False

Answers: 1. True; 2. False; 3. (d); 4. (b); 5. True; 6. (a); 7. False; 8. (d); 9. False; 10. True.

REFERENCES

Bayley, N., & Aylward, G. P. (2019a). *Bayley Scales of Infant and Toddler Development* (4th ed.). Pearson.

Bayley, N., & Aylward, G. P. (2019b). *Bayley Scales of Infant and Toddler Development* (4th ed.): *Administration manual.* Pearson.

Bayley, N., & Aylward, G. P. (2019c). *Bayley Scales of Infant and Toddler Development* (4th ed.): *Technical manual.* Pearson.

Flanagan, D. P., & Alfonso, V. C. (2017). *Essentials of WISC-V assessment.* John Wiley & Sons, Inc.

Individuals with Disabilities Education Improvement Act, Pub. L. 108-446, 118 Stat. 2647 (2004).

NCS Pearson, Inc. (2021, February). *Bayley Scales of Infant and Toddler Development, Fourth Edition.* https://www.pearsonassessments.com/store/usassessments/en/Store/Professional-Assessments/Cogniton-%26-Neuro/

Bayley-Scales-of-Infant-and-Toddler-Development-%7C-Fourth-Edition/p/1000001996.html?tab=faq.

Sattler, J. M. (2018). *Assessment of children: Cognitive foundations and applications* (6th ed.). Author.

Four

HOW TO INTERPRET THE BAYLEY–4

Vincent C. Alfonso, Joseph R. Engler, and Andrea D. Turner
Gonzaga University and Pearson Assessments

Interpretation of young children's (i.e., infants and toddlers) performance on assessments is different from interpretation of school-aged children or adolescents' performance on assessments. For example, item development for infants and toddlers is a challenging, if not daunting, task. Test authors and developers must have much experience working with young children and understand the "mind" of the young child for whom they are creating items. Pioneers such as Drs. Nancy Bayley and Dorothea McCarthy are great examples of psychologists who worked with young children for decades and thus developed two of the best assessments for young children, the Bayley Scales and the *McCarthy Scales of Children's Abilities* (MSCA; McCarthy, 1972).

There are myriad reasons why assessing young children differs from assessing older children and adolescents. For example, many assessments for school-aged children such as the *Wechsler Intelligence Scale for Children–Fifth Edition* (WISC–V; Wechsler, 2014) or adolescents such as the *Kaufman Adolescent and Adult Intelligence Test* (KAIT; Kaufman & Kaufman, 1993) include several subtests, scales, and composites because they tap individuals' multiple cognitive abilities and processes, have long traditions dating back to the *Stanford–Binet* (SB; Terman, 1916) and *Wechsler–Bellevue Intelligence Scale* (WBIS; Wechsler, 1939), and are

DON'T FORGET 4.1

Interpretation of young children's (i.e., infants and toddlers) performance on assessments is different from interpretation of school-aged children or adolescents' performance on assessments.

≡ Rapid Reference 4.1

Some of the Differences Between Assessments for Infants and Toddlers and School-Aged Children and Adolescents

- Item development for infants and toddlers is particularly challenging given their nature as young children (e.g., limited attention span, distractibility, impulsivity, limited expressive language, etc.) (Bracken & Theodore, 2020).
- Many assessments for school-aged children and adolescents have long traditions dating back to the SB (Terman, 1916) and WBIS (Wechsler, 1939) and as such continue to be templates or blueprints for today's assessments.
- Assessments for school-aged children and adolescents such as the WISC–V (Wechsler, 2014) and KAIT (Kaufman & Kaufman, 1993) typically tap multiple, separate cognitive abilities and processes because of substantial brain differentiation in older children relative to young children (Aylward, 2020).
- Nearly all cognitive assessments today refer to the Cattell–Horn–Carroll (CHC) theory of cognitive abilities and processes (Flanagan & McDonough, 2018; Schneider & McGrew, 2018) whereas infant and toddler assessments tend to be atheoretical.
- Infant and toddler assessments require additional education and training, which is very difficult to find even today (Alfonso et al., 2020; Nagle et al., 2020).
- The purposes of infant and toddler assessment (e.g., screening, early intervention services, etc.) may differ greatly from those of school-aged children and adolescents (e.g., classification under Public Laws 99-457, 101-476, 105-17, and 108-446).

administered to individuals who typically sit still for long periods of time, pay attention, and comply with practitioners' requests! Rapid Reference 4.1 lists some of the differences between assessments for young children and school-aged children and adolescents that practitioners should keep in mind when assessing and interpreting young children's test performance.

In this chapter we present an integrated model of Bayley–4 (Bayley & Aylward, 2019a) performance interpretation based on the following: (a) the interpretive method discussed in Chapter 5 of Bayley and Aylward (2019c), (b) the interpretive method discussed and applied in Aylward (2020), and (c) the present authors' interpretive method that is a traditional approach highlighting reliability as a foundational psychometric property of all assessments. There is certainly overlap among these three individual interpretive methods and one interpretive method is not necessarily better than another interpretive method. We believe that all three interpretive methods have merit and as such integrated them for ease of reading and understanding. Practitioners may decide to use one interpretive method over another instead of using the integrated model based on several variables including experience working with young children, familiarity with assessments for young children as well as for school-aged children and adolescents, and report-writing skills to name a few. Whatever interpretive method a practitioner chooses is not as important as how the practitioner communicates the results of the assessment and an evaluation of performance to caregivers and other adults (e.g., teachers) in the young child's life. Thus, verbal and written communication should be "caregiver" friendly, devoid of as much psychological jargon as possible, and meaningful such that caregivers understand well their young child's functioning.

Prior to reviewing the integrated model of Bayley–4 performance interpretation, practitioners should know that assessment and interpretation (evaluation of all assessment results) of young children is an iterative process that is best conducted via a multi-method, multi-source, and multi-setting approach (Alfonso, Engler, et al., 2020). For example, assessment methods include standardized, norm-referenced tests such as the Bayley–4, systematic direct observations, and interviews. Multiple sources include caregivers, siblings, grandparents, teachers, and neighbors, as all of them may have an understanding of the young child's functioning and may impact that functioning (e.g., Blair, 2002; Bronfenbrenner, 1977, 1986; Bronfenbrenner & Ceci, 1994; Bulotsky-Shearer et al., 2020; Ladd et al., 1999). Multiple settings include the home, school, playground, and even the practitioner's office (Ferretti & Bub, 2017; Fomby & Mollborn, 2017). Indeed, according to Bayley and Aylward (2019c), "developmental evaluation using the Bayley–4 is a three-part process: historical information provided by the caregiver, behavioral observation, and item administration" (p. 57). They continue to state that other sources of information are usually available including "medical and psychosocial history, previous test scores, and qualitative aspects of the test" (p. 57).

> **DON'T FORGET 4.2**
>
> Assessment and interpretation (evaluation of all assessment results) of young children is an iterative process that is best conducted via a multi-method, multi-source, and multi-setting approach.

Here we focus on interpretation of the young child's Bayley–4 performance, keeping in mind the above information regarding the multi-method, multi-source, multi-setting assessment. Our integrated model has three major components: (a) theoretical underpinnings or assessment content, (b) quantitative interpretation of test performance, and (c) qualitative interpretation of test performance. All three are important and should not be viewed as mutually exclusive. Rather, they should be understood as interdependent components that affect each other and when integrated paint a clinically rich picture of the young child.

THEORETICAL UNDERPINNINGS AND ASSESSMENT CONTENT

Traditionally, the Bayley Scales have been atheoretical but have always included items that tap multiple developmental domains such as cognition, language, and motor because the goal has been to provide reliable and valid indicators of an infant or toddler's current developmental functioning. The *Bayley Scales of Infant Development* (Bayley, 1969) and *Bayley Scales of Infant Development–Second Edition* (BSID–II; Bayley, 1993) were comprised of two scales that yielded two indexes, the Mental Development Index and the Psychomotor Development Index (see Chapter 1 and Table 1.1). When the *Bayley Scales of Infant and Toddler Development– Third Edition* (Bayley–III; Bayley, 2006) was published, it was comprised of five scales but remained atheoretical for the most part. The clarity around cognitive, language, and motor items plus the addition of the Social–Emotional and Adaptive Behavior Scales were received positively by practitioners.

The Bayley–4 has the same scales as the Bayley–III, but has a theory or integrated model underlying the items on the Cognitive, Language, and Motor Scales in particular. It is called the integrated neuro-environmental synthesis model of development that reflects the interaction of external biological and environmental influences and internal brain development (Aylward, 2020). As such, this model is not one theory, per se, but rather an integration of several lines of thinking and research, particularly in brain development, environmental influences, and their interaction. The Bayley–4 items were designed or modified to reflect neuro-developmental functions and early forms of executive functioning. Indeed, there is a veritable explosion of research in neurology, neuropsychology, executive functions, and developmental psychology that is impossible to cover in one volume. However, as stated in Chapter 1, practitioners are encouraged to read Aylward (2020), Bayley and Aylward (2019b, 2019c), and Chapter 6 for details regarding Bayley–4 item development, and Chapters 2 and 3 for details on item administration and scoring, as this provides practitioners with foundational information on what the Bayley–4 items and their corresponding scales measure. Table 4.1 provides a summary of the underlying skills assessed by the various Bayley–4 scales culled from the sources mentioned above. It is important to reiterate that there is some item-type overlap across the scales, given the challenge of creating scale-specific items and the nature of the developing young child.

Table 4.1 Summary of Underlying Skills Assessed by the Bayley—4

Cognitive Scale	Language Scale	Motor Scale	Social–Emotional Scale	Adaptive Behavior Scale
• Attention • Imitation • Habituation • Basic concepts • Acquired knowledge • Working memory • Problem solving • Learning • Numerical concepts • Classification • Planning • Cause and effect • Processing speed • Imagination	• Concrete terms • Abstract terms • Social interaction • Complex concepts • Verbal working memory • Non-specific vocalizations • Sophisticated sounds • Articulation • Gesturing • Vocabulary knowledge	• Visual tracking and focus • Sensorimotor behaviors and reflexes • Grasping • Visual-motor integration • Writing skills such as imitating, tracing, and copying • Fine motor speed • Head and trunk control • Motor planning • Locomotion such as walking, running, hopping, etc. • Throwing (e.g., a ball)	• Sensory processing • Self-regulation • Engaging in relationships • Using emotions purposely • Communicating via emotional signals or gestures • Using emotional signals or gestures to solve problems • Using symbols or ideas to convey intentions/feelings • Using symbols or ideas to express complex needs • Creating bridges between emotions and ideas	• Listening • Understanding • Talking • Self-care • Relating to others • Playing

Sources: Aylward (2020), Bayley and Aylward (2019b, 2019c), and Chapters 2 and 3

QUANTITATIVE INTERPRETATION OF TEST PERFORMANCE

Table 1.1 indicated that the Bayley–4 includes several scores such as scaled, standard, percentile ranks, confidence intervals, developmental age equivalents, and growth scale values. Each of these scores has its strengths and limitations that are detailed in Bayley and Aylward (2019c). As we provide quantitative interpretive guidelines, we also mention some of these strengths and limitations. In addition, it is incumbent upon practitioners to review Table 1.3 and Chapter 6 to become familiar with the evaluation of the Bayley–4 quantitative characteristics so they can make sound interpretations of infants' and toddlers' performance.

Our quantitative interpretive guidelines follow from an internal consistency reliability-based foundation. That is, internal consistency reliability sets the ceiling on validity and, as such, is absolutely necessary to consider when interpreting performance (American Educational Research Association et al., 2014; Crocker & Algina, 1986; Urbina, 2014). Typically, the score that has the highest internal consistency reliability is the composite score. In the case of the Bayley–4, this is the standard score or overall score for each scale. Indeed, these standard scores have good average internal consistency reliability across the ages of the Bayley–4. The score with the next highest internal consistency reliability is the scaled score, and again these are rated as having good average internal consistency reliability across the ages of the Bayley–4. Given that standard and scaled scores have the highest internal consistency reliability, we have great confidence in interpreting them, especially when using confidence intervals.

Interpreting and Reporting Bayley–4 Standard and Scale Scores

One way of presenting interpretation of young children's performance is by scale. For example, practitioners may want to discuss the child's performance on the Cognitive Scale followed by the Language, Motor, Social-Emotional, and Adaptive Behavior. We agree with Bayley and Aylward (2019c) and Aylward (2020) that practitioners should report first the child's standard and scaled scores. As a reminder, standard scores have a mean of 100 and standard deviation of 15 while scaled scores have a mean of 10 and standard deviation of 3. This is important information to convey to caregivers and may be done more easily via the Caregiver Report of the Bayley–4 that has a subtest/subdomain score profile.

> **DON'T FORGET 4.3**
>
> Standard scores have a mean of 100 and standard deviation of 15 while scaled scores have a mean of 10 and standard deviation of 3.

When reporting a standard score it is a common practice to provide the percentile rank associated with that score as well as the confidence interval. Percentile ranks indicate "the percentage of children in the standardization sample at a given age who obtained scores less than or equal to a given subtest scaled score or standard score" (Bayley & Aylward, 2019c, p. 62). For example, a standard score of 90 is associated with a percentile rank of 25, indicating that the child earned a standard score at or higher than 25% of same-aged children included in the standardization sample. Confidence intervals are used to convey the precision of the standard score and indicate "a child's score as an interval that is likely to contain the child's true score" (Bayley & Aylward, 2019c, p. 63). Confidence intervals for the Bayley–4 standard scores are readily calculable by adding and subtracting a number to and from the observed standard score. These numbers, which are based on the estimated true score and standard error of estimation from the standardization sample, are available for the 90 and 95% confidence intervals and are found on the bottom right-hand corners of Tables A.4 and A.5 in Bayley and Aylward (2019b). For example, if a child earned a standard score of 90 on the Cognitive Scale and the practitioner wanted to use the 95% confidence interval for that standard score, the practitioner would add and subtract 7 from 90 as noted in Table A.4 of Bayley and Aylward (2019b, p. 308). Thus, the confidence interval would be 83–97, indicating that 95 times out of 100, the child's true score would be between 83 and 97.

In addition to percentile ranks and confidence intervals associated with standard scores, it is typical to use a descriptive category with that standard score. There are several descriptive classification systems including the one found in Bayley and Aylward (2019c), and there has been a fair amount of debate in recent years regarding which one or ones are correct. For example, on one test a score of 90 may be considered "average," whereas on another test it may be considered "low average." Flanagan and Alfonso (2017) discuss the debate around various classification systems and state, "What is most important is that all scores be classified based only on one classification system to avoid confusion" (p. 174). We espouse using a more traditional classification system found in many assessment manuals including Bayley and Aylward (2019c) and Rapid Reference 4.2.

Interpreting and Reporting Bayley–4 Developmental Age Equivalents and Growth Scale Values

Developmental or test age equivalents are available for all subtests on the Cognitive, Language, and Motor Scales as well as the subdomains of the Adaptive Behavior Scale. "Age equivalents are obtained by computing the average raw scores obtained

≡ Rapid Reference 4.2

Recommended Descriptive Classification System for Bayley–4 Standard and Scaled Scores

Standard Score Range	Scaled Score Range	Percentile Rank Range	Descriptive Classification
≥130	16-19	≥98	Extremely High
120-129	14-15	91st-97th	Very High
110-119	12-13	75th-90th	High Average
90-109	8-11	25th-74th	Average
80-89	6-7	9th-24th	Low Average
70-79	4-5	2nd-8th	Very Low
≤69	1-3	≤2nd	Extremely Low

Note: Percentile ranks associated with specific standard scores are found in Tables A.4 and A.5 in Bayley and Aylward (2019b). Although rarely reported, percentile ranks associated with specific scaled scores are found in Table 5.1 in Bayley and Aylward (2019c) and Chapter 2. Sources: Bayley and Aylward (2019c) and Flanagan and Alfonso (2017).

on a test by children at different ages" (Sattler, 2018, p. 107). There is a fair amount of controversy surrounding the use of age equivalents given their potential to be misleading because they are not psychometrically sound. Sattler (2018) and Bayley and Aylward (2019c) provide good discussions regarding the limitations of age equivalents and some of these limitations are listed in Rapid Reference 4.3. Although several limitations exist and practitioners should be cautious when interpreting age equivalents, they "place performance in a developmental context, and they provide information that consumers of the findings (e.g., caregivers and the public) can easily understand" (Sattler, 2018, p. 108). Also, some of the limitations associated with age equivalents are mitigated "when test items are distributed uniformly over a wide range of difficulty, when students [children] are administered the subset of items centered on their level of ability, and when the test has been normed on an appropriately selected sample of students [children] across a wide grade [age] range" (McGrew et al., 1991, p. 40).

CAUTION 4.1

There is a fair amount of controversy surrounding the use of age equivalents given their potential to be misleading because they are not psychometrically sound.

≡ *Rapid Reference 4.3*

Some Limitations of Developmental or Test Age Equivalents

- Provide little information regarding a child's standing relative to same-age peers.
- Small changes in raw scores (on which age equivalents are based) may result in large changes in age equivalents.
- An extreme age equivalent does not mean the child is similar to the extreme age group in every way.
- Distributions of age equivalents may not be in equal units.
- Developmental skills may not be reflected accurately by age equivalents.
- Important statistical measures cannot be computed because age equivalents are on an ordinal scale.

Sources: Bayley and Aylward (2019c) and Sattler (2018).

An example of a statement regarding a child's age equivalent on the Receptive Communication subtest is the following: Julie, a 12-month-old female child, scored similarly to an average 10-month-old child (age equivalent of 10 months) on the Receptive Communication subtest, indicating slightly below performance relative to her age peers. It is important to note that it is not accurate to make general statements regarding Julie's communication skills (e.g., pragmatic communication skills), her performance on other assessments of receptive communication skills (e.g., Adaptive Behavior Scale), or her performance in other developmental domains (e.g., fine motor skills) based on her age equivalent of 10 months on the Receptive Communication subtest of the Language Scale. Age equivalents for the Cognitive, Language, and Motor Scales are found in Table B.1 on page 312 in Bayley and Aylward (2019b). Age equivalents for the Adaptive Behavior Scale are found in Table B.7 on page 317 in Bayley and Aylward (2019b).

Growth scale values (GSVs) allow practitioners to track or monitor a child's growth over time, have a mean of 500 and standard deviation of 25, measure skills on an absolute, equal-interval scale, and cannot be meaningfully compared between subtests and subdomains (Bayley & Aylward, 2019c). Effectively, these values increase as the child's skill level grows, even if the child's scaled or standard score does not increase. This is important information to convey to caregivers and teachers because a young child may be improving or growing over time despite not appearing to be when interpreting other scores (i.e., scaled or standard).

For example, if a child were assessed at 12 months of age and then again at 18 months of age, GSVs may be the same at time one and time two, there may be an increase from time one to time two, or there may be a decrease from time one to time two. It is important to determine if the GSVs are statistically significantly different from each other rather than occurring by chance. In order to determine if two GSVs are statistically significant from each other, practitioners look for the critical values found in Table B.5 on page 316 in Bayley and Aylward (2019b). The critical value for the Cognitive and Gross Motor subtests is 5 and the critical value for the Receptive, Expressive, and Fine Motor subtests is 6. In other words, a 5 or 6 GSVs difference on the same subtest between two assessments is needed in order to state that a child performed significantly higher at test time one compared to test time two.

An example may assist in understanding how to interpret and report GSVs. James earned a GSV of 523 on the Receptive Communication subtest when he was 30 months of age and a GSV of 532 on the same subtest when he was 36 months of age. The difference between his GSVs at time one and time two is 9 and this difference exceeds the critical value of 6 (mentioned above). Thus, James demonstrated significant growth in his receptive communication skills from age 30 months to age 36 months, even though his scaled score remained the same at time one and time two (i.e., 8). According to Aylward (2020), "The GSV is more sensitive to small developmental gains than are scaled scores" (p. 32). GSVs and critical values for the Adaptive Behavior subdomains are found in Tables B.8 and B.11 on pages 318 and 321, respectively, in Bayley and Aylward (2019b).

> ### DON'T FORGET 4.4
> Growth scale values increase as the child's skill level grows, even if the child's scaled or standard score does not increase.

Supplemental Quantitative Analyses

Practitioners may be interested in conducting additional quantitative analyses regarding the young child's Bayley–4 performance. For example, practitioners may want to compare the child's performance on the two subtests that comprise the Language Scale or the Motor Scale to determine if the child performed similarly or significantly higher or lower on one subtest than the other. Similarly, practitioners may want to determine if a child performed significantly higher or lower on one scale versus another (e.g., Cognitive versus Language or Motor or Language versus Motor). When comparing a child's performance on one subtest versus another or one scale versus another, statistical significance and base rate data are suggested to assist with interpretation. A statistically significant difference indicates that the child performed significantly higher or lower on one subtest or one scale versus another and is based on probability and critical values. If one subtest scaled score or one scale standard score is significantly higher or lower than the comparison scaled score or standard score, then the difference is real or true as opposed to occurring by chance. Practitioners may choose the .10 or .05 significance level depending on at least two factors.

First, selecting the .10 versus .05 significance level makes it more likely that a significant difference is found because the magnitude of the difference score needed for statistical significance (i.e., the critical value) is less at the .10 level than at the .05 level. For example, 8.42 standard score points are required for a .10 level of statistical difference between the Cognitive and Language Scales whereas more than 10 standard score points are required for a .05 level of statistical significance (see Bayley & Aylward, 2019b, p. 315). In this example there is increased statistical power using the .10 significance level, but also an increased likelihood of a Type 1 error or stating there is a statistically significant difference when there really is not one (Cohen, 2013). Some researchers, statisticians, and practitioners believe making a Type II error is worse than making a Type I error because a Type II error indicates that there is not a statistically significant difference when there really is one.

Second, and related to the first reason, practitioners have to weigh whether "there is more harm in the error of interpreting a chance difference as significant or in the error of failing to interpret a true difference as significant" (Bayley & Aylward, 2019c, p. 65). For example, if making a Type II error prevents a child from receiving services that is worthy of much concern. Whatever significance level the practitioner chooses (i.e., .10 or .05), it should be the same one for all comparisons. In addition, it is prudent for the practitioner to determine a priori what pairwise comparisons to make because the more comparisons conducted, the greater the probability of a significant finding by chance alone (Grégoire et al., 2011; Kaufman, 1994; Silverstein, 1982, 1993). The .05 significance level typically guards against errors associated with multiple comparisons, especially when few comparisons are made. Practitioners can determine a priori what pairwise comparisons to make based on the reason for referral, background information, and prior assessment data.

> # CAUTION 4.2
>
> It is prudent for the practitioner to determine a priori what pairwise comparisons to make because the more comparisons conducted, the greater the probability of a significant finding by chance alone.

It is generally agreed that statistical significance alone is not sufficient when interpreting young children's performance on more than one subtest or scale because statistical significance simply tells practitioners that the child performed higher on one subtest or scale than the other. Therefore, base rate data are required to interpret how clinically meaningful is the difference in performance. Base rate data inform practitioners how frequent a difference of a specific magnitude occurs in the standardization sample. Typically, and almost always, if two scores are not statistically significant then the magnitude of the difference in the scores occurs often in the general population or age group of the child. If, however, two scores are statistically significantly different then it is possible that the magnitude of the difference in the scores does not occur often in the general population or age group of the child. A general rule of thumb popularized by Kaufman (1994), based on the work of Silverstein (1993), is 10% rarity or uncommonness. In other words, if two scores (scaled or standard) are statistically significantly different and the magnitude of the difference occurs in about 10% (or less) of the general population or age group of the child, then practitioners should try to determine why the difference occurred and its clinical relevance. Bayley and Aylward (2019c) state "In addition to the base rate statistics, clinical judgment and factors, such as the child's cultural background, relevant medical history, or physical condition, must be evaluated to determine what level of occurrence is considered rare" (p. 65).

Two examples are in order to demonstrate statistical significance and base rate. In the first example, the practitioner wanted to determine if Robert's motor skills are significantly better than his language skills based on Robert's mother's report that Robert, who is three years of age, is highly active but not very verbal. Robert earned a standard score of 97 on the Motor Scale and a standard score of 87 on the Language Scale. These scores are regarded as Average and Low Average, respectively. An examination of Table B.4 on page 315 in Bayley and Aylward (2019b) indicated that the magnitude of the difference in Robert's standard scores is statistically significant at the .05 level of significance because the critical value is 9.9 points. Thus, this difference is real for Robert and his motor skills are significantly higher than his language skills. However, a difference of 10 standard score points between the Language and Motor Scales occurs in about 15–25% of children his age, which is higher than the 10% rule of thumb. As such, Robert's performance and the difference between his language and motor skills are rather common. Nevertheless, a standard score of 87 on the Language Scale is at the 19th percentile and there is a 90% chance that his true standard score is between 81 and 93. Consequently, the practitioner may want to recommend some language activities to Robert's mother, a more comprehensive language assessment, or a follow-up language assessment in 6–12 months.

In the second example, the practitioner wanted to know if Shirley's Interpersonal Relationships subdomain scaled score is significantly different from her Play and

Leisure subdomain scaled score on the Adaptive Behavior Scale and if the difference in her scaled scores is rare or uncommon because Shirley's father described Shirley as highly relational, but at times preferred to play alone or not at all. Shirley's scaled scores on the Interpersonal Relationships and Play and Leisure subdomains, based on her father's ratings, were 10 and 9, respectively. An examination of Table B.9 on page 320 in Bayley and Aylward (2019b) indicated that the magnitude of the difference in Shirley's scaled scores is not statistically significant at the .05 level because the critical value is 2.35 points. Thus, the 1-point difference in scaled scores occurred by chance. The practitioner also noted that the 1-point scaled score difference between Shirley's Interpersonal Relationships and Play and Leisure skills is very common, occurring in at least 25% of children Shirley's age. Therefore, Shirley's Interpersonal Relationships and Play and Leisure skills as measured by the Adaptive Behavior Scale are regarded as Average and developing evenly.

QUALITATIVE INTERPRETATION OF TEST PERFORMANCE

Practitioners should be familiar with the evaluation of the qualitative characteristics of the Bayley–4 found in Table 1.4, Chapter 1, and Chapter 6. This evaluation is helpful in interpreting a young child's performance in general, at a global level, or from a validity lens. That is, the Bayley–4 is appealing to young children, includes a variety of tasks, and does not require complex verbal responses unless measuring language skills. As important as this information is, it does not tell us much about the young child's specific assessment performance. Therefore, practitioners are strongly encouraged to be familiar with as many test items as possible, including their administration, record detailed behavioral observations, engage with the child's caregiver to gain important information, and integrate information from the Bayley–4 manuals such as the autism spectrum disorder checklist, accommodations and modifications, and developmental risk indicators in order to describe the young child's performance qualitatively. Practitioners who combine an understanding of theoretical underpinnings and assessment content, quantitative characteristics, and qualitative characteristics of the Bayley–4 in their interpretation of the young child's performance will provide caregivers with an excellent summary of their child's functioning and developmental status.

DON'T FORGET 4.5

Practitioners are strongly encouraged to be familiar with as many test items as possible, including their administration, record detailed behavioral observations, engage with the child's caregiver to gain important information, and integrate information from the Bayley–4 manuals such as the autism spectrum disorder checklist, accommodations and modifications, and indicators of abnormality in order to describe the young child's performance qualitatively.

Types of Items and Their Administration

As detailed in Chapter 2, the Bayley–4 has demonstration, sample, and multiple trial items. Each item type can provide valuable information regarding the young child's learning, reaction to new stimuli, management of frustration or stress, reactions to success, and other qualitatively rich behavior observations. In addition, the Bayley–4 has series items, related items, and timed items. Similar to demonstration, sample, and multiple trial items, these items can provide practitioners with information about how the young child generalizes, makes connections, and solves problems. Timed items can provide information on the young child's efficiency, automatization, and perseverance. Guidance on scoring items qualitatively is found throughout Bayley and Aylward (2019b) and is included with every item given the new polytomous scoring approach. Practitioners should also observe the child's affect while performing certain items. For example, does the child seem to enjoy manipulatives and motor activities more than language-based items or items that do not involve manipulatives?

Record Behavioral Observations

Practitioners are strongly encouraged to record detailed observations of the child before, during, and after the formal assessment. For example, how does the child separate from the caregiver and react to the "toys" (stimuli)? Does the child maintain focus during the assessment or is the child "all over the place" and difficult to engage? When the formal assessment is completed, does the child seem happy, sad, relieved, or indifferent? All of these behavior observations are important when describing and interpreting the young child's performance. Completing the Behavior Observation Inventory (BOI) on the back page of the Bayley–4 Record Form may be particularly helpful in describing the child's behavior during the assessment and comparing it with the caregiver's ratings. The BOI is easy to complete, provides a breadth of descriptors of the child's behaviors, and allows the practitioner to make generalizations of the child's behavior across settings. In addition, practitioners can and should record item behaviors as much as possible, especially on related items, as this information can be used to suggest activities for the caregiver to do with their child (see Caregiver Report).

> ### DON'T FORGET 4.6
>
> Completing the BOI on the back page of the Bayley–4 Record Form may be particularly helpful in describing the child's behavior during the assessment and comparing it with the caregiver's ratings.

Engage with the Child's Caregiver

One of the Bayley–4 revision goals was to include caregivers in the evaluation process, and that is accomplished via 51 structured items that include Caregiver Questions across the Cognitive, Language, and Motor Scales. These questions require the caregiver to provide valuable information regarding the child's behavior, skills, and temperament. Perhaps even more valuable is the interaction between the practitioner and caregiver. Including Caregiver Questions provides the opportunity for adults in the room to engage dynamically, establish rapport, and increase the validity of the assessment. In addition, the interaction between the practitioner and caregiver is consistent with family-focused assessment that is critical when determining the developmental status of children and with the Individuals with Disabilities Education Improvement Act (IDEIA, 20 U.S.USC. §1400, 2004), Part C, and The American Academy of Pediatrics (2006). Finally, in our professional opinion, including the caregiver throughout the assessment process is simply the right thing to do.

Autism Spectrum Disorder Checklist, Accommodations and Modifications, and Developmental Risk Indicators

The Autism Spectrum Disorder (ASD) Checklist consists of 26 items across the Cognitive and Language Scales that may be indicators of ASD. Two examples are "responds to name" and "uses gestures." In addition, there are 10 observational items that can be suggestive of ASD. For example, the child stares blankly on several occasions during the assessment. Bayley and Aylward (2019c) and Aylward (2020) make it clear that the ASD Checklist and observational items do not yield a diagnosis; however, "the more positive indicators noted during testing and information provided by the caregiver, the greater the likelihood of ASD" (Bayley & Aylward, 2019c, p. 85). Also, these items provide critical information that may be used to generate hypotheses, make referrals for more in-depth assessment, or suggest recommendations for activities for the caregiver and child. Practitioners may also find useful information regarding the potential for ASD by reviewing the items on the Social–Emotional Scale.

Bayley and Aylward (2019b) discuss the difference between accommodations and modifications, explain how the Bayley–4 embedded many accommodations within test administration, and provide information about general approaches to children with various disabilities. Practitioners are strongly encouraged to read pages 323–328 in order to gain useful information when assessing young children in general as well as those with disabilities, including visual impairment, hearing impairment, motor impairment, and those who perform behaviors in a different way because of a disability. It is critical to keep in mind that although accommodations are embedded in the Bayley–4, practitioners may make additional accommodations as long as these accommodations do not change the construct of the administered item. In the latter case of changing the construct, the practitioner would be making a modification. In other words, a modification "is a change in the construct being measured, versus a change in the administration format" (p. 323). When practitioners make accommodations or modifications, they should explain what they did, why, and how the changes affected the child's performance. If a practitioner makes too many modifications, "it is best to report the child's strengths and areas of need rather than evaluate the child's performance using the normative data" (p. 323). All quantitative and qualitative data are important to integrate when assessing young children. Therefore, it is incumbent upon practitioners to "maintain the integrity of the test, elicit a child's best performance, and gather thorough and meaningful information about the child" (p. 324).

> ### CAUTION 4.3
>
> It is critical to keep in mind that although accommodations are embedded in the Bayley–4, practitioners may make additional accommodations as long as these accommodations do not change the construct of the administered item.

Finally, practitioners may find the developmental risk indicators on the Bayley–4 helpful. Although these indicators are not included in the Bayley–4 item set per se, they are important to note when they are observed, especially if a child has a documented disability or is suspected of having one. Appendix A in Bayley and Aylward (2019c, pp. 81–86) provides practitioners with succinct information on these indicators, including those associated with the following: delay, dissociation, and deviance; movement and muscle tone; eye movement and coordination; hand movements; ASD (see above); and attention/executive function deficit. The authors caution, however, that practitioners should "not make a diagnosis based on them; rather, use these findings to raise concerns to communicate with the child's physician for further, more specific evaluation" (p. 86).

SUMMARY OF BAYLEY–4 INTERPRETATION

This chapter presented an integrated model of Bayley–4 assessment performance interpretation based on three different, but related methods and described how theoretical and assessment content, quantitative data, and qualitative information can be combined to describe the young child's developmental status. In addition, a multi-method, multi-source, multi-setting approach to assessment and evaluation was espoused and emphasized. Examples of quantitative interpretive statements and qualitative questions to ask were provided to assist new and seasoned practitioners with the language that may best explain a young child's performance and functioning. Readers may turn to the illustrative case examples in Chapter 7 for the application of many suggestions found in this chapter.

TEST YOURSELF

1. **Two great examples of psychologists who worked with young children for decades and thus developed two of the best assessments for young children were:**
   a) Alfred Binet and Louis Terman
   b) David Wechsler and Alan Kaufman
   c) Nancy Bayley and Dorothea McCarthy
   d) Collin Elliott and Jack Naglieri
2. **The assessment approach espoused and emphasized in this chapter includes:**
   a) Multiple methods
   b) Multiple sources
   c) Multiple settings
   d) All of the above
3. **The theoretical model underlying the Bayley–4 is the:**
   a) Eclectic Theory
   b) Integrated neuro-environmental synthesis model of development
   c) Three Stratum Theory
   d) Cattell–Horn–Carroll Theory
4. **The Bayley–4 includes several scores except:**
   a) Stanines
   b) Scaled
   c) Standard
   d) Percentile ranks
5. **When making decisions what error is generally worse to make?**
   a) Type I
   b) Type III
   c) Type II
   d) None of the above
6. **All of the following are true except:**
   a) Scaled scores have a mean of 10
   b) Standard scores have a standard deviation of 15

   c) Growth scale values have a mean of 500

   d) Growth scale values have a standard deviation of 15

7. **Statistical significance and base rate data are important to report:**

   a) Always

   b) Most times

   c) Sometimes

   d) Never

8. **Qualitative information regarding a child's performance on the Bayley–4:**

   a) Is not very important

   b) May be obtained from many methods, sources, and settings

   c) Cannot be obtained from the child's caregiver

   d) Is more important than quantitative information

9. **The following are true regarding the Autism Spectrum Disorder Checklist except:**

   a) It includes 26 items

   b) It does not include a separate record form

   c) It can be used to assist practitioners in thinking about Autism Spectrum Disorder

   d) It should be used alone to diagnose Autism Spectrum Disorder

10. **The Bayley-4 allows for accommodations during the assessment as long as:**

   a) They are embedded in the Bayley–4

   b) They are explained to the child

   c) They do not change the underlying construct

   d) They change the underlying construct

Answers: 1. (c); 2. (d); 3. (b); 4. (a); 5. (c); 6. (d); 7. (a); 8. (b); 9. (d); 10. (c)

REFERENCES

Alfonso, V. C., Engler, J. R., & Lepore, J. C. C. (2020). Assessing and evaluating young children: Developmental domains and methods. In V. C. Alfonso & G. J. DuPaul (Eds.), *Healthy development in young children: Evidence-based interventions for early education* (pp. 13–44). American Psychological Association. https://doi.org/10.1037/0000197-002

Alfonso, V. C., Ruby, S., Wissel, A. M., & Davari, J. (2020). School psychologists in early childhood settings. In F. C. Worrell, T. L. Hughes, & D. D. Dixson (Eds.), *The Cambridge handbook of applied school psychology* (pp. 579–597). Cambridge University Press.

The American Academy of Pediatrics. (2006). Identifying infants and young children with developmental disorders in the medical home: An algorithm for developmental surveillance and screening. *Pediatrics, 118*, 405–420.

American Educational Research Association, American Psychological Association, & National Council on Measurement in Education. (2014). *Standards for educational and psychological testing*. American Educational Research Association.

Aylward, G. P. (2020). *Bayley 4 clinical use and interpretation*. Academic Press.

Bayley, N. (1969). *The Bayley Scales of Infant Development: Manual*. Psychological Corporation.

Bayley, N. (1993). *Bayley Scales of Infant Development* (2nd ed.): *Manual*. Psychological Corporation.

Bayley, N. (2006). *Bayley Scales of Infant and Toddler Development* (3rd ed.). Pearson.

Bayley, N., & Aylward, G. P. (2019a). *Bayley Scales of Infant and Toddler Development* (4th ed.). Pearson.

Bayley, N., & Aylward, G. P. (2019b). *Bayley Scales of Infant and Toddler Development* (4th ed.): *Administration manual*. Pearson.

Bayley, N., & Aylward, G. P. (2019c). *Bayley Scales of Infant and Toddler Development* (4th ed.): *Technical manual*. Pearson.

Blair, C. (2002). School readiness: Integrating cognition and emotion in a neurobiological conceptualization of children's functioning at school entry. *American Psychologist, 57*(2), 111–127. https://doi.org/10.1037/0003-066X.57.2.111

Bracken, B. A., & Theodore, L. A. (2020). Observation of preschool children's assessment-related behaviors. In V. C. Alfonso, B. B. Bracken, & R. J. Nagle (Eds.), *Psychoeducational assessment of preschool children* (5th ed., pp. 32–54). Routledge.

Bronfenbrenner, U. (1977). Toward an experimental ecology of human development. *American Psychologist, 32*(7), 513–531. https://doi.org/10.1037/0003-066X.32.7.513

Bronfenbrenner, U. (1986). Ecology of the family as a context for human development: Research perspectives. *Developmental Psychology, 22*(6), 723–742. https://doi.org/10.1037/0012-1649.22.6.723

Bronfenbrenner, U., & Ceci, S. J. (1994). Nature-nurture reconceptualized in developmental perspective: A bioecological model. *Psychological Review, 101*(4), 568–586. https://doi.org/10.1037/0033-295X.101.4.568

Bulotsky-Shearer, R., Futterer, J., Bailey, J., & Morris, C. (2020). Leveraging the developmental strengths of young children in context. In V. C. Alfonso & G. J. DuPaul (Eds.), *Healthy development in young children: Evidence-based interventions for early education* (pp. 167–189). American Psychological Association. https://doi.org/10.1037/0000197-009

Cohen, B. H. (2013). *Explaining psychological statistics* (4th ed.). John Wiley & Sons.

Crocker, L., & Algina, J. (1986). *Introduction to classical and modern test theory.* Harcourt.

Ferretti, L. K., & Bub, K. L. (2017). Family routines and school readiness during the transition to kindergarten. *Early Education and Development, 28*(1), 59–77. https://doi.org/10.1080/10409289.2016.1195671

Flanagan, D. P., & Alfonso, V. C. (2017). *Essentials of WISC-V assessment.* John Wiley & Sons.

Flanagan, D. P., & McDonough, E. M. (2018). *Contemporary intellectual assessment: Theories, tests, and issues.* Guilford Press.

Fomby, P., & Mollborn, S. (2017). Ecological instability and children's classroom behavior in kindergarten. *Demography. 54*(5), 1627–1651. https://doi.org/10.1007/s13524-017-0602-2

Grégoire, J., Coalson, D. L., & Zhu, J. (2011). Analysis of WAIS-IV index score scatter using significant deviation from the mean index score. *Assessment, 18*(2), 168–177. https://doi.org/10.1177/1073191110386343

Individuals With Disabilities Education Improvement Act, 20 U.S.C. § 1400 (2004).

Kaufman, A. S. (1994). *Intelligent testing with the WISC-III.* John Wiley & Sons.

Kaufman, A. S., & Kaufman, N. L. (1993). *Kaufman Adolescent & Adult Intelligence Test: Manual.* American Guidance Service.

Ladd, G. W., Birch, S. H., & Buhs, E. S. (1999). Children's social and scholastic lives in kindergarten: Related spheres of influence? *Child Development, 70*(6), 1373–1400. https://doi.org/10.1111/1467-8624.00101

McCarthy, D. (1972). *The McCarthy Scales of Children's Abilities: Manual.* The Psychological Corporation.

McGrew, K. S., Werder, J. K., & Woodcock, R. W. (1991). *Technical Manual. Woodcock-Johnson Psycho-Educational Battery-Revised.* Rolling Meadows, IL: Riverside.

Nagle, R. J., Gagnon, S. G., & Kidder-Ashley, P. (2020). Issues in preschool assessment. In V. C. Alfonso, B. B. Bracken, & R. J. Nagle (Eds.), *Psychoeducational assessment of preschool children* (5th ed., pp. 29–48). Routledge.

Sattler, J. M. (2018). *Assessment of children: Cognitive foundations and applications* (6th ed.) J. M. Sattler.

Schneider, W. J., & McGrew, K. S. (2018). The Cattell–Horn–Carroll theory of cognitive abilities. In D. P. Flanagan & E. M. McDonough (Eds.),

Contemporary intellectual assessment: Theories, tests, and issues (3rd ed., pp. 73–163). Guilford Press.

Silverstein, A. B. (1982). Pattern analysis as simultaneous statistical inference. *Journal of Consulting and Clinical Psychology, 50*(2), 234–240. https://doi. org/10.1037/0022-006X.50.2.234

Silverstein, A. B. (1993). Type I, Type II, and other types of errors in pattern analysis. *Psychological Assessment, 5*(1), 72–74. https://doi. org/10.1037/1040-3590.5.1.72

Terman, L. M. (1916). *The measurement of intelligence: An explanation of and a complete guide for the use of the Stanford revision and extension of the Binet– Simon Intelligence Scale.* Houghton Mifflin.

Urbina, S. (2014). *Essentials of psychological testing* (2nd ed.). John Wiley and Sons.

Wechsler, D. (1939). *Wechsler-Bellevue Intelligence Scale.* Psychological Corporation.

Wechsler, D. (2014). *Wechsler Intelligence Scale for Children* (5th ed.). Pearson.

Five

CLINICAL APPLICATIONS OF THE BAYLEY–4

Vincent C. Alfonso, Joseph R. Engler, and Andrea D. Turner
Gonzaga University and Pearson Assessments

The landscape of early childhood assessment has changed throughout the years. Much of the change can be directly related to increases in infancy research, increases in life expectancy for children born prematurely or medically fragile, changes in laws (e.g., Individuals with Disabilities Education Improvement Act, 2004, Part C), growth of professional organizations (e.g., National Association for the Education of Young Children), and a commitment toward early intervention to remediate threats to the healthy development of young children (Black & Matula, 2000; Raines et al., 2020). Consequently, a call for a broader scope of assessment and measurement to inform the decision-making process for young children has concurrently occurred (Walker et al., 2008). This includes screening tools to identify if a young child is at risk for developing future difficulties, progress monitoring tools to measure growth and evaluate the effectiveness of interventions, and tools that can be used for diagnostic purposes.

The *Bayley Scales of Infant and Toddler Development–Fourth Edition* (Bayley–4; Bayley & Aylward, 2019a) was designed with the primary purpose of identifying developmental delays in young children while also providing valuable information for intervention planning. In doing so, the Bayley–4 has extended its clinical application from its predecessors to include a standalone and built-in screening mechanism. In addition, the Bayley–4 now includes a score called a Growth Scale Value (GSV) that can be used for progress monitoring. Lastly, the Bayley–4 can be used to help inform diagnostic decisions for young children with medical conditions. As a result, the Bayley–4 is more versatile than the *Bayley Scales of Infant and Toddler Development–Third Edition* (Bayley–III; Bayley, 2006).

Therefore, a thorough discussion of the clinical application of the Bayley–4 as a screening, progress monitoring, and diagnostic tool follows.

CLINICAL USE OF THE BAYLEY–4 AS A SCREENING TOOL

Screening, especially during early childhood, allows practitioners to identify areas of potential concern. Identifying areas of concern can then be monitored and intervened upon to prevent further problems throughout development. The Bayley–4 has two built-in mechanisms that can be used for screening. The first is a standalone screening test (Bayley–4 Screening Test; Bayley & Aylward, 2019b) and the second is an Autism Spectrum Disorder (ASD) checklist that is embedded within the full Bayley–4 (Bayley & Aylward, 2019a). While a comprehensive review of the Bayley–4 Screening Test is precluded from the chapter due to space limitations, a brief overview is provided. Readers who are interested in using the Bayley–4 Screening Test are encouraged to read the manual thoroughly to determine its appropriate use within practical settings. After providing a brief overview of the Bayley–4 Screening Test, a description of the ASD Checklist follows.

Bayley–4 Screening Test

The Bayley–4 Screening Test was created as part of the overall Bayley–4 developmental process (see Chapter 6 for overview of the Bayley–4 development). The primary purpose of the Bayley–4 Screening Test is to determine quickly and accurately whether a young child is at risk of developing a delay in one or more developmental domain areas (Aylward, 2020). The Bayley–4 Screening Test includes a subset of items from the Cognitive, Language, and Motor Scales. Specifically, 30 items from the Cognitive Scale, 45 items from the Language Scale (22 Receptive Communication and 23 Expressive Communication subtests), and 54 items from the Motor Scale (27 Fine Motor and 27 Gross Motor subtests) were included in the Screening Test. While practitioners are not required to administer all scales and/or subtests, Aylward (2020) recommends screening all five subtest areas to provide the practitioner with a comprehensive overview of the child's developmental performance.

The Bayley–4 Screening Test includes a subset of items from the full Bayley–4. Therefore, the administration procedures including start points, item administration, polytomous scoring, and discontinue rules remain similar between both instruments. That said, there are a couple of differences. The first, and most noticeable difference, is the overall administration time needed to administer the instrument. The Bayley–4 Screening Test is estimated to take approximately 15–20 minutes for children 12–24 months of age and approximately 30 minutes for children

25 months of age and older. In comparison, the full Bayley–4 takes approximately 35–68 minutes to administer depending on the age of the child. Therefore, there is approximately a 50% reduction in overall time spent administering the Bayley–4 Screening Test. As a result, the Bayley–4 Screening Test is relatively easy to administer, especially if the practitioner is familiar with the full Bayley–4.

The second noticeable difference is the scores provided by the instrument. After administering the Bayley–4 Screening Test, the practitioner then calculates the total raw score for each subtest. The total raw score is transferred to a summary sheet and then is used to determine a corresponding risk category when compared to other children within a similar age range. The Bayley–4 Screening Test uses three risk categories: High Risk, Borderline Risk, and Low Risk. A High Risk category is assigned when the total raw score is equivalent to the raw score obtained by 0–2% of the normative sample. A Borderline Risk category is assigned when the total raw score is equivalent to the raw score obtained by 3–25% of the normative sample. A Low Risk category is assigned when the total raw score is equivalent to the raw score obtained by 26–100% of the normative sample. In this way, the Bayley–4 Screening Test is relatively easy to score and interpret.

In addition to being easy to administer, score, and interpret, the Bayley–4 Screening Test is psychometrically sound. The internal consistency, as measured by split-half reliability coefficient averages across ages, ranged from .86 to .92. Further, reliability coefficients were consistently within the .80s and .90s with the exceptions of the Receptive Communication subtest at four to six months of age ($r = .79$), Cognitive subtest at 37–42 months of age ($r = .76$), and Fine Motor subtest at 37–42 months of age ($r = .75$). As such, the internal consistency generally meets an acceptable standard of .80 and above for screening measures (Salvia et al., 2013). Additionally, test–retest reliability coefficients were provided for 152 children with a mean delay between administrations of 11.8 days. Test–retest reliability coefficients were in the .80s and .90s across all subtests and ages with one exception. At 21–42 months of age, the test–retest reliability for the Gross Motor subtest was .78. In general, the Bayley–4 Screening Test appears to be highly stable over time. The Bayley–4 Screening Test Manual provides evidences for the validity of the instrument. Overall, the evidences for the validity of the instrument are similar to that of the full Bayley–4. The one exception is that the Bayley–4 Screening Test provides more evidence regarding classification accuracy than the full Bayley–4, which is necessary for any screening measure.

CAUTION 5.1

The evaluative criteria differ between instruments used for screening purposes and those used for high-stakes decision making.

The Bayley–4 test authors provided classification accuracy data between the Bayley–4 Screening Test and the full test. On the screening test, test authors used the classification risk categories (e.g., High, Borderline, and Low) and compared them to corresponding scaled score ranges (e.g., 1–4, 5–7, 8+), respectively, on the full Bayley–4. The classification accuracy for the High Risk group ranged from 54% on the Cognitive subtest to 67.4% on the Gross Motor subtest. The classification accuracy for the Borderline Risk group ranged from 70.8% on the Gross Motor subtest to 87.3% on the Expressive Communication subtest. The classification accuracy for the Low Risk Group ranged from 78.6% for the Receptive Communication subtest to 84.3% for the Fine Motor subtest. Additionally, very few (i.e., < .7%) of children who obtained a subtest scaled score above 8 were misidentified in the High Risk group.

In addition to providing classification accuracy data with the full Bayley–4, data were provided regarding the classification accuracy between the Bayley–4 Screening Test and special group studies. There are a number of terms that are important when interpreting these studies. The first is sensitivity, which refers to an instrument's ability to identify correctly individuals with a condition (Sheldrick et al., 2015). For example, if a child had a developmental delay, high sensitivity would suggest that the instrument correctly identifies it. The second is specificity, which refers to an instrument's ability to identify correctly an individual without a condition (Sheldrick et al., 2015). For screening instruments, it is more important to have high sensitivity, although this may result in more Type I errors (Aylward, 2020). Further, it is better to say that someone is at risk, when they truly are not at risk (Type I error) than to say they are not at risk when they truly are at risk (Type II error) because a Type I error will often be ruled out during a more comprehensive evaluation. It is important to note that sensitivity and specificity are inversely related (Parikh et al., 2008) and that it is important to balance the two with regard to the context of the situation.

Across all special group studies, sensitivity increases dramatically when combining the High and Borderline Risk groups. Doing so, however, lowers the specificity, which may result in an increase of Type I errors. That said, the inclusion of the Borderline Risk group will also significantly increase the number of children needing follow-up. For example, Aylward (2020) recommends that practitioners administer a full Bayley–4 when one or more scores fall within the High Risk range. If one score falls within the Borderline Risk range, Aylward recommends monitoring that area and

DON'T FORGET 5.1

The Bayley–4 Screening Test is purchased separately from the full Bayley–4.

possibly screening again in a couple of months. If two or more scores fall within the Borderline Risk range, he recommends rescreening in a couple of months, administering the full Bayley–4 in the areas of concern, or administering the full Bayley–4 in all developmental areas. Consequently, it is important for practitioners to understand these tradeoffs when making decisions about the proper use of risk categories.

ASD Checklist

In addition to the Bayley–4 Screening Test, the ASD Checklist is embedded within the full Bayley–4 that can be used as a screening tool. The need for screening ASDs during early childhood has grown as the prevalence rates have increased. Current estimates suggest that 1 in 59 children in the United States are diagnosed with ASD (Baio et al., 2018). As such, an increased emphasis has been placed on early childhood screening for ASD in hopes of earlier identification and, consequently, specialized early interventions (Hogan et al., 2020). Aylward (2020) described two levels of screening seen in early childhood development. The first, which he referred to as Level I screening, involves screening an entire population of young children. For example, Level I screening may involve screening an entire preschool classroom. Level II screening, however, is more targeted and is recommended when a child's development is already a concern. Moreover, Aylward recommends using the ASD Checklist for Level II screening concerns.

The ASD Checklist is comprised of 26 items and 10 incidentally observed items. The 26 items involve nine items from the Cognitive Scale, five items from the Receptive Communication subtest, and 12 items from the Expressive Communication subtest. The incidentally observed items include items that may be "red flags" for developing ASD. For example, items such as atypical vocalizations, echolalia, repetitive and/or restricted use of test items, etc., would be considered "red flags" of ASD (Aylward, 2020). After the 26 items on the ASD Checklist have been administered, the practitioner simply adds up the total number of items rated as a "0" and that number becomes the total score. Currently, the ASD Checklist does not have a cut-point. Rather, the authors contend that the more items indicated by the checklist, the more probable that the child should be referred for a more comprehensive ASD evaluation. It should be noted, however, that the authors recommend

> **CAUTION 5.2**
>
> The ASD Checklist does not have a cut-point to determine whether young children are at risk for developing autism. Thus, it should be used with clinical judgment and other sources of data prior to making a decision.

using the checklist, incidental observations, and Social–Emotional and Adaptive Behavior Questionnaire for the case conceptualization for the child. Additionally, practitioners are recommended to compare the aforementioned against contraindicative behaviors throughout the screening process (see Chapter 7, Case Study Susie, for an example of how the ASD Checklist can be used in practice).

SUMMARY OF THE BAYLEY–4 AS A SCREENER

The Bayley–4 shows much promise in the area of early childhood screening through the Bayley–4 Screening Test and ASD Checklist. The Bayley–4 Screening Test is an easy to administer, score, and interpret tool with good psychometric properties. The Bayley–4 Screening Test has good specificity (e.g., identifying children without developmental delays) and adequate sensitivity when combining children who are High Risk and Borderline Risk. In doing so, however, the number of children needing additional follow-up may be cumbersome and will likely yield many Type I errors. Thus, these considerations must be taken into account prior to using the test for screening purposes. The main drawback of the Bayley–4 Screening Test is that it is a standalone test and would therefore need to be purchased separately from the full Bayley–4. Despite this drawback, there are a multitude of reasons why practitioners may want to purchase the test and use it for screening purposes.

The ASD Checklist also shows promise in early identification of children at risk for having ASD. The checklist is quick and easy to administer and score as it is comprised of 26 items from the Bayley–4, along with 10 incidental items identified as "red flags" for ASD. The ASD Checklist provides qualitatively rich data regarding behaviors that may be seen in young children with ASD. There are two main drawbacks to the ASD Checklist. First, there is no cut-point to identify young children needing a more comprehensive evaluation or monitoring. As a result, it is likely to work best in conjunction with clinical judgment and behavioral observations to make such decisions. Second, we believe that the ASD Checklist would be enhanced by having a social–emotional and adaptive behavior component. This would provide the practitioner with a more comprehensive view of the young child's developmental abilities.

CLINICAL USE OF THE BAYLEY–4 FOR PROGRESS MONITORING

When a young child has been identified as at-risk for emerging developmental difficulties, it may be necessary to intervene in the area(s) of concern. The hope, then, would be that intervening in the area(s) of concern would provide improved functioning and better outcomes for young children (VanDerHeyden & Snyder, 2006). The use of progress monitoring tools is a viable option for determining whether a young child is making sufficient progress, or if an intervention needs to be modified or abandoned altogether. Generally speaking, progress monitoring tools fall into two categories: skill mastery and general outcome measures (McConnell et al., 2002). While an in-depth discussion of progress monitoring tools is precluded from this chapter, the main takeaway for readers is that progress monitoring tools are designed to measure behaviors quickly and efficiently that can be linked to future positive outcomes (Greenwood et al., 2011). In addition, progress monitoring tools have gained favor in early childhood settings because of their ease of use, sensitivity to change, and frequency in which they can be administered (i.e., weekly). Several of these characteristics were lacking within traditional standardized, norm-referenced instruments.

The Bayley–III was the first instrument in the *Bayley Scales of Infant and Toddler Development* lineage to discuss "measuring growth" or what has become known as progress monitoring. In the Bayley–III Technical Manual, Bayley (2006) briefly discusses the ability to convert a raw score to a "growth score." Then, she discusses plotting the "growth score" on a chart to show progress (or lack thereof) that is made over multiple administrations. Since then, the Bayley–4 has further conceptualized and operationalized its use as a progress monitoring tool through Growth Scale Values (GSVs). GSVs for the Bayley–4 are created on a developmental ability continuum and represent a young child's skill acquisition on a particular measure. In this way, GSVs can be useful for measuring, tracking, and monitoring individual growth on repeated measurements. The GSVs for the Bayley–4 have a mean of 500 and a standard deviation of 25. GSVs have a number of strengths that make them particularly appealing for progress monitoring.

First, GSVs represent an equal interval scale. As such, a growth of 10 represents the same amount of growth at the bottom of the scale as at the top of the scale. Therefore, GSVs can be more accurately compared over time than raw scores or percentile ranks, which do not represent equal interval scales. Second, GSVs are focused on an individual's performance so that direct comparisons between past performance and current performance can be made easily. Third, GSVs can help inform the effectiveness of an intervention on a young child. For example, if a young child is making growth, but the amount of growth is not enough to close a gap between individual and peer performance, the intervention may need to be modified, or discontinued in order to try a different intervention.

While there are clear benefits of using the Bayley–4 GSVs for progress monitoring purposes, there are also drawbacks. First, GSVs are only useful when an instrument has been administered multiple times. Therefore, a young child would need multiple administrations to calculate a GSV. Multiple administrations may present challenges. For example, the administration time and resources needed (i.e., protocols, scheduling, access, etc.) may not be suited for cases where frequent progress monitoring is necessary. Second, the GSV represents a young child's growth over time, plus measurement error. As a result, practitioners would want to determine whether the change in GSVs was statistically significant (Bayley & Aylward, 2019c), rather than using the GSV in isolation. Third, GSVs are dependent on the instrument. As such, making direct comparisons between GSVs on different instruments, or between subtests/subdomains, is not appropriate.

> **DON'T FORGET 5.2**
> ....
> GSVs cannot be compared across instruments.

SUMMARY OF THE BAYLEY–4 FOR PROGRESS MONITORING

The Bayley–4 is the first edition of the venerable Bayley Scales to include a formal score for measuring progress. The Bayley–4 utilizes a GSV to measure change over time and also to determine whether an intervention is facilitating "adequate" growth. The GSV accomplishes both; however, the Bayley–4 must be administered multiple times to the same young child to do so. Given the time and resources needed to administer the Bayley–4, it seems logical that the GSV is best used to monitor progress for young children who are identified as Low Risk, or for young children who may need monitoring on a monthly basis (or perhaps less frequently). In contrast, it is recommended to use a general outcome measure such as Individual Growth and Developmental Indicators (IGDIs; Walker et al., 2008) for young children who are identified as Borderline or High Risk because they are quick and easy to administer. Additionally, young children at Borderline or High Risk will likely need frequent progress monitoring (i.e., weekly), making a general outcome measure the more appropriate choice in such cases.

CLINICAL USE OF THE BAYLEY–4 AS A DIAGNOSTIC TOOL

One of the primary uses of the Bayley–4 is to identify children as having a developmental delay in one or more area(s) of functioning (Bayley & Aylward, 2019c). To identify whether a child has a developmental delay requires a comparison of the child's performance on the Bayley–4 to the standardization sample. In an effort to increase the instrument's sensitivity, Aylward (2020) reported that children who were considered "at risk" were not included in the standardization sample. Therefore, the standardization sample is comprised of children who could be described as "typically developing" (see Chapter 6 for a further description of the standardization sample). To provide evidence of special group performance, the test authors offered data to show how children with one or more disabling conditions performed on the Bayley–4. Further, special group study data were provided in the Technical Manual (Bayley & Aylward, 2019c) for children with: (1) Autism Spectrum Disorders (ASD), (2) Developmental Delay (DD), (3) Down Syndrome (DS), (4) Language Delay/Specific Language Impairment (LD/SLI), (5) Premature Birth, (6) Motor Impairment (MI), and (7) Prenatal Drug/Alcohol Exposure.

Autism Spectrum Disorders

According to the *Diagnostic and Statistical Manual of Mental Disorders* (5th ed.; DSM-5; American Psychiatric Association, 2013), ASDs are characterized by deficits in social communication and interactions, and engagement in restricted, repetitive patterns of behavior, interests, or activities. Therefore, language delays are a primary characteristic of children with an ASD. Researchers, however, have also identified other developmental domains thought to be impacted by ASDs. For example, Ray-Subramanian and colleagues (2011) found that young children with ASDs perform approximately 1 SD below the mean on a measure of cognitive abilities and approximately 1.5 SD below the mean on a measure of adaptive behavior. In addition, Li et al. (2020) found that boys with ASDs were reported by their parents as having higher externalizing and internalizing problems as compared to typically developing peers. The authors also found that young children with ASDs had lower levels of emotional functioning when compared to typically developing peers. Consequently, research suggests that many, if not all, of the developmental domains measured by the Bayley–4 are likely to be negatively affected by having an ASD.

To test these hypotheses, the Cognitive, Language, and Motor Scales of the Bayley–4 were administered to 31 children with a primary classification of ASDs. Additionally, children with a secondary classification of a DD, LD, SLI, or motor impairments were allowed to participate in the study. Children who met the inclusionary criteria for DS and children with low speech intelligibility (<50%) were excluded from the study. The results of the study showed that children with ASD scored significantly lower across the Cognitive, Language, and Motor Scales. Thus, children with ASD displayed global delays across the aforementioned scales. Within the scales, children with ASD performed lowest on the Receptive Communication and Expressive Communication subtests (ss = 3.4 and 3.7, respectively) and performed highest on the Fine Motor and Gross Motor subtest (ss = 4.6 and 5.5, respectively). It should be noted, however, that no information was provided in the Technical Manual (Bayley & Aylward, 2019c) for the Social–Emotional and Adaptive Behavior Scales. Consequently, important information was missing that could further support the use of the Bayley–4 for children with ASD.

Developmental Delay

The test authors also provided a special group study on children with DD. Although the definition of DD differs across states, the evaluative criteria typically involves standard scores at least 1.5 or 2.0 standard deviations below the mean in one or more developmental domains (Shackelford, 2006). Therefore, it is expected that children with DD would perform within that range on the Bayley–4. Children were included in this study if they had a primary classification of DD and/or they received services in two or more developmental domains. In contrast, children were excluded from this study if they met the criteria for DS, ASD, or prenatal drug/alcohol exposure. Additionally, children were excluded from the study if they were diagnosed with one or more genetic disorders. A total of 57 children with DD were administered the Bayley–4 Cognitive, Language, and Motor Scales and scored, on average, between 1.0 and 1.5 standard deviations below the mean of a matched control. Classification accuracy was provided on the Cognitive, Language, and Motor Scales for the sample. The classification accuracy was .82, which is considered very good (Johnson & Sinharay, 2018). The Adaptive Behavior Scale was also administered to 32 children with DD. Across all subdomains, children with DD scored significantly lower than a matched control. On average, subdomain and domain scores were approximately 1.0 to 1.5 standard deviations below the matched control. The results of this study show strong evidence that the Bayley–4 is an appropriate instrument for identifying DD in early childhood.

Down Syndrome

DS is a chromosomal abnormality where children are born with an additional 21st chromosome (Kim et al., 2017). Often, children born with DS have corresponding mild to moderate intellectual disabilities as well as other developmental deficits (Patterson et al., 2013). As such, the Bayley–4 test authors hypothesized that children with DS would score between 2 and 3 standard deviations below a matched control. In sum, 54 children were included in this special group study because they were diagnosed with DS. Children with DS were also included in the study if they had a secondary classification of DD, LD, SLI, MI, or were born premature. Children who met the inclusionary criteria for ASD or prenatal drug/alcohol exposure were excluded from this study. The sample was given the Cognitive, Language, and Motor Scales of the Bayley–4. Children with DS scored approximately 2 standard deviations below the matched control on all scales. More specifically, scaled scores ranged from 3.3 on the Gross Motor subtest to 4.6 on the Fine Motor subtest. Therefore, children with DS performed within a predictable pattern on the Bayley–4, which supports its use in similar cases.

Language Delay/Speech Language Impairment

The test authors of the Bayley–4 provided data on 50 children with either a Language Delay (LD; n = 25) or a Specific Language Impairment (SLI; n = 25). Children were included in the LD sample if they had a primary classification of LD and/or were receiving language services, or were suspected of having a language delay. In addition, children were included if they met criteria for the MI group but the child's language delay is considered a primary classification. Children were excluded from the LD study if they had DS, ASD, were diagnosed with an articulation disorder, or met the inclusionary criteria as a primary classification of another special group. Children with an LD were administered the Cognitive, Language, and Motor Scales of the Bayley–4. Children with LD performed significantly lower than the matched control on all subtests with the exception of Fine Motor. Children with an LD performed the lowest on the Expressive Communication subtest (5.5), which would be expected. The classification accuracy of the Language Scale for children with an LD was .86, which is considered very good (Johnson & Sinharay, 2018).

The authors of the Bayley–4 provided a special group study on children with SLI. To be included in this study, children had to be diagnosed with an SLI. If they met the criteria for the MI special group study, but the SLI was a primary classification, they were also included in this study. To be excluded from the study, children could not have DS or ASD, have an IQ below 70, or have a primary classification matching one of the other special groups. The 25 children in this study were administered the Cognitive, Language, and Motor Scales of the Bayley–4. They performed significantly lower on all subtest and composite scores than a matched control, with the lowest performance on the Expressive Communication subtest. The classification accuracy for distinguishing SLI group membership was .80, which is considered good accuracy. As such, there is support for the use of the Bayley–4 for children with language delays and speech and language impairments.

Children Born Prematurely

Current estimates suggest that approximately 10% of all births in the United States are considered premature (e.g., <37 weeks gestation). Consequently, babies born prematurely may experience a number of deficits that negatively affect their development. For example, research has shown that children born prematurely may have lower cognitive and communication scores than those born full-term (Matson et al., 2010). In addition, Gidley Larson et al. (2011) found that children born prematurely may have motor difficulties later in life. These findings are increasingly evident in children who are born extremely prematurely (Marlow et al., 2005). The Cognitive, Language, and Motor Scales of the Bayley–4 were administered to 136 children born prematurely. Of the total sample, 70 were born moderate/late prematurely whereas 66 were born very/extremely prematurely. The test authors defined moderate/late premature as a child being born between 32 weeks 0 days and 36 weeks 6 days gestation. Children were considered very/extremely premature if they were born prior to 32 weeks 0 days gestation.

The test authors predicted that those born very/extremely prematurely would perform significantly lower than a matched control and lower than the moderate/late premature sample. Children within the moderate/late premature group performed approximately .5 to 1 SD lower than a matched control. While performance across subtests and scales was considered in the low average to average range of functioning, it is noteworthy that children in the moderate/late premature group performed statistically significantly lower than a matched control across all subtests and scales. Children within the very/extremely premature group performed approximately 1 to 1.5 SD lower than a matched control. This was statistically significantly lower than the matched control. Additionally, children born very/extremely prematurely scored significantly lower than the moderate/late premature group. The results of this study support previous research demonstrating the effects of premature birth on developmental domains throughout early childhood. Additionally, the results support the use of the Bayley–4 for children who were born prematurely.

Children with Motor Impairment

Data were provided in the Technical Manual (Bayley & Aylward, 2019c) on 40 children who were identified as having either Cerebral Palsy (CP) or a developmental coordination disorder. According to the Center for Disease Control and Prevention (2020), CP encompasses a range of disorders that primarily affect one's motor ability, balance, and posture. Children with CP may also experience difficulties related to cognition, seizures (Center for Disease Control and Prevention, 2020), and speech (Novak et al., 2017). Developmental coordination disorders are characterized by difficulties in acquiring and executing coordinated muscle movements (American Psychiatric Association, 2013). Collectively, this group was identified by the Bayley–4 test authors as having a motor impairment. The Cognitive, Language, and Motor Scales were administered to 40 children who were identified as having an MI. Inclusionary criteria included being diagnosed with mild to moderate CP, developmental coordination disorder, or having a documented motor delay. Children with a secondary classification of LD/SLI, premature birth, prenatal drug/alcohol exposure, and DD were included in the study. Children with severe CP, DS, and ASD were excluded from the study.

The Bayley–4 authors predicted that children with a motor impairment would demonstrate deficits in fine motor, gross motor, and cognitive tasks that include motor skills. The motor impairment sample performed significantly lower than the matched control across all areas, with the lowest performance on the Gross Motor subtest ($M = 4.2$) and the Cognitive subtest ($M = 5.5$). This demonstrates the relationship between Gross Motor skills and several of the items on the Cognitive subtest. Interestingly, children with motor impairments performed the highest on the Fine Motor subtest ($M = 6.5$), which was tied with performance on the Expressive Communication subtest. Although children with motor impairments performed the highest on the Fine Motor and Expressive Communication subtests, it should be noted that their performance was still greater than 1 SD below the national average. The Motor Scale was associated with a .90 classification accuracy, suggesting that the Motor Scale distinguishes children with and without motor impairments with a high degree of accuracy. Further, the results of the special group study support the use of the Bayley–4 for children with motor impairments.

Children with Prenatal Drug/Alcohol Exposure

When a pregnant woman consumes drugs and/or alcohol, the drugs and/or alcohol can pass through the placenta and affect prenatal brain development (Ross et al., 2015). As a result, children born after prenatal exposure may experience myriad difficulties. For example, cognitive, self-regulation, emotional, and adaptive behavior deficits may exist and persist throughout early childhood development (Hagan et al., 2016). As such, the Bayley–4 authors provided a special group study to examine the performance of children with prenatal drug/alcohol exposure on the Cognitive, Language, and Motor Scales. To be eligible for the special group study, there was a history of prenatal drug or alcohol exposure, even if the child met inclusionary criteria for DD, LD, SLI, MI, or was born prematurely. Children, however, who met the inclusionary criteria for DS or ASD were excluded from the study. The Bayley–4 Cognitive, Language, and Motor Scales were administered to 44 children who met inclusionary criteria for the study. Results showed that children with prenatal drug/alcohol exposure performed significantly lower than a matched control on all areas assessed. Specifically, children with prenatal drug and/or alcohol exposure performed approximately 1 to 1.5 SD below the matched control on all subtests and scales measured. Consistent with previous research, children with prenatal drug/alcohol exposure performed the lowest on the Cognitive subtest. The results of the study support the use of the Bayley–4 for children with prenatal drug/alcohol exposure.

> ## CAUTION 5.3
>
> Including young children with multiple disabling conditions may deflate all developmental domains measured in the special group studies.

SUMMARY OF SPECIAL GROUP STUDIES

When standardizing the Bayley–4, the authors intentionally excluded children with disabling conditions from the normative sample. The purpose of doing so was to improve the diagnostic sensitivity and clinical utility of the test (Bayley & Aylward, 2019c). Consequently, the test authors collected and provided data, in the way of special group studies, on seven conditions/impairments that can disrupt the typical developmental pattern for young children. Across all special group studies, children with disabling conditions performed within a predictable pattern based upon current research and commonly known correlates of each condition. As such, the special group studies provide emerging support of the Bayley–4's clinical utility. That said, as with all special group studies, there are limitations that must be taken into account to ensure practitioners are using the Bayley–4 in a responsible way.

One, and most notable, limitation of the special group studies is the inclusion of children with secondary classifications in each special group study. For example, all of the special group studies, with the exception of the DD study, included children with secondary classifications in one or more of the other disabling conditions. As a result, the secondary classifications may attenuate subtest and composite scores in different areas than the primary classification. A good example of this is in the LD study. If the LD study included children with language deficits *only*, one might expect the Expressive Communication, Receptive Communication, and Cognitive subtests to be significantly lower than the matched control, but not the Fine Motor and Gross Motor subtests. In the study, however, children with a secondary classification of MI were included. Consequently, children in the study performed significantly lower on the Gross Motor subtest than the matched control. Thus, by including children with multiple conditions, one would anticipate the results to show more global delays than a pronounced profile if only one condition was included (e.g., LD only).

A second limitation was that the Social–Emotional and Adaptive Behavior Scales were not included in the majority of the special group studies as they were normed with different instruments than the Bayley–4. For example, the Social–Emotional Scale was unchanged from the Bayley–III (Bayley, 2006), and the Adaptive Behavior Scale was created using the *Vineland Adaptive Behavior Scales (3rd ed.), Comprehensive Parent/Caregiver Form* (Vineland–3; Sparrow et al., 2016). Therefore, these two scales were not collected as part of the development phase of the Bayley–4. In other words, data on the majority of special groups were collected using the Cognitive, Language, and Motor Scales only. As a result, the special group studies provide an incomplete picture regarding performance across all five developmental domains.

Although the Bayley–4 clinical utility may be enhanced by having purer special groups and data across all developmental domains, it should be noted that no instrument is perfect. The Bayley–4 continues to be the gold standard instrument for assessing young children across developmental domains. Keeping in mind that the primary purpose of the Bayley–4 is to help identify developmental delays amongst young children (Bayley & Aylward, 2019c), the Bayley–4 does so very well. Therefore, it is our opinion that the strength of the Bayley–4 is its ability to identify developmental delays in young children as well as delays in one or more of the five developmental domains it assesses. When, however, a delay in one or more of the five developmental domains is found, we recommend that practitioners consider referring young children to a professional with expertise in diagnoses in that particular area (e.g., Speech–Language Pathologist, Occupational Therapist, Physical Therapist, etc.).

≡ Rapid Reference 5.1

Strengths and Limitations of the Bayley–4 Clinical Applications

Strengths
- Breadth of the Bayley–4 includes screening and progress monitoring tools.
- Bayley–4 Screening Test has good psychometric characteristics.
- Has an increased emphasis on early identification of ASD.
- Provides useful data when evaluating young children with medical or other early childhood conditions.

(Continued)

Limitations
- Bayley–4 Screening Test is a separate purchase.
- ASD Checklist would be enhanced with a cut-score.
- Special group studies may be more informative with more restrictive inclusionary criteria.
- Information on the Social–Emotional and Adaptive Behavior Scales was not provided in several special group studies.

SUMMARY

The Bayley–4 represents the most comprehensive and clinically useful instrument in the history of the Bayley Scales. The Bayley–4 now includes multiple screening measures and GSVs for monitoring individual growth and measuring intervention efficacy. The inclusion of screening measures and their application for progress monitoring adds value and appeal to those who work in early childhood settings, as well as for clinicians, practitioners, and interventionists. As the Bayley–4 broadens its scope, however, there are considerations and recommendations made throughout this chapter that may enhance and further strengthen its application for screening and progress monitoring purposes. While the aforementioned are of *added value*, the strength and main purpose of the Bayley–4 is to identify accurately developmental delays in young children. The Bayley–4 succeeds in its purpose and delivers on its promise. Additionally, the Bayley–4 provides valuable data when assessing young children with medical conditions or who are experiencing other conditions that impact healthy development. As such, the Bayley–4 continues to remain the gold standard in early childhood assessment.

TEST YOURSELF

1. **Which of the following has not directly affected the changing landscape of early childhood assessment?**
   a) Infancy research
   b) Change in laws
   c) Part B of IDEIA
   d) Growth of professional organizations
2. **It is recommended to use the ASD Checklist for Level I screening only.**
   a) True
   b) False

3. **The Bayley–4 score that can be used for progress monitoring is called**
   a) Growth Score Value
   b) Growth Scale Value
   c) Growth Rate
   d) Growth Quotient
4. **The ASD Checklist is comprised of**
   a) 26 items from the Bayley–4 Cognitive, Language, and Motor Scales and 10 incidental observations
   b) 22 items from the Bayley–4 Cognitive, Language, and Motor Scales and 10 incidental observations
   c) 26 items from the Bayley–4 Cognitive, Language, and Motor Scales and 8 incidental observations
   d) 22 items from the Bayley–4 Cognitive, Language, and Motor Scales and 8 incidental observations
5. **On the Bayley–4 Screening Test, the Borderline Risk category corresponds to what percentage of the normative sample?**
   a) > 50%
   b) 40–49%
   c) 30–39%
   d) 3–25%
6. **Down syndrome involves an additional 21st chromosome.**
   a) True
   b) False
7. **Approximately 25% of all births in the U.S. are considered premature.**
   a) True
   b) False
8. **Current estimates suggest the prevalence rate for ASD is 1 in.**
   a) 28
   b) 40
   c) 51
   d) 59
9. **Including children with multiple disabling conditions in special group studies enhances overall performance.**
   a) True
   b) False
10. **Cerebral palsy primarily affects an individual's motor ability, balance, and posture.**
    a) True
    b) False

Answers: 1. (c); 2. (b); 3. (b); 4. (a); 5. (d); 6. (a); 7. (b); 8. (d); 9. (b); 10. (a)

REFERENCES

American Psychiatric Association (2013). *Diagnostic and statistical manual of mental disorders* (5th ed.). Author.

Aylward, G. P. (2020). *Bayley–4 clinical use and interpretation.* Academic Press.

Baio, J., Wiggins, L., Christensen, D. L., Maenner, M. J., Daniels, J., Warren, Z., …, Dowling, N. F. (2018). Prevalence of ASD among children aged 8 years – Autism and developmental disabilities monitoring network, 11 sites, United States, 2014. MMWR. *Surveillance Summaries, 67,* 1–23. DOI: 10.15585/mmwr.ss6706a1 and DOI: 10.15585/mmwr.ss6707a1

Bayley, N. (2006). *Bayley Scales of Infant and Toddler Development* (3rd ed.): *Technical manual.* Pearson.

Bayley, N., & Aylward, G. P. (2019a). *Bayley Scales of Infant and Toddler Development* (4th ed.). Pearson.

Bayley, N., & Aylward, G. P. (2019b). *Bayley Scales of Infant and Toddler Development* (4th ed.). *Screening test technical manual.* Pearson.

Bayley, N., & Aylward, G. P. (2019c). *Bayley Scales of Infant and Toddler Development* (4th ed.). *Technical manual.* Pearson.

Black, M. M., & Matula, K. (2000). *Essentials of Bayley Scales of Infant Development–II assessment.* John Wiley & Sons, Inc.

Center for Disease Control and Prevention (2020, December). *What is cerebral palsy?* https://www.cdc.gov/ncbddd/cp/facts.html.

Gidley Larson, J. C., Baron, I. S., Erickson, K., Ahronovich, M. D., Baker, R., & Litman, F. R. (2011). Neuromotor outcomes at school age after extremely low birth weight: Early detection of subtle signs. *Neuropsychology, 25*(1), 66–75. https://doi.org/10.1037/a0020478.

Greenwood, C. R., Carta, J. J., & McConnell, S. (2011). Advances in measurement for universal screening and individual progress monitoring of young children. *Journal of Early Intervention, 33*(4), 254–267. https://doi.org/10.1177/1053815111428467.

Hagan, J. F., Jr., Balachova, T., Bertrand, J., Chasnoff, I., Dang, E., Fernandez-Baca, D., …, Zubler, J. (2016). Neurobehavioral disorder associated with prenatal alcohol exposure. *Pediatrics, 138*(4), 1–23. https://doi.org/10.1542/peds.2015-1553.

Hogan, A. L., Hills, K. J., Wall, C. A., Will, E. A., & Roberts, J. (2020). Screening and diagnosis of ASD in preschool-aged children. In V. C. Alfonso, B. A. Bracken, & R. J. Nagle (Eds.), *Psychoeducational assessment of preschool children* (5th ed., pp. 323–345). Routledge.

Johnson, M. S., & Sinharay, S. (2018). Measures of agreement to assess attribute-level classification accuracy and consistency for cognitive diagnostic assessments. *Journal of Educational Measurement, 55*(4), 635–664. DOI: 10.1111/jedm.12196

Kim, H. I., Kim, S. W., Kim, J., Jeon, H. R., & Jung, D. W. (2017). Motor and cognitive developmental profiles in children with Down syndrome. *Annals of Rehabilitation Medicine, 41*(1), 97–103. https://doi.org/10.5535/arm.2017.41.1.97.

Li, B., Bos, M., Stockmann, L., & Rieffe, C. (2020). Emotional functioning and the development of internalizing and externalizing problems in young boys with and without ASD. *Autism, 24*(1), 200–210. https://doi.org/10.1177/1362361319874644.

Marlow, N., Dieter Wolke, D. M., Bracewell, M. A., & Samara, M. (2005). Neurologic and developmental disability at six years of age after extremely preterm birth. *The New England Journal of Medicine, 352*(1), 9–19. DOI: 10.1056/NEJMoa041367

Matson, J. L., Hess, J. A., Sipes, M., & Horovitz, M. (2010). Developmental profiles from the Battelle Developmental Inventory: A comparison of toddlers diagnosed with Down Syndrome, global developmental delay, and premature birth. *Developmental Neurorehabilitation, 13*(4), 234–238. DOI: 10.3109/17518421003736032

McConnell, S. R., McEvoy, M. A., & Priest, J. S. (2002). "Growing" measures for monitoring progress in early childhood education: A research and development process for individual growth and development indicators. *Assessment for Effective Intervention, 27*(4), 3–14. DOI: 10.1177/073724770202700402

Novak, I., Spirit-Jones, A., & Morgan, C. (2017). First words: Speech and language interventions in cerebral palsy. *Developmental Medicine and Child Neurology, 4*, 343. https://doi.org/10.1111/dmcn.13383.

Parikh, R., Mathai, A., Parikh, S., Sekhar, G. C., & Thomas, R. (2008). Understanding and using sensitivity, specificity and predictive values. *Indian Journal of Ophthalmology, 56*(1), 45–50. https://doi.org/10.4103/0301-4738.37595.

Patterson, T., Rapsey, C. M., & Glue, P. (2013). Systematic review of cognitive development across childhood in Down syndrome: Implications for treatment interventions. *Journal of Intellectual Disability Research, 57*(4), 306–318. https://doi.org/10.1111/j.1365-2788.2012.01536.x.

Raines, T. C., Malone, C. M., Biedleman, L. M., & Bowman, N. (2020). National policies and laws affecting children's health and education. In V. C.

Alfonso & G. J. DuPaul (Eds.), *Healthy development in young children: Evidence-based interventions for early education* (pp. 319–335). American Psychological Association. https://doi.org/10.1037/0000197-016.

Ray-Subramanian, C. E., Huai, N., & Weismer, S. E. (2011). Brief report: Adaptive behavior and cognitive skills for toddlers on the autism spectrum. *Journal of Autism and Developmental Disorders, 41(5)*, 679–684. https://doi.org/10.1007/s10803-010-1083-y.

Ross, E. J., Graham, D. L., Money, K. M., & Stanwood, G. D. (2015). Developmental consequences of fetal exposure to drugs: What we know and what we still must learn. *Neuropsychopharmacology Reviews, 40(1)*, 61–87. https://doi.org/10.1038/npp.2014.147.

Salvia, J., Ysselkyke, J. E., & Bolt, S. (2013). *Assessment in special and inclusive education* (12th ed.). Wadsworth.

Shackelford, J. (2006). State and jurisdictional eligibility definitions for infants and toddlers with disabilities under IDEA (NECTAC Notes No. 20). The University of North Carolina, FPG Child Development Institute, National Early Childhood Technical Assistance Center.

Sheldrick, R. C., Benneyan, J. C., Kiss, I. G., Briggs-Gowan, M. J., Copeland, W., & Carter, A. S. (2015). Thresholds and accuracy in screening tools for early detection of psychopathology. *The Journal of Child Psychology and Psychiatry, 56(9)*, 936–948. https://doi.org/10.111/jcpp.12442.

Sparrow, S. S., Cicchetti, D. V., & Saulnier, C. A. (2016). *Vineland Adaptive Behavior Scales* (3rd ed.). Pearson.

VanDerHeyden, A. M., & Snyder, P. (2006). Integrating frameworks from early childhood intervention and school psychology to accelerate growth for all young children. *School Psychology Review, 35(4)*, 519–534. DOI: 10.1080/02796015.2006.12087959

Walker, D., Carta, J. J., Greenwood, C. R., & Buzhardt, J. F. (2008). The use of individual growth and developmental indicators for progress monitoring and intervention decision making in early education. *Exceptionality, 16(1)*, 33–47. https://doi.org/10.1080/09362830701796784.

Six

TECHNICAL REVIEW INCLUDING STRENGTHS AND LIMITATIONS OF THE BAYLEY–4

Vincent C. Alfonso, Joseph R. Engler, and Andrea D. Turner

Gonzaga University and Pearson Assessments

The Bayley Scales research team utilized literature reviews in childhood development and expert panels (e.g., practitioners, individuals familiar with previous versions, etc.) to identify revision goals for the *Bayley Scales of Infant and Toddler Development–Fourth Edition* (Bayley–4; Bayley & Aylward, 2019a). As such, the research team set forth seven major goals for this revision. These goals were to maintain the basic qualities and format of the *Bayley Scales of Infant and Toddler Development–Third Edition* (Bayley–III; Bayley, 2006), develop polytomous scoring rather than dichotomous scoring, include caregivers in the evaluation, simplify administration to reduce testing time, improve content coverage, improve diagnostic sensitivity and clinical utility, and update the normative data. This chapter begins by describing the developmental process for the Bayley–4. From there, we evaluate the quantitative characteristics and qualitative characteristics of the Bayley–4. This chapter concludes with a discussion of the major strengths and limitationes of the Bayley–4 in relation to the revision goals provided in the Bayley–4 Technical Manual (Bayley & Aylward, 2019c). The identified strengths and limitationes are determined using a review of existing literature, examination of the quantitative and qualitative characteristics of the instrument using the Bayley–4 Technical Manual (Bayley & Aylward, 2019c) and Bayley–4 Administration Manual (Bayley & Aylward, 2019b), and the authors' and colleagues' experiences.

CONTENT COVERAGE

Prior to beginning the test developmental phases, the Bayley Scales research team reviewed the test content of the Bayley–III to maintain its qualities and format while improving the content coverage and reducing the administration time of the instrument. To accomplish these goals, items with a correlation coefficient of > .79 and measuring overlapping constructs were recommended for removal from the Bayley–4. In addition, items were added to increase the content coverage to subtest floors (see the Floors section). In total, 18 items were excluded and eight items were added to the Cognitive Scale, 28 items were excluded and four items were added to the Language Scale, 46 items were excluded and 12 items were added to the Motor Scale, the Social–Emotional Scale remained unchanged, and 120 items were used from the *Vineland Adaptive Behavior Scales–Third Edition Comprehensive Parent/Caregiver Form* (Vineland–3; Sparrow et al., 2016) for the Adaptive Behavior Scale. As a result, administration takes approximately 35 minutes for children less than 12 months of age, 63 minutes for children 13–24 months of age, and 68 minutes for children 25 months of age and older. In comparison, the estimated administration time for the Bayley–III was approximately 50 minutes for children 12 months of age and under, and 90 minutes for children 13 months of age and over (Bayley, 2006). Therefore, administration times were reduced by approximately 30%. This significant reduction in administration time represents a considerable strength of the Bayley–4.

TEST STRUCTURE AND DEVELOPMENT

Consistent with its goal of maintaining the basic qualities of the Bayley–III, the Bayley–4 has maintained the overall structure of the instrument. The structure of the Bayley–4 continues to include a Cognitive Scale, Language Scale (i.e., Receptive and Expressive Communication subtests), Motor Scale (i.e., Fine and Gross Motor subtests), Social–Emotional Scale, and Adaptive Behavior Scale. Thus, it continues to measure the five core areas necessary to identify developmental disabilities in young children.

The creation of the Bayley–4 involved expert guidance and feedback throughout several phases of development. The first phase of development was a conceptual phase. During this phase, a literature review was conducted and information was obtained from experts across a variety of related fields. Then, the development of the Bayley–4 transitioned into assessment labs and focus groups. The purpose of this phase was to ensure that test directions and scoring criteria were easily understood across delivery modalities (e.g., paper, digital, and rating scales). Next, a pilot research phase commenced. The purpose of this phase was twofold. First, it was used to ensure that test items could be administered in a standardized manner. Second, it was used to determine reliable and valid item sets for each of the subtests using newly designed items and a polytomous scoring system.

After completing the pilot research phase, the Bayley–4 research team began a tryout research phase. During this phase, a nationally representative sample was used to evaluate the administration and psychometric properties of the instrument. The research team concluded that the reliability data were generally acceptable. Following this phase, an advisory panel, experts, and consultants evaluated the data and made final recommendations for the Bayley–4 prior to moving into the standardization phase of development.

QUANTITATIVE CHARACTERISTICS

Standardization

For any instrument, it is necessary to evaluate critically the standardization sample to ensure that the normative sample is representative of the population at large (Salvia et al., 2017). With respect to the standardization sample, there are several quantitative characteristics that should be evaluated. They include the size of the normative group, recency of normative data, age division of norm tables, and the match of the demographic characteristics of the normative group when compared to the United States population (see Alfonso & Flanagan, 2009; Engler & Alfonso, 2020 for a further discussion). Collectively, these quantitative characteristics provide useful information regarding practitioners' ability to generalize assessment results.

The Bayley–4 was published in 2019 and included 1700 typically developing children ages 16 days to 42 months in the normative sample for the Cognitive, Language, and Motor Scales. The normative sample was divided into approximately one month increments through seven months of age, three month increments through 28 months of age, and four to six month increments through 42 months of age. In total, there were 17 age divisions with 100 participants per division. The normative sample was matched with the 2017 U.S. Census data according to age, parent education level, race/ethnicity, region, and sex. Overall, the normative sample matched the U.S. population on the majority of demographic variables with only slight variations. Asian children from lower parent education levels, however, were not represented after 12 months of age. Based upon the information provided in the Technical Manual (Bayley & Aylward, 2019c), the Bayley–4

> ## CAUTION 6.1
>
> A rating of *inadequate* on a test characteristic does not indicate that the test is bad or should not be used. Always consider all technical data when determining the appropriateness of a test for a given circumstance.

Cognitive, Language, and Motor Scales are considered *adequate* to *good* across standardization characteristics.

The normative sample for the Social–Emotional Scale included 320 children of ages 16 days to 42 months. The normative sample was divided into approximately two to four month increments through nine months of age, four to six month increments from 10 months to 30 months of age, and a 12 month increment from 31 to 42 months of age. There was a total of eight age divisions with 40 participants per division. The normative sample for the Social–Emotional Scale was matched with the 2017 U.S. Census data according to age, parent education level, race/ethnicity, region, and sex. The normative sample matched the U.S. population on the majority of demographics with only slight variations. There were no Asian children included in the normative population for children of ages 15 to 18 months. As a result, the standardization characteristics for the Social–Emotional Scale ranged from *inadequate* to *good*. Moreover, a major limitation of the Social–Emotional Scale is it only included 320 children, making it difficult to generalize the results of this scale to the population at large.

The normative sample for the Adaptive Behavior Scale was collected from the Vineland–3 (Sparrow et al., 2016) standardization sample. The normative sample included 750 children and was divided into four month increments through 23 months of age, six month increments from 24 to 35 months of age, and seven month increments from 36 to 42 months of age. There was a total of nine age divisions with 80–90 participants per division. The normative sample for the Adaptive Behavior Scale was matched with the 2014 U.S. Census data according to age, parent education level, race/ethnicity, region, and sex. There was an under-representation of children eight to 23 months of age from the lowest parental education level. Collectively, the standardization characteristics of the Adaptive Behavior Scale were generally *adequate* to *good* across ratings with the exception of the normative group size, which was *inadequate*.

Evidences of Reliability

The *Standards for Educational and Psychological Testing* (American Educational Research Association et al., 2014) recommend that test developers provide evidences of reliability for test users. There were three evidences of reliability provided in the Bayley–4 Technical Manual (Bayley & Aylward, 2019c). The first evidence was test–retest reliability, which provides an estimate of an instrument's stability. In sum, 152 children were administered the Cognitive, Language, and Motor Scales within a range of 1–43 days ($M = 11.8$). The test–retest sample was matched to the U.S. population according to age, parental education level, race/ethnicity, region, and sex. Overall, there was a slight under-representation of

African American children and a slight over-representation of Hispanic children. The size and representativeness of the test–retest sample and interval length were rated as *good* across the Cognitive, Language, and Motor Scales. The test–retest sample was divided into children zero to seven months of age, eight to 20 months of age, and 21 to 42 months of age. As a result, the test–retest sample age range for the Cognitive, Language, and Motor Scales received an *inadequate* rating. The corrected correlation coefficients (*r*) were generally *adequate* across all ages (e.g., above .80). The major exception was at the zero to seven months of age range where the Motor Scale, Expressive Communication, and Fine Motor subtests were rated as *inadequate*. Regarding the Social–Emotional Scale, test–retest reliability was not provided, and thus could not be rated. Test–retest reliability data were provided for the Adaptive Behavior Scale. Sixty-seven children were included in the test–retest sample ranging from zero to three years of age. The sample was matched to the U.S. population on age, parent education level, race/ethnicity, region, and sex. There was a slight over-representation of White children included in the sample and no Asian children were included. Corrected correlation coefficients ranged from .72 to .87, which is considered *inadequate* to *adequate*. Specifically, the Personal subdomain and Daily Living Skills domain were the two areas rated as *inadequate*, whereas all other subdomains and domains were rated as *adequate*.

The second evidence of reliability provided was internal consistency. Internal consistency provides an estimate of consistency within an instrument and is used to calculate the standard error of measurement (SEM) and confidence intervals. The average SEMs for all Bayley–4 subtests and subdomains are <1.0 and for all Bayley–4 scales <4.0 (Bayley & Aylward, 2019c, p. 34). Confidence intervals are addressed in Chapter 4. The authors of the Bayley–4 utilized a split-half reliability coefficient as evidence for internal consistency. The Cognitive and Motor Scales have split-half reliability coefficients of .90 or above across all ages, whereas the Language Scale has coefficients in the .80s and above. Therefore, the Cognitive and Motor Scales were rated as *good* and the Language Scale was rated as *adequate*. Within the Language Scale, split-half reliability coefficients are significantly lower for the Receptive and Expressive Communication subtests prior to eight months of age.

The authors of the Bayley–4 also provide reliability coefficients of special group samples across the Cognitive, Motor, and Language Scales. Across all groups, with the exception of the Fine Motor subtest for children with Language Delay (*r* = .88), reliability coefficients meet or exceed .90. In addition, data were provided regarding the reliability coefficients on the Social–Emotional Scale. Reliability coefficients were generally *adequate* (e.g., .80 or above) for all ages, with the exception of children aged six to nine months (*r* = .79). Lastly, reliability coefficients were provided on the Adaptive Behavior Scale. Within the Adaptive Behavior Scale, the Communication and Socialization domains had *good* internal consistency across ages whereas the Daily Living Skills had *adequate* internal consistency for children aged four to seven months and *good* internal consistency across all other ages. Within the Adaptive Behavior Scale, subdomains had *adequate* to *good* internal consistency across all ages.

> ## DON'T FORGET 6.1
> ....
> When evaluating critically the reliability of a test, key areas to consider are consistency, stability, and interrater reliability.

Evidences of Validity

The American Educational Research Association et al. (2014) recommends that test developers provide validity evidence about their test scores. Further, there are six different validity evidences that may be provided. Those are content-oriented evidence, evidence regarding cognitive processes, evidence regarding internal structure, evidence regarding relationships with conceptually related constructs, evidence regarding relationships with criteria, and evidence based on consequences of tests (see American Educational Research Association et al., 2014 for further details). The Bayley–4 Technical Manual (Bayley & Aylward, 2019c) specifically addresses several types of validity evidences.

The first validity evidence provided in the Technical Manual (Bayley & Aylward, 2019c) is evidence based on test content. Unlike many of the other validity evidences, evidence based on test content does not involve the use of statistical analyses or empirical findings. Rather, evidence based on test content involves ensuring that the test items represent appropriately the content being measured. The Bayley–4 test authors provide evidence based on test content established by extensive literature and expert reviews. When independently reviewing the Bayley–4, the test content appears to match the intended constructs well. This is further substantiated by reviewing the changes made between the content of the Bayley–III and Bayley–4. The changes in item content appear to be focused better on the scales they measure. Additionally, the way in which the items are worded, the administration procedures, and the scoring all demonstrate consistency between test content and measuring developmental processes for young children. Further, Sattler (2018) recommends evaluating the content validity of a test by asking the following four questions: (1) Does the test measure the domain of interest? (2) Are the test questions appropriate? (3) Does the test contain enough information to cover appropriately what it is supposed to measure? (4) What is the level of mastery at which the content is being assessed? (p. 118). Based upon the information provided in the Technical Manual and a thorough review of the test content, the Bayley–4 appears to have *good* support for test content validity evidence. Table 4.1 provides lists of the underlying skills assessed by the Bayley–4.

The second validity evidence provided in the Technical Manual (Bayley & Aylward, 2019c) is evidence based on response processes. The test authors provide evidence for this based upon review by the development staff and advisory panel. Moreover, the development staff and advisory panel collected information on the expected response patterns of young children. When collecting this information, reviewers looked for the following: (1) the task focused on the intended skill, (2) the task did not require skills that were not acquired by children at the target ages, (3) the task included supports to minimize confounding processes, and (4) the content of the task was focused on child-friendly and child-familiar themes. While these areas of review can provide validity evidence, the Technical Manual did not provide the results of this review. Further, it would be helpful for test users to know how this information was confirmed or used to enhance the content within the Bayley–4.

The third validity evidence provided in the Technical Manual (Bayley & Aylward, 2019c) is evidence based on the internal structure. This validity evidence can be difficult to evaluate given that the internal structure is based upon psychological constructs that cannot be directly observed (Sattler, 2018). The test authors include subtest intercorrelations for the Cognitive, Language, and Motor Scales to demonstrate that each subtest was measuring different constructs. Overall, the subtests were moderately correlated with each other, demonstrating some overlap; however, the subtests appear to measure separate and distinct constructs. Given that the overall structure of the Bayley–4 did not differ from the Bayley–III, the test authors did not conduct a confirmatory factor analysis to provide evidence for the internal structure. Rather, the test authors cite the confirmatory factor analysis conducted on the Bayley–III to support the use of a three-factor model (e.g., Cognitive, Language, and Motor Scales). While there is a significant amount of consistency between the Bayley–III and Bayley–4, it would be helpful for an updated factor analytic analysis to assess this evidence of validity.

The fourth evidence of validity provided in the Technical Manual (Bayley & Aylward, 2019c) is evidence based on the relation to other variables. The authors divide this section into two parts: the relation between the Bayley–4 and other measures and special group studies. First, however, they compared the average Bayley–III and Bayley–4 Cognitive, Language, and Motor subtest and scale scores. Correlations ranged from a high of .75 for the Motor Scale to a low of .69 for the Receptive Communication subtest, indicating that these instruments are measuring similar constructs (Bayley & Aylward, 2019c, p. 44). The authors compared the Bayley–4 to the *Wechsler Preschool and Primary Scale of Intelligence – Fourth Edition* (WPPSI-IV; Wechsler, 2012) and the *Peabody Developmental Motor Scales–Second Edition* (PDMS-2; Folio & Fewell, 2000) to provide evidence of concurrent validity. As expected, the Cognitive Scale was highly correlated with the Verbal Comprehension Index (.71), Working Memory Index (.71), and the Full Scale IQ (.79) on the WPPSI-IV. The Language Scale was highly correlated with the Verbal Comprehension Index (.64), Working Memory Index (.66), and the Full Scale IQ (.72).

When compared to the PDMS-2 (i.e., test of motor development), the Bayley–4 Fine Motor subtest was correlated with the Fine Motor Quotient (.42) and the Total Motor Quotient (.50) of the PDMS-2. The Bayley–4 Gross Motor subtest was highly correlated with the Gross Motor Quotient (.64) and the Total Motor Quotient (.63) of the PDMS-2. Lastly, the Bayley–4 Motor Scale was correlated at .66 with the PDMS-2 Total Motor Quotient. Additionally, the means and standard deviations of each test were relatively consistent.

An additional validity evidence provided in the Technical Manual (Bayley & Aylward, 2019c) is evidence based on special group studies. In particular, validity evidence was provided for children with: (1) Autism Spectrum Disorder (ASD), (2) Developmental Delay (DD), (3) Down Syndrome (DS), (4) Language Delay/ Specific Language Impairment (SLI), (5) Premature Birth, (6) Motor Impairment, and (7) Prenatal Drug/Alcohol Exposure. A thorough description of the special group studies is found in Chapter 5. Overall, the special group studies support the emergence of predictive validity for the Bayley–4. That is, the participants in the special group studies performed as one would expect given their disabling condition. There were, however, some noticeable limitations within the special group studies.

First, the participant sample for children diagnosed with ASD did not include information from the Social–Emotional and Adaptive Behavior Scales. Given the criteria for an ASD diagnosis/classification, it is recommended that data within these developmental domains be provided. Second, several of the special group studies included participants with multiple disabling conditions (e.g., Language Delay and the history of prenatal drug and/or alcohol exposure). As such, special group studies including participants with multiple disabling conditions showed general delays across developmental domains rather than more pronounced deficits in one or more of the expected developmental areas (e.g., Receptive Communication). Therefore, it is recommended to include participants with only one disabling condition in the special group studies so the sample is a purer measure of expected performance. The inclusion of multiple disabling conditions is likely to confound the results of the special group studies.

In summary, evidence of a test's validity is not an all-or-nothing phenomenon. Further, it is not inherent to a test (Sireci, 2009). Rather, the concept of validity refers to several sources of evidence that support the interpretation of a test based upon its test scores. The Technical Manual (Bayley & Aylward, 2019c) provides evidence regarding the Bayley–4's content, response processes, internal structure, relation to other variables, and special group studies. Based upon the information provided within this chapter, the Bayley–4 provides support for the interpretation of the test and was rated as *good*. That said, it is important to know that evidences for a test's score validity continue to accrue over time. Moreover, what has been provided in the chapter serves as a starting point in understanding the clinical utility of the Bayley–4. Readers are encouraged to read and examine critically future research and clinical studies on the Bayley–4 to add to the evidences already provided.

> **DON'T FORGET 6.2**
> ....
> Evidence for validity increases over time.

Test Floors

When assessing young children, it is imperative to have adequate test floors (Bracken & Theodore, 2020; Gregory, 2016). Test floors are necessary to ensure that a young child's performance is not overestimated at the lower level of functioning. This is accomplished by having a sufficient number of "easy" items so that performance amongst examinees may be differentiated at the lowest levels (Alfonso & Flanagan, 2009). An adequate test floor is obtained when a raw score of 1 is associated with a standard score greater than two standard deviations below the mean (see Alfonso & Flanagan, 1999; Bracken, 1987 for more details). In the Bayley–4, an *adequate* floor was not achieved until one month, six days to one month, 15 days of age. At that age, the Cognitive and Receptive Communication subtests were the only two with *adequate* floors. It was not until one month, 26 days to two months, five days of age where all five subtests obtained *adequate* floors. That said, all scales and domains were rated as having *adequate* floors.

With respect to the Social–Emotional Scale, *adequate* floors were obtained at all age intervals. The Adaptive Behavior Scale is comprised of a Receptive Communication, Expressive Communication, Personal, Interpersonal Relationships, and Play and Leisure subdomains. The first subdomain to obtain an *adequate* floor was Interpersonal Relationships at two months of age. The Play and Leisure and Receptive Communication subdomains obtained *adequate* floors at seven and nine months of age, respectively. The Expressive Communication and Personal subdomains did not have *adequate* floors until 13 and 14 months of age, respectively.

Test Ceilings

Similar to test floors, it is necessary for tests to have adequate ceilings. An adequate ceiling ensures that the test performance is not under-represented at the higher level of functioning (Engler & Alfonso, 2020). An adequate ceiling is established when the highest obtained raw score is associated with a standard score greater than two standard deviations above the mean. The Cognitive and Fine Motor subtests had *adequate* ceilings across all age ranges. The Expressive Communication subtest had an *adequate* ceiling until 27 months, 15 days of age and had an *inadequate* ceiling thereafter. The Receptive Communication subtest had an *adequate* ceiling until 30 months, 15 days of age and the Gross Motor subtest had an *adequate* ceiling until 33 months, 15 days of age.

The Social–Emotional Scale had *adequate* ceilings for five of eight age ranges. Specifically, *adequate* ceilings were identified at zero to three, six to nine, 10 to 14, 15 to 18, and 31 to 42 months of age. The remaining age ranges (e.g., four to five, 19 to 24, 25 to 30) all had *inadequate* ceilings. On the Adaptive Behavior Scale, all subdomains had *adequate* ceilings through 22 months, 30 days of age. From 23 to 42 months of age, the Interpersonal Relationships subdomain had *inadequate* ceilings. From 24 to 42 months of age, the Receptive and Expressive subdomains had *inadequate* ceilings. The Play and Leisure subdomain had *inadequate* ceilings from 26 to 42 months of age and the Personal subdomain had *inadequate* ceilings from 34 to 42 months of age.

Item Gradients

Item gradients are a way to measure the incremental change associated with the conversion of raw scores to scaled or standard scores (Bracken & Theodore, 2020). Moreover, item gradients are used to differentiate examinee performance. Bracken (1988) recommended that a raw score increase of 1 point should be associated with no greater than a 1/3 standard deviation difference. For example, if a raw score of 14 is associated with a scaled score ($M = 10$, $SD = 3$) of 7, a raw score increase to 15 (e.g., 1 point) should correspond with a scale score of no greater than 8 (e.g., 1/3 SD). An increase of greater than 1/3 standard deviation would be considered an item gradient violation. Alfonso and Flanagan (2009) furthered this recommendation and provided guidance regarding the total number of item gradient violations within a test. Alfonso and Flanagan note that tests where no item gradient violations occur, or all item gradient violations occur between two and three standard deviations below the mean, or the total number of item gradient violations is less than 5% receive an evaluation classification as *good.*

To evaluate the item gradient violations within the Bayley–4, a thorough review of the normative tables is provided. When reviewing the normative tables for the Cognitive, Language, and Motor Scales, very few item gradient violations were found. In total, there were less than 5% item gradient violations, which suggests that the Bayley–4 Cognitive, Language, and Motor Scales appropriately differentiate subtle performance differences amongst examinees, which was rated as *good*. Within these scales, the majority of item gradient violations were found within the Expressive Communication subtest for children from birth through three months, 15 days of age. After that age, relatively few item gradient violations were found. On the Social–Emotional Scale, there was less than 5% item gradient violations rendering a *good* rating. All violations were at the higher end of performance and occurred in children four to nine months of age with one additional violation for children 15–18 months of age. The total number of item gradient violations was also calculated for the Adaptive Behavior Scale. Similar to all other scales, there was less than 5% item gradient violations, which is considered *good*. In total, the Bayley–4 has few item gradient violations, which allows examiners the ability to differentiate performance uniformly across examinees.

≡ Rapid Reference 6.1

**Strengths and Limitations of the Bayley–4
Quantitative Characteristics**

Strengths

- The Bayley–4 Cognitive, Language, and Motor Scales are considered adequate to good across standardization characteristics. Likewise, standardization characteristics of the Adaptive Behavior Scale were generally adequate to good across ratings with the exception of the normative group size.
- The size and representativeness of the test–retest sample and interval length were rated as good across the Cognitive, Language, and Motor Scales.
- Regarding internal consistency, the Cognitive and Motor Scales were rated as good and the Language Scale was rated as adequate.
- Based upon the information provided in the Technical Manual and a thorough review of the test content, the Bayley–4 appears to have good support for test content validity evidence.
- With respect to the Social–Emotional Scale, adequate floors were obtained at all age intervals.
- In total, the Bayley–4 has few item gradient violations, which allows examiners the ability to uniformly differentiate performance across examinees. All five Bayley–4 Scales were rated as good in this area.

Limitations

- Within the Cognitive, Language, and Motor Scales normative sample, Asian children from lower parent education levels were not represented after 12 months of age. Relatedly, the normative sample for the Social–Emotional Scale did not include Asian children between ages 15 to 18 months.
- The normative sample for the Social–Emotional Scale included only 320 children, making it difficult to generalize the results of this scale to the population at large.
- There was an under-representation of children eight to 23 months of age from the lowest parental education level within the Adaptive Behavior Scale normative sample.
- The age range of the test–retest sample was rated as inadequate for all five scales.
- Regarding the Social–Emotional Scale, test–retest reliability was not provided and thus could not be rated.
- The Technical Manual did not provide the results of the response process validity review.
- Given that the overall structure of the Bayley–4 did not differ from the Bayley–III, the test authors did not conduct a confirmatory factor analysis to provide evidence for the internal structure. Rather, the test authors cite confirmatory factor analysis conducted on the Bayley–III to support the use of a three-factor model (e.g., Cognitive, Language, and Motor Scales).

QUALITATIVE CHARACTERISTICS

In addition to examining the quantitative characteristics of a test, it is important to examine the qualitative characteristics of an instrument as well. Although examining qualitative characteristics has not received as much attention in the literature as evaluating the quantitative characteristics of instruments, it is a necessary component of early childhood assessment because early children's development is unlike many other developmental periods (e.g., adolescence, adulthood) and necessitates special attention (Bulotsky-Shearer et al., 2020). For example, young children may have shorter attention spans, limited language capacities, and motivational constraints that can be addressed as parts of the assessment process (Bracken & Theodore, 2020). Therefore, examiners should evaluate whether tests are designed to minimize the negative influences of the aforementioned. If so, the probability of obtaining valid results may increase. While a thorough review of all qualitative considerations is precluded from this chapter due to space limitations (see Alfonso & Flanagan, 2009 for a more detailed review), our review of the qualitative characteristics of the Bayley–4 focuses on the following: Administrative and Scoring Directions, Test Kit Materials, Manipulatives, and Printed Materials.

Administrative and Scoring Directions

The administration and scoring directions play a vital role in the assessment of young children. First, simplified administration and scoring directions allow the examiner to spend less time on administration and scoring, and more time engaging young children. This can increase motivation and attention for the examinee while fostering a brisk administration for the examiner. Consequently, simplified administration and scoring directions can dramatically reduce the overall test administration time. Second, as previously mentioned, young children are not equipped with the language capabilities of older children. Therefore, tests for young children should attempt to minimize the receptive and expressive language demands on children. Doing so may facilitate a better understanding of the test demands, while minimizing confounding variables, which is necessary when assessing children with cultural and/or linguistical differences. Third, simplified administration and scoring directions increase standardization and facilitate objectivity of an assessment. When directions are long and cumbersome, it may be more likely for the examiner to miss key details or components. Similarly, when scoring directions are difficult to follow, it increases variability in scoring and leads to unreliable results.

The Bayley–4 included several improvements over the Bayley–III to enhance the administration procedures. First, the Bayley–4 Administration Manual (Bayley & Aylward, 2019b) now includes detailed pictures to guide the Cognitive Scale administration procedures. This provides the examiner with a better understanding on how to organize and set up the materials as well as how to position the examinee. Second, the Bayley–4 retained the Series Items, or items including the same directions, and added Related Items. Related Items include the same manipulatives. Thus, examiners are able to administer items that use the same materials, which can reduce administration time. Third, the Bayley–4 added a Caregiver Report that can be used to ascertain information from the parent rather than having to observe the desired task during an administration. Thus, the inclusion of caregivers in the administration enhances the flow of the administration and also reduces the overall testing time. Fourth, the Bayley–4 now includes a digital administration (see Chapter 8), which allows the examiner to administer and score the entire test on a virtual platform. Not only does this increase the ease of administration, it also increases the accuracy of scoring and limits the probability of making errors when transferring raw scores to scaled/standard scores.

The Bayley–4 included improvements over the Bayley–III regarding scoring procedures. First, the Bayley–4 Administration Manual (Bayley & Aylward, 2019b) includes a dedicated section on quantitative- and qualitative-based scoring. In particular, the test authors listed several items where qualitative or clinical judgement is needed. In addition to the item list, the test authors provided examples to aid clinical judgement. Second, the Bayley–4 now includes polytomous scoring (e.g., mastery, emerging, not present). Prior editions relied heavily on dichotomous scoring (e.g., mastery, not present), which did not reflect a full continuum of developmental skills (Aylward, 2020). Third, the inclusion of a digital administration greatly enhances the accuracy and ease of scoring the Bayley–4.

While the Bayley–4 includes several improvements to aid in the administration of the test, there were two identifiable limitations that should be noted. First, the significant number of manipulatives requires a substantial amount of training by the examiner prior to administering the test. Second, Aylward (2020) noted that items that may increase the ceiling were reduced or eliminated to reduce testing time. The Bayley–4 is typically used to identify developmental delays in young children; however, not including higher end items limits its clinical utility to only young children at the lower end of functioning.

Test Kit Materials

The Bayley–4 includes 43 items (23 of which are manipulatives) and are packaged in a rolling case. The rolling case can be used like a suitcase and includes an extension handle for ease of rolling. Within the test kit, the manipulatives are arranged in three large plastic zip lock bags and several of the manipulatives are individually wrapped. The test kit also includes a pegboard and a pink/blue board. The Bayley–4 now includes an introductory online training option as well as an observation checklist that can be used to become more familiar with items that can be scored through incidental observations. The online training takes approximately 1.5 hours to complete and comes with a Certificate of Completion. Similar to previous versions, the print version of the Bayley–4 is heavy, cumbersome, and can be difficult to pack into the rolling kit.

Manipulatives

There are 23 manipulatives that come with the Bayley–4 test kit. The manipulatives appear to be strong and durable, which is a dramatic upgrade since the original *Bayley Scales of Infant Development* (Black & Matula, 2000). The one exception is the clear box, which is breakable and can result in sharp edges that could injure a young child. In addition to being durable, the majority of manipulatives are large enough so that they are not easily lost or ingested. The two exceptions are the bottle without a lid and the coins. Due to the cost of replacement, examiners will want to be cognizant so that manipulatives are not lost or broken. In previous editions of the Bayley Scales, manipulatives could be purchased individually. This is no longer the case as the Bayley–4 sells the manipulatives as a complete set. Therefore, if one or two items are lost, it will be expensive to replace the manipulatives and an examiner will end up with more replacements than are necessary. In general, the majority of the manipulatives are made out of plastic, which allows them to be easily cleaned. Given that young children put toys in their mouth, having manipulatives that are easily sanitized is important. There are two manipulatives (button sleeve and shoelace) that are made of fabric, which may be difficult to clean if a young child puts them in their mouth. That said, given where that item occurs in a standardized administration, it is unlikely that a young child will put either of these in their mouth.

Printed Materials

The Bayley–4 paper administration test kit includes several printed materials. The Administration Manual (Bayley & Aylward, 2019b) is soft covered and contains a spiral binding. With consistent use, the pages within the Administration Manual can easily rip. While the ends of the spiral binding are bent in, the use of spiral binding allows the Administration Manual to "walk" away from the binding over time. The printed materials within the Administration Manual are clear, easy to follow, and enhance the ease of administration. For example, many items include a picture demonstrating the material setup for the task. The Bayley–4 includes a thin Technical Manual, which includes information on the development, standardization, and psychometric properties of the test. The Technical Manual (Bayley & Aylward, 2019c) is well laid out and provides the necessary components to support the test.

The Record Forms are color coded and easy to follow. The Record Form for the Cognitive, Language, and Motor Scales includes the item number, materials needed, and scoring criteria. It also lists the Caregiver Question, when necessary. While each individual scale (e.g., Cognitive, Language, and Motor) is color-coded separately, the colors assigned to the Language and Motor Scale are difficult to differentiate. Therefore, an examiner may not be able to navigate between these scales as quickly. The Social–Emotional and Adaptive Behavior Questionnaire is included in one booklet. This is helpful for examiners as it requires less materials to bring to the testing session. The Stimulus Book includes a variety of pictures that are appropriately sized, colorful, and engaging.

Overall, the Bayley–4 has several qualitative characteristics that make it an ideal instrument for assessing young children. For example, the administration and scoring procedures are easy to follow for the examiner. The Bayley–4 has opportunities to teach tasks to ensure that items accurately measure the ability to perform a task, rather than the ability to understand directions. There are alternative stopping rules that can be applied to limit the amount of time spent assessing an examinee. In addition to administrative and scoring procedures, the Bayley–4 has a number of characteristics to engage appropriately young children in the assessment process. In particular, the test materials are attractive, colorful, and contain several developmentally appropriate manipulatives that are engaging.

Collectively, these qualitative characteristics should enhance the assessment session with young children.

≡ Rapid Reference 6.2

Strengths and Limitations of the Bayley–4 Qualitative Characteristics

Strengths

- The Bayley–4 included several improvements over the Bayley–III to enhance the administration procedures, including detailed pictures to guide the Cognitive Scale administration procedures, Series Items that include the same directions, Related Items that include the same manipulatives, a Caregiver Report, and a digital administration.
- The Bayley–4 also included improvements over the Bayley–III regarding scoring procedures, including a dedicated section on quantitative- and qualitative-based scoring within the Administration Manual, polytomous scoring, and a digital administration.
- The majority of the manipulatives that come with the Bayley–4 appear to be strong, durable, and large enough so that they are not easily lost or ingested.
- The printed materials within the Administration Manual are clear, easy to follow, and enhance the ease of administration.
- The Record Forms are individually color coded and easy to follow.

Limitations

- The Bayley–4 includes a significant number of manipulatives, requiring a substantial amount of training prior to administering the test.
- Aylward (2020) noted that items that may increase the ceiling were reduced or eliminated to reduce testing time. Failing to include higher end items limits the Bayley–4's clinical utility to only young children at the lower end of functioning.
- The print version of the Bayley–4 is heavy and cumbersome, so it can be difficult to pack into the rolling kit.
- Manipulatives cannot be purchased individually. Therefore, if one or two items is lost, it will be expensive to replace the manipulatives and practitioner will end up with more replacements than are necessary.
- With consistent use, the pages within the Administration Manual can easily rip. Additionally, despite the ends of the spiral binding being bent in, the use of spiral binding allows Administration Manual to "walk" away from the binding over time.
- The colors assigned to the Language and Motor Scales are difficult to differentiate.

SUMMARY OF STRENGTHS AND LIMITATIONS

The Bayley–4 has a number of strengths related to its revision goals. The Bayley–4 maintains the basic qualities and format of the Bayley–III by retaining the same five scales as the Bayley–III, which eliminated reconciliation efforts by the research team. In particular, the Bayley–4 maintains the scales that are necessary for identifying and diagnosing developmental delays in young children, which remains one of its primary uses. An identified limitation, however, is that the test authors did not provide a confirmatory factor analysis to support the overall structure of the Bayley–4. One of the most significant upgrades to the Bayley–4 is the inclusion of polytomous scoring rather than dichotomous scoring, which also represents a considerable strength of the instrument. Doing so now allows practitioners to give credit for skills that are "emerging." This better represents the current literature that developmental skills should not be dichotomized as either "mastered" or "not developed."

The Bayley–4 was also designed to include caregivers in the evaluation and to simplify administration in an effort to reduce testing time. Authors of the Bayley–4 are commended for incorporating caregivers in the assessment process by using Caregiver Questions. This allows caregivers to participate actively in the assessment process, assists in building rapport, and reduces the overall administration time by not having to observe all items. Through the inclusion of Caregiver Questions and other efforts (e.g., eliminating redundant items, removing items near the ceiling, having a digital platform) the overall testing time was reduced by approximately 30%. While this is a significant reduction in time, a limitation of the Bayley–4 is that it is more limited to assessing young children at the lower level of functioning.

Quantitatively, the Bayley–4 serves as the gold standard in early childhood assessment. The majority of quantitative characteristics were rated as *adequate* to *good* across standardization, reliability, test–retest sample, floors, ceilings, item gradients, and validity evidences. One area, however, that was rated as *inadequate* across all five scales was the age range of the test–retest sample. Further, it may be beneficial to include a test–retest sample that spans no more than 1 year in future editions of the Bayley Scales. Qualitatively, the Bayley–4 has many strengths. The Bayley–4 contains attractive materials with manipulatives that are engaging for young children, limited expressive and receptive language requirements on subtests not assessing language, and opportunities to teach tasks. One qualitative limitation is that the replacement materials are very expensive and cannot be purchased individually.

TEST YOURSELF

1. **Which of the following was not one of the development team's seven major revision goals for the Bayley–4?**
   a) Maintain the basic qualities and format of the Bayley–III
   b) Develop polytomous scoring
   c) Exclude caregivers from the evaluation
   d) Update normative data
2. **Administration times for the Bayley–4 were reduced by approximately 30% compared to the Bayley–III.**
   a) True
   b) False
3. **What two subtests make up the Language Scale?**
   a) Fine Motor and Receptive Communication
   b) Cognitive and Expressive Communication
   c) Cognitive and Receptive Communication
   d) Expressive Communication and Receptive Communication
4. **How many children were included in the normative sample for the Cognitive, Language, and Motor Scales?**
   a) 1600
   b) 1700
   c) 1900
   d) 2000
5. **How many children were included in the normative sample for the Social–Emotional Scale?**
   a) 300
   b) 320
   c) 500
   d) 750
6. **The authors of the Bayley–4 utilized a split-half reliability coefficient as evidence for internal consistency.**
   a) True
   b) False
7. **The Technical Manual provides validity evidence based on test content, response processes, internal structure, relation to other variables, and special group studies.**
   a) True
   b) False

8. **Which scale obtained adequate floors at all age intervals?**
   a) Cognitive
   b) Motor
   c) Adaptive Behavior
   d) Social–Emotional
9. **Each of the Bayley–4 scales had less than 5% item gradient violations, rendering ratings of good for all five scales.**
   a) True
   b) False
10. **Similar to previous editions of the Bayley, Bayley–4 manipulatives can be purchased individually.**
    a) True
    b) False

Answers: 1. (c); 2. (a); 3. (d); 4. (b); 5. (b); 6. (a); 7. (a); 8. (d); 9. (a); 10. (b)

REFERENCES

Alfonso, V. C., & Flanagan, D. P. (1999). Assessment of cognitive functioning in preschoolers. In E. V. Nuttall, I. Romero, & J. Kalesnik (Eds.), *Assessing and screening preschoolers* (2nd ed., pp. 186–217). Allyn & Bacon.

Alfonso, V. C., & Flanagan, D. P. (2009). Assessment of preschool children: A framework for evaluating the adequacy of the technical characteristics of norm-referenced instruments. In B. Mowder, F. Rubinson, & A. Yasik (Eds.), *Evidence based practice in infant and early childhood psychology* (pp. 129–166). John Wiley & Sons.

American Educational Research Association, American Psychological Association, & National Council on Measurement in Education (2014). *Standards for educational and psychological testing*. American Educational Research Association.

Aylward, G. P. (2020). *Bayley 4 clinical use and interpretation*. Academic Press.

Bayley, N. (2006). *Bayley Scales of Infant and Toddler Development* (3rd ed.): *Administration manual*. Pearson.

Bayley, N., & Aylward, G. P. (2019a). *Bayley Scales of Infant and Toddler Development* (4th ed.). Pearson.

Bayley, N., & Aylward, G. P. (2019b). *Bayley Scales of Infant and Toddler* (4th ed.): *Administration manual*. Pearson.

Bayley, N., & Aylward, G. P. (2019c). *Bayley Scales of Infant and Toddler Development* (4th ed.): *Technical manual.* Pearson.

Black, M. M., & Matula, K. (2000). *Essentials of Bayley Scales of Infant Development-II assessment.* John Wiley & Sons, Inc.

Bracken, B. A. (1987). Limitations of preschool instruments and standards for minimal levels of technical adequacy. *Journal of Psychoeducational Assessment, 5*(4), 313–326. DOI: 10.1177/073428298700500402

Bracken, B. A. (1988). Ten psychometric reasons why similar tests produce dissimilar results. *Journal of School Psychology, 26*(2), 155–166. DOI: 10.1016/0022-4405(88)90017-9

Bracken, B. A., & Theodore, L. A. (2020). Creating the optimal preschool testing situation. In V. C. Alfonso, B. A. Bracken, & R. J. Nagle (Eds.), *Psychoeducational assessment of preschool children* (5th ed., pp. 55–76). Routledge.

Bulotsky-Shearer, R., Futterer, J., Bailey, J., & Morris, C. (2020). Leveraging the developmental strengths of young children in context. In V. C. Alfonso & G. J. DuPaul (Eds.), *Healthy development in young children: Evidence-based interventions for early education* (pp. 167–189). American Psychological Association.

Engler, J. R., & Alfonso, V. C. (2020). Cognitive assessment of preschool children: A pragmatic review of theoretical, quantitative, and qualitative characteristics. In V. C. Alfonso, B. A. Bracken, & R. J. Nagle (Eds.), *Psychoeducational assessment of preschool children* (5th ed., pp. 226–249). Routledge.

Folio, R. M., & Fewell, R. R. (2000). *Peabody Developmental Motor Scales* (2nd ed.). Pro-Ed.

Gregory, R. J. (2016). *Psychological testing: History, principles, and applications* (7th ed.). Pearson.

Salvia, J., Ysseldyke, J. E., & Witmer, S. (2017). *Assessment in special and inclusive education* (13th ed.). Cengage.

Sattler, J. M. (2018). A primer on statistics and psychometrics. In J. M. Sattler (Ed.), *Assessment of children: Cognitive foundations and applications* (Jerome M. Sattler, 6th ed., pp. 91–136). Author.

Sireci, S. G. (2009). Packing and unpacking sources of validity evidence. In R. W. Lissitz (Ed.), *The concept of validity* (pp. 19–38). Information Age Publishing, Inc.

Sparrow, S. S., Cicchetti, D. V., & Saulnier, C. A. (2016). *Vineland Adaptive Behavior Scales* (3rd ed.). Pearson.

Wechsler, D. (2012). *Wechsler Preschool and Primary Scale of Intelligence* (4th ed.). Pearson.

Seven

ILLUSTRATIVE CASE EXAMPLES AND REPORTS

Vincent C. Alfonso, Joseph R. Engler, and Andrea D. Turner
Gonzaga University and Pearson Assessments

Chapters 1 through 6 provided an overview of the *Bayley Scales of Infant and Toddler Development–Fourth Edition* (Bayley–4; Bayley & Aylward, 2019) as well as detailed information regarding the administration, scoring, interpretation, clinical applications, and technical review of the instrument. The culmination of this information is represented within three illustrative case examples and reports in this chapter. The first illustrative case example of Arie involves a young child who was born prematurely and is experiencing motor difficulties. The case of Arie is interpreted through a leveled framework discussed by Aylward (2020). Within the case of Arie, an example of how to incorporate age-adjustments for prematurity into a developmental evaluation is provided. In addition, several interpretive strategies from Chapter 4 are included (e.g., pairwise comparisons, base rates).

The second illustrative case example of Susie involves a young child suspected of autism spectrum disorder (ASD). In Susie's case, the evaluator uses the Autism Spectrum Disorder Checklist as part of the developmental evaluation process to rule out ASD. The third illustrative case example of Carol involves a parent who is concerned that her young child is developing slower than peers. The developmental assessment uses an integrated model of Bayley–4 interpretation first discussed in Chapter 4 to determine whether Carol is on a healthy developmental trajectory. Collectively, the illustrative case examples provide three different approaches to a developmental evaluation using a plethora of strategies and tools provided by the Bayley–4.

Essentials of Bayley™–4 Assessment, First Edition. Vincent C. Alfonso,
Joseph R. Engler and Andrea D. Turner.
© 2022 John Wiley & Sons, Inc. Published 2022 by John Wiley & Sons, Inc.

Case Example #1: Arie

CONFIDENTIAL DEVELOPMENTAL EVALUATION REPORT

Name: Arie P.
Date of Birth: March 21, 2020
Age: 11 months, 1 day
Adjusted age: 9 months, 21 days (expected date of birth: May 1, 2020)
Evaluator: Shawnda W. Layton, PhD
Dates of Assessment: February 20 and 22, 2021
Date of Report: March 1, 2021

Reason for Referral

Arie is an 11-month, 1-day-old child referred by his pediatrician for a developmental assessment for concerns regarding "neurological soft signs" and to determine if his development is progressing as expected given he was born prematurely. Arie's mother, Tonia, expressed concerns to the pediatrician that Arie was not crawling like his cousins who are close in age.

Background Information

An interview was conducted on February 22, 2021 with Tonia prior to the testing session with Arie. All information included in the medical history, developmental history, and social history was provided by Tonia.

Medical History

Arie was born at 35 weeks gestation. He required an oxygen hood for 7 hours after he was born and was in an incubator for two days in the Neonatal Intensive Care Unit (NICU). Because of his small size, the main priority was having Arie gain weight via a feeding tube for three days. Arie was in the NICU for approximately two weeks. Arie was a slow eater during his first six months; he took 45 minutes to drink 2–3 ounces of milk, and thus had difficulty maintaining a healthy weight. Once his pediatrician prescribed breast milk fortifier, he started to gain weight more consistently. Arie has been generally healthy since, except for a cold in December 2020, and respiratory syncytial virus when he was 5 months old that was successfully treated without hospitalization. Otherwise, his medical history is unremarkable.

Developmental History

Arie appears to be doing well in most developmental domains with the exception of motor. Arie is not crawling and he sometimes pushes himself backwards when he tries. His ankles and legs are stiff, and he has difficulty being supported in a standing position and putting his full weight on his legs. His legs are held out stiffly during tummy time as well. Arie has been showing some signs of progress in the motor domain, and Tonia hopes that with intervention he will "get around" like his cousins. Tonia and Arie's father, Renae, use baby signs that they learned at a parenting class at church to communicate with Arie, and he knows the signs for sleep, eat, drink, more, all done, mommy, and daddy. He is making babbling sounds such as "mamama" and is starting to try "da" but does not consistently say "dada." Arie says "bah" when he sees the family dog, whose name is Bandit; Tonia said she is not sure if Arie is trying to say "dog" or "Bandit."

Social History

Arie is Tonia's only child and Renae's second child. Arie's parents do not live together and are no longer in a romantic relationship, but Tonia and Renae co-parent well. Renae comes to Tonia's house to interact with Arie almost daily and sometimes spends the night to be part of the night-time routine. Arie sees his 5-year-old brother twice a week and they get along well and play together. Both parents frequently read to Arie and try to take him on walks and to events within the community that they think Arie will enjoy. The extended family is very large, and Tonia and Arie have a substantial support system. Tonia is employed as a care-taker for an older woman who cannot care for herself. Tonia said that it is difficult to meet her monthly financial obligations at times, but she is part of the Women, Infants, and Children program and receives Supplemental Nutrition Assistance Program benefits, as well. Renae pays child support and assists with other expenses when he can. Tonia is able to take Arie to work with her, and she has not yet had the need for daycare. Tonia and Arie have a strong support system within their faith community that provides many opportunities for interaction and learning, and Tonia has friends in that community who also have children Arie's age.

Behavioral Observations

Arie and Tonia arrived on time for the assessment, dressed casually and appropri-ately for the weather. Tonia had everything available to meet Arie's needs during the assessment. The assessment took place in a testing room within the evalua-tor's clinic. Testing was completed in one session, and Arie was generally coopera-tive and exhibited a pleasant demeanor throughout the testing session. Two breaks were taken, one to change Arie's diaper and another to give Arie a break when he appeared tired. Arie needed support when sitting for longer than a few seconds, and he did not move around on his own when placed on the floor. Tonia reported that Arie's behavior and responses were similar to his everyday behavior; therefore, the results of the assessment are valid indicators of Arie's functioning.

TEST ADMINISTERED/RESULTS

The Bayley Scales of Infant and Toddler Development–Fourth Edition (Bayley–4) was administered to Arie to assess his Cognitive, Language, Motor, Social–Emotional, and Adaptive Behavior functioning. His age was adjusted for prematurity to 9 months, 21 days in order to make developmentally appropriate performance comparisons to his peers in the standardization sample. Tonia completed the Social–Emotional and Adaptive Behavior Questionnaire electronically and submitted her responses two days before the testing session.

Findings (Level I)

Arie obtained a Cognitive subtest scaled score of 11, which is in the average range for his adjusted age and corresponds with an age equivalent of 10 months. His Cognitive Scale standard score was 105 (63rd percentile; 95% confidence interval = 98–112). Thus, Arie's cognitive abilities (e.g., alertness, awareness) are equal to or better than 63% of same-aged children in the Bayley–4 standardization sample.

Arie's Receptive Communication subtest scaled score was 11, which is in the average range and corresponds with an age equivalent of 11 months, indicating appropriate functioning for his adjusted and chronological age. His Expressive Communication subtest scaled score was 10, which is also in the average range, and corresponds to an age equivalent of 10 months, indicating appropriate functioning for his adjusted age. Collectively, the scores yielded a Language Scale standard score of 105 (63rd percentile; 95% confidence interval = 98–112). Further, Arie's receptive and expressive communication skills were the same or better than 63% of children in his adjusted age range in the standardization sample.

On the Fine Motor subtest, Arie obtained a scaled score of 9. This score is in the average range and corresponds with an age equivalent of 9 months, indicating appropriate functioning for his adjusted age. His Gross Motor subtest scaled score of 5 is in the very low range with an age equivalent of 7 months. Arie had difficulty on items that required him to sit unsupported for long periods of time, items related to appropriate crawling behavior, and items that are precursors to walking, including early stepping movements and supporting his own weight. His Motor Scale standard score was 82 (12th percentile; 95% confidence interval of 75–89). Arie's performance on the Motor Scale is equal to or better than 12% of peers in his adjusted age range and indicates a 36% delay based on his chronological age.

Regarding social–emotional functioning, Arie obtained a scaled score of 10 on the Social–Emotional subtest, which yields a Social–Emotional Scale standard score of 100 (50th percentile; 95% confidence interval = 98–102). The age adjusted scores are within the average range, suggesting his social-emotional abilities are developing consistent with 50% of children from the standardization sample.

On the Adaptive Behavior Scale, Arie obtained a standard score of 102 (55th percentile; 95% confidence interval = 98–106), which is in the average range for his adjusted age. All of his domain and subdomain scores are also within the average range, suggesting even development across domains. The Communication domain, on which Arie obtained a standard score of 104 (61st percentile; 95% confidence interval = 99–109), is made up of the Receptive and Expressive subdomains. Arie obtained a scaled score of 11 on the Receptive subdomain, which yields an age equivalent of 10 months, 15 days. On the Expressive subdomain, he obtained a scaled score of 10, which corresponds with an age equivalent of 9 months, 15 days. Additionally, the Daily Living Skills domain is made up of the Personal subdomain. Arie obtained a Personal scaled score of 11, which is at an age equivalent of 10 years, 15 months, and his Daily Living Skills domain standard score is 105 (63rd percentile; 95% confidence interval = 97–113). Finally, Arie obtained a Socialization domain standard score of 100 (50th percentile; 95% confidence interval = 94–106). The Socialization domain is comprised of the Interpersonal Relationships subdomain (scaled score = 10; age equivalent of 9 months, 15 days) and the Play and Leisure subdomain (scaled score = 10; age equivalent of 8 months, 15 days).

Score Analysis and Developmental Risk Indicators (Level II)

Arie's performance on the Bayley–4 was consistently within the average range for his adjusted age except the Gross Motor subtest, which is in the very low range. Thus, it is not surprising that a significant difference emerged between the Fine Motor and Gross Motor subtests, with only 5% or less of children demonstrating this difference in the standardization sample. This suggests that Arie's fine motor skills are better developed than his gross motor skills. Regarding standard scores, significant differences emerged between the Cognitive Scale and Motor Scale and the Language Scale and Motor Scale. In all cases, the Motor Scale was significantly lower than the others, which is likely to be attributed to the deflation on the Gross Motor subtest. There was no significant difference between the Cognitive and Language Scales, suggesting evenly developed skills in these areas.

Arie's performance on the Gross Motor subtest, paired with Tonia's report of muscle stiffness in the legs and ankles may be a result of hypertonia. Further, hypertonia is more commonly reported in preterm infants. This indicates some developmental risk; however, there were no other developmental risk factors present, and the other skills assessed are progressing on an expected developmental trajectory for Arie's adjusted age.

Synthesis and Discussion (Level III)

In general, Arie is exhibiting age-appropriate developmental functioning in most areas for his adjusted age. His performance indicates a possible delay in gross motor skills, and this delay appears linked to hypertonia, which is consistent with Tonia's and the pediatrician's referral. The hypertonia Arie is experiencing is affecting his ability to carry out age-appropriate ambulatory behaviors and learn new ones. Arie's hypertonia has improved slightly in the past month without intervention, which is a positive sign for improved development; however, this problem may need to be assessed and treated by a physical therapist soon if the condition does not continue to improve.

Reports of Arie's parents co-parenting well, a consistent daily routine that includes enrichment activities, a strong extended family network, and a strong tie to a faith community provide opportunities for growth that should contribute positively to Arie's development. Continued positive interaction with his family and community, coupled with intervention to address possible gross motor delays, will be assets for continued favorable development.

RECOMMENDATIONS

Based on the results of the developmental assessment, the following recommendations are made:

1. A follow-up developmental assessment in 3 months to monitor Arie's growth, especially in the motor domain.
2. Consider sharing this evaluation report with Arie's pediatrician, other professionals, and interventionists supporting Arie's development to ensure coordination of care.
3. Parents should continue positive interactions that encourage development including reading, frequent labeling of objects with words and signs, and providing enriching activities such as outdoor walks, visits to the library for infant story time, etc., that are part of their daily routines and interactions with family and community.
4. Tonia was given a list of activities at the feedback session that she and Renae may use with Arie to promote gross motor development.
5. Arie's parents may benefit from training in infant massage to help loosen and soothe Arie's tight muscles in his lower extremities. Infant massage is also a way to build the infant–caregiver bond, which is essential for healthy development.

Shawnda W. Layton, PhD
Licensed Psychologist
Infant Mental Health Specialist

Case Example #2: Susie

CONFIDENTIAL PSYCHOEDUCATIONAL REPORT

NAME: Susie R.
DATE OF BIRTH: XX.XX.XXXX
AGE: 28 months, 4 days
EVALUATOR: David L., PhD
DATE OF ASSESSMENT(S): XX.XX.XXXX
DATE OF REPORT: XX.XX.XXXX

Reason for Referral

Susie is currently 28 months of age and was referred for a developmental evaluation by her pediatrician, Dr. Jones. In her referral, Dr. Jones noted that during Susie's last annual physical examination, her mother reported that she suspected Susie has an autism spectrum disorder. More specifically, Dr. Jones requested the evaluation to determine whether Susie would qualify for an Individual Family Service Plan through her school district.

Background Information

(Background information was obtained via a semi-structured interview with Susie's mother, Gwen on XX.XX.XXXX.)

Developmental History: Gwen reported that Susie was born full-term after an uneventful pregnancy. Moreover, Gwen noted that she was under prenatal care throughout her pregnancy and did not report emotional or medical difficulties during this time. Gwen stated that Susie weighed 7 pounds, 14 ounces and measured 19.5 inches at birth. Susie's birth was unremarkable and Gwen was discharged after a 24-hour stay in the hospital. After Susie's birth, Gwen noted that she experienced postpartum depression for approximately two or three months after Susie was born. During this time, Susie's maternal grandmother came from out-of-state to help care for her. Gwen stated that when her postpartum depression subsided, Susie's grandmother returned to her home. Gwen reported that Susie met all of her developmental milestones within normal limits with the exception of a delay in speech and language functioning. More specifically, Gwen noted that Susie did not say her first word until 16 months of age and continues to have difficulty stringing more than two words together. Gwen noted that Susie was able to stand at 10 months of age, and walk independently at 11 months of age. Gwen reported that Susie is able to throw a ball and walk upstairs without any assistance. Susie currently sleeps through the night, is toilet trained, and is described as an "easy baby."

Susie resides with her biological mother, father, and 9-year-old brother who was diagnosed with an autism spectrum disorder at 3 years of age. Gwen reported that Susie's father manages a bank and she stays at home to care for her children. Gwen noted, however, that she previously worked as a high school math teacher for five years, but decided to leave her job when her son was diagnosed with an autism spectrum disorder. Gwen reported that she does not usually take her children out of the house due to her son's behavioral difficulties. She stated that since her son's diagnosis, there has been a tremendous amount of stress in the household. Moreover, Gwen stated that she and her husband have been receiving marriage and family counseling for the past five years to manage family stress. Gwen reported that she has seen a significant decrease in household dysfunction since the start of counseling. For example, Gwen stated that she has learned several behavioral techniques that assist her in parenting. She noted that the family attends church services two to three times per month and this has given her a social outlet.

Medical History: Susie has been under the care of her primary pediatrician, Dr. Jones, since birth. Gwen reported that Susie regularly attends routine medical appointments and is a healthy child. Gwen noted, however, that Susie had her first ear infection at 12 months of age and has had chronic double ear infections since. Susie is currently being seen by an ear, nose, and throat specialist to determine whether tubes may be necessary to alleviate the ear infections. Approximately four months ago at Susie's two-year check-up, Gwen brought concerns to Dr. Jones regarding the possibility of Susie having an autism spectrum disorder. Moreover, Gwen reported that Susie's older brother (age 9) was diagnosed with an autism spectrum disorder at age 3. Gwen has noticed similarities between Susie and her brother, prompting this referral. Specifically, Gwen stated that Susie and her brother were delayed in speech and language and are disengaged from others socially. Besides Susie's older brother, the family does not have any reported history of autism spectrum disorders nor other mental health disorders per Gwen's report.

Social History: As previously mentioned, Susie is the youngest child of two in her family. Gwen reported that Susie has a typical relationship with her brother and both parents. Due to the age gap between children (6 years), Gwen stated that the two children do not play together much. Gwen noted that Susie enjoys playing in her room with stuffed animals and her imaginary friend, Amelia. Gwen reported that Susie does not have a preoccupation with a particular toy or subject area. Rather, Susie was described as having a great imagination for her age. Gwen reported that Susie has limited opportunities to play with other children her age. Specifically, prior to Susie's birth, Gwen and her family relocated due to her husband's job and they do not have any family within a three-state radius. Additionally, because Susie stays at home with her mother, she has never attended daycare or another childcare facility, which limits her potential interactions with peers. When asked if her church has a children's program, Gwen noted that the church does, but she prefers to have her children with her in the sanctuary during the church service. Gwen reported that when the entire family is together, they enjoy playing board games and watching movies. That said, she noted that they have not had many opportunities to do so over the last year or so.

Behavioral Observations

Susie and Gwen arrived on time for the assessment. Susie was casually dressed and appropriately groomed for her age. Prior to the evaluation, rapport was established with Susie through informal conversations. At first, Susie appeared to be guarded and stayed close to Gwen. After approximately 15 minutes, Susie appeared to warm up and engaged in subtle conversation with the examiner. Further, she briefly introduced the examiner to Amelia (her imaginary friend). During the initial session, Susie demonstrated a number of behaviors contraindicative of autism spectrum disorders. For example, she frequently made eye contact with the examiner and her mother throughout the evaluation session. Additionally, she displayed age-appropriate social responses. For example, the examiner began the initial meeting with a joke and Susie appeared to understand the joke and appropriately laughed at the end. During informal conversations, it was noticed that Susie typically provided only a one- or two-word response. Her speech was moderately intelligible. When asked specific questions, Susie preferred to point to pictures rather than verbalize her response. During the evaluation, Susie demonstrated age-appropriate fine and gross motor skills as well as good balance and posture. Based upon the aforementioned observations and Gwen describing the evaluation session as "typical," the results appear to represent a valid assessment of Susie's current development.

TEST ADMINISTERED/RESULTS

Bayley Scales of Infant and Toddler Development–Fourth Edition (Bayley–4).

Scale	Composite standard score	Percentile rank	Qualitative description
Cognitive	85	16	Low Average
Motor	106	66	Average
Language	68	2	Extremely Low
Adaptive Behavior	83	13	Low Average
Social–Emotional	95	37	Average

Scores < 70 indicate extremely low, 70–79 very low, 80–89 low average, 90–109 average, 110–119 high average, 120–129 very high, > 129 extremely high

Scale Breakdown	
Motor:	Score
Fine Motor	(11)
Gross Motor	(11)
Language:	
Expressive	(3)
Receptive	(5)
Adaptive Behavior:	
Communication	**69**
• Expressive	(3)
• Receptive	(5)
Daily Living Skills	**110**
• Personal	(12)
Socialization	**88**
• Interpersonal Relationships	(8)
• Play and Leisure	(8)

*Standard scores (M = 100, SD = 15) indicated with **bold**, scaled scores (M = 10, SD = 3) indicated with ( ).*

INTERPRETATION OF ASSESSMENT RESULTS

Susie was administered the Bayley–4 on XX.XX.XXXX. The Bayley–4 is an individually administered assessment instrument that measures developmental functioning in children one to 42 months of age. Specifically, it measures the following developmental domains: Cognitive, Motor, Language, Adaptive Behavior, and Social–Emotional. Collectively, that information can be used to determine whether a child is displaying typical development for their age. It can also be used as part of a more comprehensive evaluation to determine whether a child may need treatment or early intervention in one or more developmental domain(s).

Cognitive Functioning

Susie obtained a Cognitive Scale standard score of 85. Chances are 95% that her true score would fall between 78 and 92. This is considered low average when compared to her same age peers. The Cognitive Scale measures several underlying skills that have been shown to be important in future cognitive development. The skills measured on the Cognitive Scale include: attention, problem-solving, learning, short-term working memory, planning, as well as other higher order tasks (e.g., executive functioning). Although Susie performed within the low average range on this measure, a further review of specific items administered demonstrated inconsistencies within performance. Further, the Cognitive Scale can be affected by language impairments, particularly with regard to receptive language. There were several instances throughout the test administration where Susie did not appear to comprehend the instructions. As such, her performance may have been negatively affected. Therefore, her performance on the Cognitive Scale is likely to underestimate her current cognitive functioning when ruling out the effects of language on her performance.

Language

Susie obtained a Language Scale standard score of 68 with a 95% confidence interval of 61–75. A score of 68 falls at the 2nd percentile rank. This means that Susie scored as high or higher than only 2% of her same age peers on this measure. The Language Scale is comprised of two subtests: Receptive Communication and Expressive Communication. Receptive communication involves the ability to comprehend what is said both verbally and non-verbally by others. In contrast, expressive communication involves the ability to communicate effectively with others through verbal and non-verbal cues. Susie performed comparably on the Receptive and Expressive Communication subtests, suggesting evenly developed skills within this domain of functioning. Although evenly developed, it should be noted that overall Susie performed well below age level expectations, indicating a significant deficit within this developmental domain.

Motor

On the Motor Scale, Susie obtained a standard score of 106 with a 95% confidence interval of 99–113. A score of 106 falls at the 66th percentile rank and is considered average when compared to her peers. The Motor Scale is comprised of two subtests: Gross Motor and Fine Motor. Gross motor skills are those requiring large muscle groups to perform (e.g., walking). In contrast, fine motor skills are those involving smaller muscles to perform (e.g., gripping a pencil). Susie performed comparably across both subtests, suggesting evenly developed motor skills. During the testing session, there were no motor difficulties noted as Susie's grasp, balance, and posture were developmentally appropriate. Further, based upon her performance, Susie is currently performing typically when compared to her same age peers within the motor developmental domain.

Social–Emotional

Gwen was asked to complete the Social–Emotional Questionnaire as a part of this evaluation. The Social–Emotional Questionnaire is a rating scale that measures functional emotional milestones in children. The milestones are age dependent and progress from showing an interest in the world to engaging in relationships to creating bridges between emotions and ideas. On this measure, Susie obtained a standard score of 95, which falls at the 37th percentile rank. This means that on this measure, Susie scored as high or higher than 37% of her peers. A standard score of 95 is considered average when compared to her peers. Therefore, there are no current concerns within this developmental domain. This is further substantiated by her ability to engage and joke with the examiner during the initial session.

Adaptive Behavior

On the Adaptive Behavior Scale, Susie obtained a standard score of 83. Chances are 95% that her true score would fall between 79 and 87. Adaptive behavior involves skills that enable a child to perform daily functional activities independently. The Adaptive Behavior Scale is comprised of three domains: Communication, Daily Living Skills, and Socialization. Due to significant differences within these domains, it is more informative to review the domains separately rather than collectively.

Susie obtained a Communication domain score of 69, which falls in the extremely low range when compared to her same age peers. The Communication domain is similar to the Language Scale in that it measures Receptive and Expressive skills. The main difference between these and the Language Scale is that the former involved Gwen's perception of Susie's performance whereas the latter directly measured these skills. On the Communication domain, Susie was rated comparably when compared to her performance on the Language Scale. This suggests that Gwen is observing similar deficits in this developmental domain, indicating a marked delay and an area of concern. On the Daily Living Skills domain, a measure of a child's ability to care for oneself, Susie obtained a standard score of 110. A score of 110 is considered high average when compared to her peers. Moreover, Susie scored significantly higher in this area than the other areas assessed, suggesting this is an iterative or personal strength.

On the Socialization domain, a measure of the ability to develop relationships and play appropriately with others, Susie obtained a score of 88. Chances are 95% that her true score would fall between 82 and 94. A score of 88 is considered low average when compared to her peers. The Socialization domain has two sub-domains: Interpersonal Relationships and Play and Leisure. Susie performed comparably in these areas, suggesting evenly developed skills. It should be noted that Susie was rated in the low average range with relatively few opportunities to interact and socialize with other children her age. Thus, with increased opportunities to interact with same age peers, Susie's abilities may increase as well.

Autism Spectrum Disorder Checklist

Embedded within the Bayley–4 is a 26-item checklist of items that are commonly seen in children with autism spectrum disorders. Of the 26 items, six were indicated during administration of the test. There is no cut-score that accurately differentiates whether a child has an autism spectrum disorder or not; however, when more items are indicated, a more thorough autism spectrum disorder evaluation may be warranted. Upon further analysis of the indicated items, the six indicated items appear to be a function of Susie's delay in language, rather than a function of an autism spectrum disorder.

SUMMARY

Susie is a 28-month-old toddler who was referred for a developmental assessment by her pediatrician due to concerns regarding autism spectrum disorders. Susie and her mother, Gwen, were administered portions of the Bayley–4 to assess five developmental domains. With respect to the referral question, autism spectrum disorders are characterized by "severe" deficits in social communication and interaction, and engagement in restrictive, repetitive behaviors. Results of the evaluation suggest a significant delay in communication; however, the delay does not appear to impact social communication nor social interaction in a negative manner. Further, Susie's performance across all developmental domains was typically within the low average to average range, with the exception of receptive and expressive language. Susie was social with the examiner and engaged in social–emotional reciprocity with her mother during the evaluation.

Additionally, there were no restricted or repetitive patterns of behavior disclosed or observed during the evaluation. Therefore, Susie's difficulties are likely to be a result of delay or impairment within the developmental domain of language.

RECOMMENDATIONS

1. A school-based team should use this information along with other pertinent information to determine whether Susie meets the eligibility requirements for an Individual Family Service Plan through her school district.
2. Chronic ear infections can cause deficits in language development. Please consult with an ear, nose, and throat specialist to determine an appropriate intervention plan moving forward.
3. When the ear infections are alleviated, it is recommended to read a minimum of 20 minutes per day with Susie. Doing so may increase Susie's vocabulary and promote both receptive and expressive language skills.
4. Consider increasing the number of opportunities for Susie to interact with her peers. This can help facilitate language development as well as enhance social skills.
5. Schedule a follow-up developmental assessment in 3–6 months to determine if Susie is making progress or falling further behind her same age peers.

Thank you for the opportunity to evaluate Susie. I hope you found the evaluation to be informative and helpful in Susie's development. If I can be of further assistance, please do not hesitate to ask.

David L., PhD

Case Example #3: Carol

CONFIDENTIAL DEVELOPMENTAL EVALUATION REPORT

Name: Carol Peters   **Date of Birth:** 2/01/2018
Address: 123 Belmont Road   **Date of Evaluation:** 2/09/2021
Somewhere, USA   **Chronological Age:** 3 years, 8 days
School: Sunshine Preschool

Reason for Referral

Carol was referred for a developmental assessment by her mother, who wanted to know if her daughter had a developmental delay that could be interfering with her behavior and learning as she becomes a preschooler in the near future. Mrs. Peters noticed that Carol was developing slower than her other children and became concerned. As such, Carol's mother was engaging in the early intervention and prevention process to ensure a healthy developmental trajectory for her daughter. Informed written consent was obtained from Mrs. Peters prior to assessing Carol.

Background Information

Carol is a three-year-old female child who resides with her mother and father in an affluent town in Somewhere, USA. She has two older siblings, a brother (age 6 years) and a sister (age 11 years), who also live with Mr. and Mrs. Peters. Mr. Peters is an investment banker and Mrs. Peters is a stay-at-home mother. Mrs. Peters reported that there is no history of developmental or early learning difficulties among her, her husband, or their other older children. Additionally, there is no history of psychological disorders for any immediate family members.

According to Mrs. Peters, Carol is generally in good health and physically fit. Carol had an eye and vision exam in October 2020, and Mrs. Peters reported that the results were normal. Additionally, Carol's hearing was assessed in November 2020; again, results were normal. Mrs. Peters indicated that Carol was born after a full-term pregnancy without complications. All of Carol's developmental milestones were reached within normal limits. Mrs. Peters recalled that Carol began speaking at the age of 8 or 9 months and walked at the age of 11 months. Carol was nursed during the first six months of her life and then bottle-fed thereafter until about 15 months of age. Presently, Carol attends preschool five mornings a week from 8:30 to 11:30 a.m. Mrs. Peters reported that Carol enjoys going to school and playing with other children her age. Additionally, Mrs. Peters described her daughter as "being strong willed and independent."

Behavioral Observations

Carol was wearing a flowered dress and pink shoes when the assessment took place in the examiner's professional office. She appeared of average height and weight relative to her age peers, and there was nothing unusual about her posture, manner, or hygiene. Carol appeared cheerful and excited to "play games" with the examiner. She followed the examiner's instructions, sat on the floor, and began playing with the toys left out for her, such as animated figures and stuffed animals. The examiner allowed her to play with the toys for several minutes in order for Carol to feel comfortable in the environment and to establish rapport.

Carol was attentive and cooperative during administration of the Cognitive and Language Scales of the Bayley–4. She complied with the instructions of the various items presented to her, demonstrating good receptive language skills. Her speech was age appropriate as she adequately expressed herself and used a variety of vocabulary words, even on the Cognitive Scale items that did not involve much verbal expression. As the formal testing proceeded, Carol asked to wash her hands. Mrs. Peters accompanied her to the bathroom, and the examiner overheard Carol crying. When the examiner asked if everything was all right, Mrs. Peters responded, "She wants to rewash her hands. She loves washing her hands." Carol refused to leave the bathroom and began rewashing her hands. The examiner encouraged her back to her seat with the promise of a snack. She returned to her seat, and the examiner resumed testing.

The administration of the Motor Scale items provided a welcome break for Carol. She enjoyed jumping, playing with the ball, and walking on the stepping path. Carol attempted to perform most of the items asked of her. She was somewhat hesitant to walk up and down the stairs without holding the handrail; however, she successfully completed the activity with some encouragement. Carol appeared to enjoy the Fine Motor subtest, as exhibited by her asking, "more" and "again" while performing scribbling and imitating strokes. Given Carol's motivation, cooperation, and seeming enjoyment of "playing" with the examiner, results of this assessment are valid indicators of her current functioning in all developmental domains assessed.

Assessment Procedures and Test Administered

Parent Interview (Mrs. Peters)
Behavioral Observations
*Bayley Scales of Infant and Toddler Development–Fourth Edition (Bayley–4)

Scale *Subtest*	Standard/ *Scaled* Score	Percentile Rank/ Classification	Age Equivalent
Cognitive	**105**/*(11)*	63rd/Average	38 months
Language	**103**	58th/Average	
Receptive	*(11)*		*38 months*
Expressive	*(10)*		*38 months*
Motor	95	37th/Average	
Fine	*(9)*		*34 months*
Gross	*(9)*		*34 months*
Social/Emotional	**105**/*(11)*	63rd/Average	
Domain *Subdomain*			
Communication	**97**	42nd/Average	
Receptive	*(10)*		*36 months*
Expressive	*(9)*		*34 months*
Daily Living Skills	**90**	25th/Average	
Personal	*(8)*		*28 months*
Socialization	**97**	42nd/Average	
Interpersonal Relationships	*(9)*		*30 months*
Play and Leisure	*(10)*		*36 months*
Adaptive Behavior	**94**	34th/Average	

*Standard scores (Mean = 100, Standard deviation = 15) indicated in **bold**, scaled scores (Mean = 10, Standard deviation = 3) indicated in ( ). The percentile rank and classification pertain to the standard score and the age equivalents are based on raw scores, which are not provided in the table. Standard scores ≤ 69 indicate extremely low, 70–79 very low, 80–89 low average, 90–109 average, 110–119 high average, 120–129 very high, and ≥ 130 extremely high functioning.*

EVALUATION OF ASSESSMENT RESULTS

Cognitive Functioning

On the Cognitive Scale of the Bayley–4 Carol earned a standard score of 105 (scaled score equivalent of 11), with a 90% confidence interval of 99–111. Her standard score is in the Average range of overall cognitive development and at the 63rd percentile, indicating that she scored as well as or higher than 63% of individuals her age included in the standardization sample. Carol's performance corresponds to an age equivalent of 38 months, suggesting her overall cognitive functioning is at least age-appropriate.

Carol earned credit for the majority of items typically administered to children her age and correctly completed the easy items administered at the beginning of testing on this scale. For example, when presented with simple puzzles such as a ball and ice cream cone, matching colors, and grouping disks based on color and size, Carol earned full credit. She seemed to enjoy these items greatly and wanted to continue to play with the "toys." When asked to complete items that required comparing masses, matching sizes, discriminating pictures, and completing simple patterns, Carol's performance was more variable. For example, when asked to sort pegs by color, Carol mixed all the pegs together. These items are more difficult for children Carol's age and thus it was not expected that she would earn full credit. Overall, Carol demonstrated Average cognitive skills and performed consistently on the Cognitive Scale in that she responded successfully to most items at the beginning of the testing and encountered some challenges as the items became more difficult. In addition, she exhibited compliance as she readily attempted all items asked of her and engaged in effective verbal and nonverbal communication with the examiner.

Language Functioning

On the Language Scale of the Bayley–4, Carol earned a standard score of 103, with a 90% confidence interval of 97–109. Her standard score is in the Average range of overall language development and is at the 58th percentile, indicating she scored as well as or higher than 58% of individuals her age included in the standardization sample. Carol earned full credit for the majority of items administered early in the language testing, as well as partial credit for several difficult items administered later. For example, on the Receptive Communication (RC) subtest, Carol earned a scaled score of 11. Carol demonstrated she understands words and sentences as well as directions. Carol earned full credit for identifying five body parts on the body of a doll, understanding part–whole relationships, and identifying actions in pictures. She did not earn any credit for understanding negatives, the past tense, or labels for masses. Carol's performance on the RC subtest corresponds to an age equivalent of 38 months, suggesting her receptive language skills are at least age-appropriate. On the Expressive Communication (EC) subtest Carol earned a scaled score of 10. Mrs. Peters told the examiner that Carol often says three-word sentences, which this examiner observed, poses questions, and uses possessives. Using prepositions and four- or five-word sentences are not in Carol's language repertoire at this time. Carol's performance on the EC subtest corresponds to an age equivalent of 38 months, suggesting her receptive language skills are at least age-appropriate. Thus, overall, Carol's language skills are clearly within normal limits and consistent with her cognitive skills as assessed with the Bayley–4.

Motor Functioning

On the Motor Scale of the Bayley–4, Carol earned a standard score of 95, with a 90% confidence interval of 89–101. Her standard score is in the Average range of overall motor development and at the 37th percentile, indicating that she scored as well as or higher than 37% of individuals her age included in the standardization sample. Carol enjoyed the items on the Fine Motor (FM) subtest. During many of the items, she talked to herself and sang aloud. Carol scribbled spontaneously, placed pellets in a small bottle, stacked blocks, and imitated horizontal and vertical strokes with a crayon. These items posed very limited challenges to Carol. A difficult item for Carol was building a train with blocks. Here, she stacked all the blocks on top of each other and made a tower. Additional difficult items for Carol included stringing three blocks together, folding paper, and building a bridge with blocks. Despite encountering difficulties performing these items successfully, Carol did not become upset or frustrated. She remained engaged, playful, and communicative. Her performance on the FM subtest corresponds to an age equivalent of 34 months, suggesting her fine motor skills are close to age-appropriate.

On the Gross Motor (GM) subtest, Carol earned full credit for the following items: walking up and down stairs with both feet on each step without support, walking backwards, kicking a ball, and jumping. She encountered difficulty when asked to walk on her tiptoes, hop, and balance on each foot without support. Overall, however, Carol enjoyed the physical activity involved in the GM subtest. Her performance on the GM subtest corresponds to an age equivalent of 34 months, suggesting her gross motor skills are close to age-appropriate. Carol appeared somewhat tired after all items were administered and requested a snack and water, which Mrs. Peters gave to her.

Adaptive Behavior Functioning

Mrs. Peters completed the Adaptive Behavior Scale, which measures a child's daily functional skills such as communication, daily living, and socialization. Each of these three domains is comprised of one or two subdomains, and all subdomain scaled scores are combined to yield an overall Adaptive Behavior standard score. Carol earned an Adaptive Behavior standard score of 94, with a 90% confidence interval of 91–97. Her standard score is in the Average range of overall adaptive behavior functioning and at the 34th percentile, indicating that she scored as well as or higher than 42% of the individuals her age included in the standardization sample.

On the Communication Domain, comprised of the Receptive Communication (RC) and Expressive Communication (EC) subdomains, Carol earned a standard score of 97, with a confidence interval of 93–101. Her standard score is in the

Average range and at the 42nd percentile, indicating that she scored as well as or higher than 42% of the individuals her age included in the standardization sample. Mrs. Peters rated Carol similarly on the two subdomains, yielding scaled scores of 10 and 9 on the RC and EC subdomains, respectively. Carol usually or often follows directions, knows at least three of her own body parts, says the names of at least three actions, and says her own name. Her age equivalents for the RC and EC subdomains are 36 and 34 months, indicating age-appropriate and near age-appropriate functioning, respectively. In addition, Carol's communication functioning, as measured by the Adaptive Scale, is consistent with her language functioning as measured by the Language Scale.

The Daily Living Skills (DLS) Domain is comprised of one subdomain, namely, Personal, and Carol earned a domain standard score of 90, with a confidence interval of 84–96. Her standard score is at the lower limit of the Average range and at the 25th percentile, indicating that she scored as well as or higher than 25% of the individuals her age included in the standardization sample. Mrs. Peters' ratings of Carol on the Personal subdomain yielded a scale score of 8. For example, Mrs. Peters indicated that Carol usually or often feeds herself, washes her hands with soap and water, and wipes her nose. Carol sometimes puts on her shoes, puts on pullover clothing, and washes her face. According to Mrs. Peters, she believes Carol can do these latter activities more often but chooses not to do so. Carol's scaled score on this subdomain was her lowest scaled score across all Bayley–4 scaled scores. Her age equivalent of 28 months is moderately below age-appropriate. Nevertheless, Mrs. Peters' ratings of her daughter and the resultant standard, scale, and age equivalents scores are not of great concern at this time.

On the Socialization Domain, comprised of the Interpersonal Relationships (IPR) and Play and Leisure (PLA) subdomains, Carol earned a standard score of 97, with a confidence interval of 92–102. Her standard score is in the Average range and at the 42nd percentile, indicating that she scored as well as or higher than 42% of the individuals her age included in the standardization sample. Mrs. Peters rated Carol similarly on the two subdomains, yielding scaled scores of 9 and 10 on the IPR and PLA subdomains, respectively. According to Mrs. Peters, Carol usually or often gives affection to people she knows, makes good eye contact when interacting with people, plays simple make-believe games with other children, and invites other children to play with her. Her age equivalents for the IPR and PLA subdomains are 30 and 36 months, indicating near age-appropriate and age-appropriate functioning, respectively. In addition, Carol's socialization functioning as measured by the Adaptive Scale is consistent with observations of Carol made by the examiner during formal testing and the assessment in general.

Overall, Mrs. Peters reported that Carol adapts to various demands of normal daily living. As such, there are no concerns regarding Carol's adaptive behavior functioning in any domain at this time.

Social–Emotional Functioning

The Social–Emotional (SE) Scale of the Bayley–4 measures a child's social–emotional milestones via the caregiver's report. Specifically, the scale measures development in infants and young children by identifying social–emotional milestones that are normally achieved by certain ages. On this measure, Mrs. Peters' responses yielded a standard score of 105 (scaled score equivalent of 11), with a 90% confidence interval of 103–107. Carol's standard score is in the Average range of overall social–emotional functioning and at the 63rd percentile, indicating that she scored as well as or higher than 63% of individuals her age included in the standardization sample.

Overall, Mrs. Peters endorsed items indicating that Carol takes action to get her needs met, imitates others in play, uses imagination in play, and uses words to communicate. Carol is a young child who forms logical bridges between her emotional ideas and those of others as well as understands the difference between fantasy and reality. Her social–emotional functioning is within normal limits as measured by this scale and consistent with this examiner's observations throughout the assessment process.

SUMMARY

Carol is a three-year-old female child who was assessed at the request of her mother, Mrs. Peters, in order to determine her daughter's current functioning in several developmental domains. She noticed that Carol was developing slower than her other children and became concerned. As such, Mrs. Peters wanted to ensure that her daughter is developing within normal limits and that there are no developmental delays interfering with her behavior and learning. According to Mrs. Peters, there is no history of developmental, learning, or psychological difficulties in the immediate family, including her, her husband, and three children. Carol was assessed in the examiner's office in her mother's presence and cooperated fully with all assessment procedures, including the administration of the Bayley–4, a standardized, norm-referenced measure of cognitive, language, motor, social–emotional, and adaptive behavior functioning. Given Carol's compliance, motivation, and prolonged engagement in the assessment process, all results are considered valid indicators of her current functioning in all developmental domains assessed.

A review of Carol's performance and ratings by her mother across all developmental domains indicates functioning within normal limits and either at or close to age-appropriate. That is, there are no developmental delays, behavior, or learning difficulties warranting immediate attention. For example, Carol earned standard scores in the Average range of functioning in cognitive, receptive and expressive language, and fine and gross motor skills. There was limited variability across these developmental domains as Carol enjoyed most items the examiner requested her to complete. Mrs. Peters rated Carol's social-emotional functioning and most adaptive behavior functioning within normal limits and age appropriate. Carol's lowest adaptive behavior functioning occurred in the Daily Living Skills Domain. Here, she earned a standard score at the lower boundary of the Average range and moderately below her age peers. Mrs. Peters believes Carol can do more for herself on a regular basis but chooses not to do so.

RECOMMENDATIONS

Based on the results of the developmental evaluation, the following recommendations are made:

1. Mrs. Peters was given the Bayley–4 Caregiver Report that provides information on what the Bayley–4 measures, a graphic representation of her daughter's test results, and lists of activities she can engage in with Carol.
2. Mrs. Peters is encouraged to share the results of this assessment with Carol's preschool teacher and immediate family members so important people in Carol's life know she has no developmental delays and is developing within normal limits.
3. As Carol ages into her preschool and school-aged years, it may be beneficial for her to have a follow-up assessment to ensure continued healthy and typical development.

Deborah B., PhD
Examiner

REFERENCES

Aylward, G. P. (2020). *Bayley 4 Clinical use and interpretation.* Academic Press.

Bayley, N., & Aylward, G. P. (2019). *Bayley Scales of Infant and Toddler Development–Fourth Edition.* Pearson.

Eight

THE BAYLEY–4 ON Q-GLOBAL

Andre C. Lane

Associate Research Director, Pearson, San Antonio, TX, The United States of America

INTRODUCTION

The Bayley–4 on Q-global (B4QG) adds a unique dimension to developmental assessment and facilitates administration and scoring of the Cognitive, Receptive Communication, Expressive Communication, Fine Motor, and Gross Motor subtests of the Bayley–4. It can be used on any device with internet access including desktops, laptops, tablets, and other mobile devices. The B4QG combines portions of the Bayley–4 Record Form and Administration Manual for easier availability during testing and more efficient administration and scoring. Examiners can also review responses prior to submitting the assessment to Q-global for scoring and reporting.

OBJECTIVES OF THE BAYLEY–4 ON Q-GLOBAL

The two primary objectives of the B4QG were to: (a) reduce testing time; and (b) reduce the complexity of administration and scoring.

Reduce Testing Time

A Bayley–4 goal was to reduce the testing time to approximately 30 minutes for ages 1–12 months and a maximum of 70 minutes for ages 13–42 months. The B4QG reduces preparation and item administration time, thereby addressing this goal. In addition, the B4QG programmatically determines the age of the child based on information entered into Q-global and adjusts for prematurity. Using the expected

Essentials of Bayley™–4 Assessment, First Edition. Vincent C. Alfonso,
Joseph R. Engler and Andrea D. Turner.
© 2022 John Wiley & Sons, Inc. Published 2022 by John Wiley & Sons, Inc.

and actual birth date, the B4QG automatically navigates to the correct starting point for each subtest. Basal and ceiling criteria are tracked and notification is provided when the reverse rule needs to be applied or the discontinue rule has been met.

Reduce the Complexity of Administration and Scoring

The B4QG reduces administration complexity by including a user interface that incorporates all elements needed to administer the item without the need for a separate manual. For each item, the materials needed, position of the child, item instructions, and the specific text to be spoken by the examiner are displayed. An integrated timer or stopwatch eliminates the need to handle a physical timing device and on some items provides an item score suggestion when the timer is stopped.

LINEAR VERSUS NONLINEAR ADMINISTRATION

Assessments similar to the Bayley–4 are intended to be administered and scored as part of a linear administration. Linear means that the first item administered to the child is set by chronological age. A basal is established and items are administered in sequential order until the discontinue rule is met or the last item of the subtest is given. Linear assessments are standardized in this manner and the results are considered invalid if the procedures are not followed. The linear administration procedure has two prime advantages: (a) assurance that all appropriate items are administered; and (b) scaled scores and standard scores can be derived. Linear administrations also ensure that the testing procedures are consistent with those used during standardization. However, linear administration mandates a rigid test administration style that can be disruptive to rapport building, resulting in invalid test results due to noncompliance. Testing time may also be longer and a linear administration on a digital application prohibits recording and scoring of items that are observation-based until the item comes up in the sequential order.

A nonlinear approach has the same requirements as the linear administration (e.g., start points, basals, ceilings), but is more flexible, permitting items and subtests to be administered in the order that best suits the child. For example, in a nonlinear administration, the start point is determined by the child's age and an attempt is made to establish the basal; however, if the caregiver spontaneously begins to describe the child's behaviors that correspond to an item much later in the item set or even in another subtest, a nonlinear administration allows that item to be scored before the basal is established. Furthermore, a nonlinear administration allows the flexibility to administer similar items that use the same test materials sequentially. The B4QG is designed to accommodate both a linear and nonlinear administration approach.

THE BAYLEY–4 ON Q-GLOBAL NAVIGATION

Start Screen

When the B4QG is launched, the start screen allows for adjustment for prematurity. The *Test Age* is determined by the information entered in Q-global prior to launching the assessment. Select *Yes or No* under *Adjustment for Prematurity?* (A in Figure 8.1). If adjustment for prematurity is needed, the expected birth date should be entered (B in Figure 8.1) to determine the *Adjusted Test Age* (C in Figure 8.1).

The start screen also allows for the selection of a default setting for the *Item Instructions* panel (D in Figure 8.1). When first learning the Bayley–4, it is

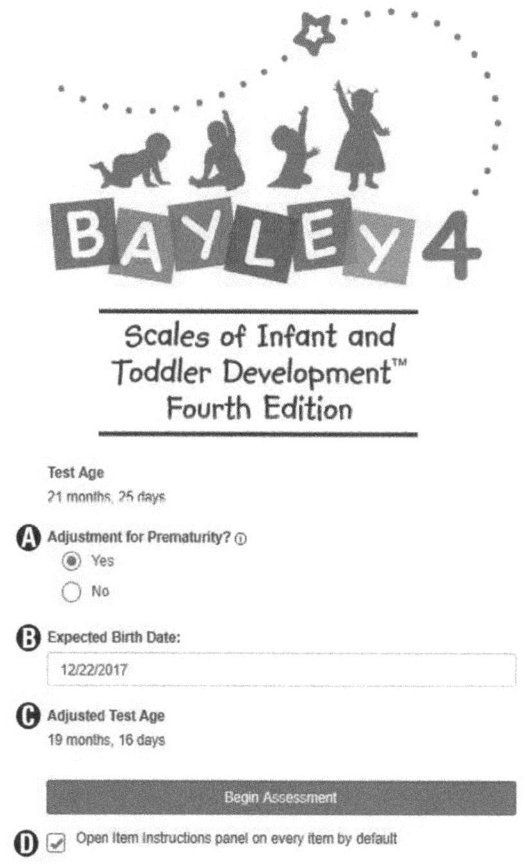

Figure 8.1   Start Screen.

advantageous to have the *Item Instructions* automatically open when selecting an item. However, once familiarity with the items is established, the panel default can be modified by deselecting the checkbox. Once the assessment begins, the start screen cannot be accessed or modified.

Subtest and Review Tabs

The B4QG includes the five subtest tabs and the *Review* tab (A in Figure 8.2). After the *Begin Assessment* button has been selected, the B4QG navigates to the *Cognitive* tab, but subtest and *Review* tabs can be selected any time. Selecting a subtest tab navigates to the start point item for the child even when other items before or after the start point have been scored.

On the *Review* tab, subtests are initially shown as not started (B in Figure 8.2). As items are scored, the subtest status icon adjusts to reflect what is occurring during testing, such as the need to establish a basal (C in Figure 8.2), which item

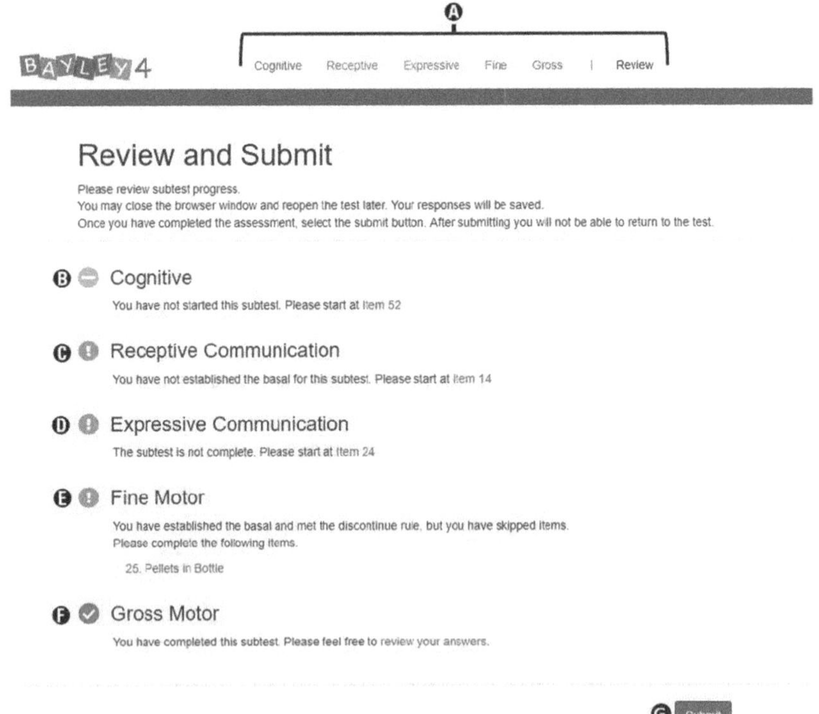

Figure 8.2   Subtest and Review Tabs.

needs to be administered next in order to complete the subtest (D in Figure 8.2) and skipped items (E in Figure 8.2). When at least one subtest is completed (F in Figure 8.2), the *Submit* button is available (G in Figure 8.2). Once the *Submit* button is selected, it is not possible to return to the subtest tabs, but all submitted data are available in Q-global.

Items Panel

The items panel displays all items for a subtest and can be used to move among the item set. This panel also contains all start point icons for the Bayley–4 age range (A in Figure 8.3). Each item is designated by an item number and title and, when selected, is made more visible by a lighter shading (B in Figure 8.3). A blue

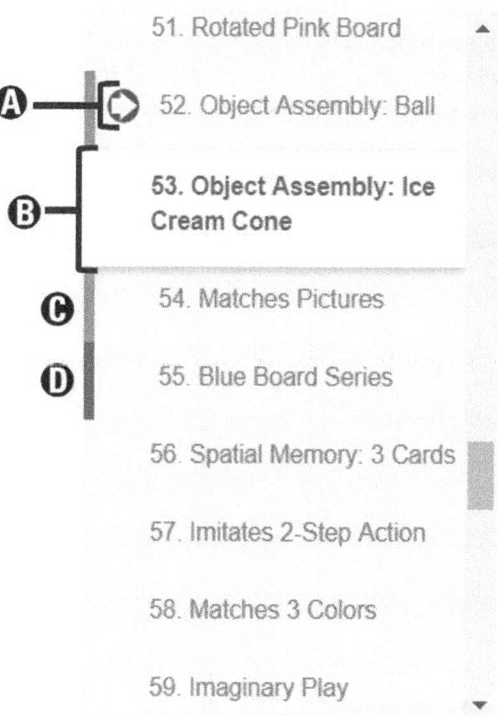

Figure 8.3   Items Panel.

or gray indicator next to the item means an item score has been assigned and saved. A blue indicator (light gray in figure; C in Figure 8.3) means the score is either a 1 or 2; a gray indicator corresponds to a score of 0 (D in Figure 8.3). These indicators can be used to manually track the reverse and discontinue rule and allow skipped items to be quickly identified.

Filters

Beneath the items panel is a section that contains various filters (A in Figure 8.4). The initial default view is the *All* filtered view. This allows all items of a subtest to be displayed in the items panel. During testing, behavioral observations may be made which allow the scores for certain items to be assigned. These items can be scored at any time using the *Obs* filter. In some circumstances, such as when scoring items based on observations made when the child and caregiver are first met, it may be more appropriate to use the Bayley–4 Observation Checklist and subsequently use the *Obs* filter to locate and assign scores.

When a related items filter is present (e.g., Blocks and cups), it appears under the *All* filter (B in Figure 8.4). Two related items filters will never appear at the same time. These filters function in the same way as the *Obs* filter, displaying only items associated with the filter (C in Figure 8.4). If the item selected before a filter is selected is not part of the items in the filter, either the next unadminis-

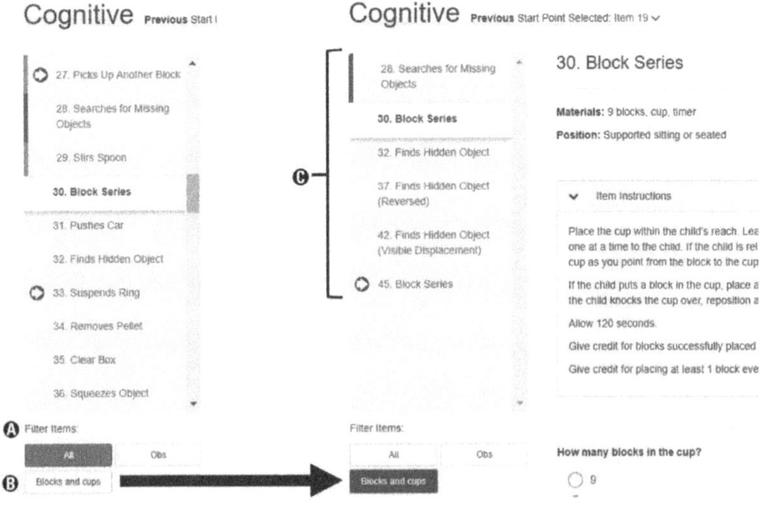

Figure 8.4   Filters.

tered item after the start point in the filtered view is displayed or the first item in the subtest is displayed, whichever is appropriate.

If a filter is used in more than one subtest (A in Figure 8.5), the filtered view will be maintained after moving to another subtest. For example, in Figure 8.5, the *Ring with string* filter is selected and the three items in the filter from the Cognitive subtest have been scored. When the *Fine Motor* tab is selected, the items using the Ring with string from the Fine Motor subtest are now displayed (B in Figure 8.5). This decreases testing duration time and maintains optimal rapport and workflow. The full utility of the filters may only be realized after becoming familiar with the Bayley–4 and mastering many of the test administration mechanics.

Next Item Button

When the *Next Item* button (see Figure 8.6) is selected, the next unadministered item in the subtest appears or the start point item for the next subtest if it is at

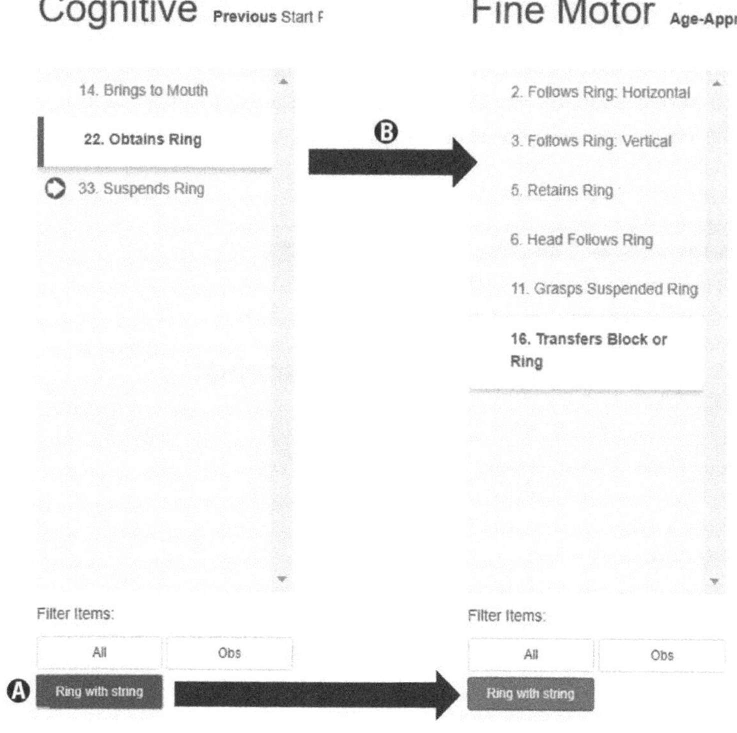

Figure 8.5   Example of Related Items Filter.

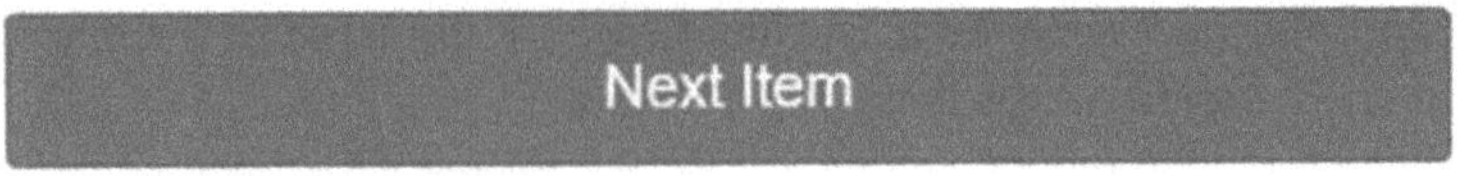

Figure 8.6   Next Item Button.

the end of a subtest. Responses, scores, and other information associated with the item are saved when: (a) the *Next Item* button is selected; (b) when selecting another item in the items panel; or (c) when selecting a subtest tab or the *Review tab*.

THE BAYLEY–4 ON Q-GLOBAL ADMINISTRATION RULES

Start Points

The start point item can be viewed in two locations (A and B in Figure 8.7). Depending on the device used, the age range associated with a start point can be displayed by selecting or hovering over the start point icon.

The *Start Point Selected* drop-down menu (B in Figure 8.7) includes both the age-appropriate start point and the previous start point (C and D in Figure 8.7). When a perfect score on the child's age-appropriate start point item is unlikely, the *Start Point Selected* drop-down menu should be used to start at the previous

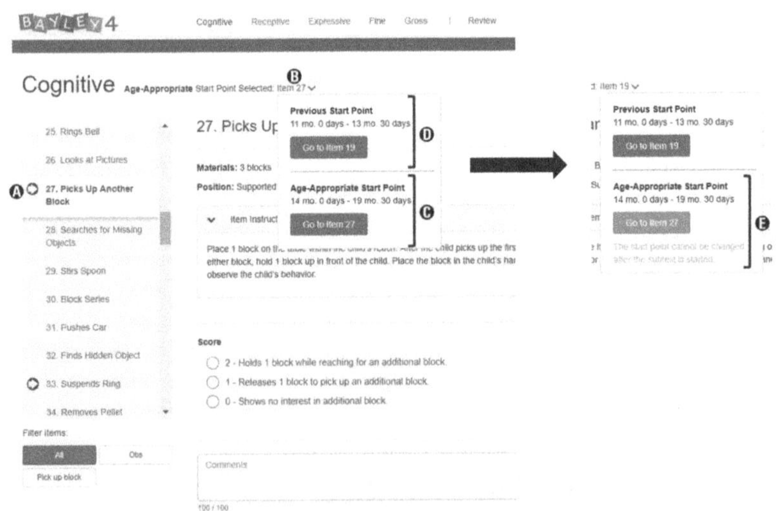

Figure 8.7   Start Points.

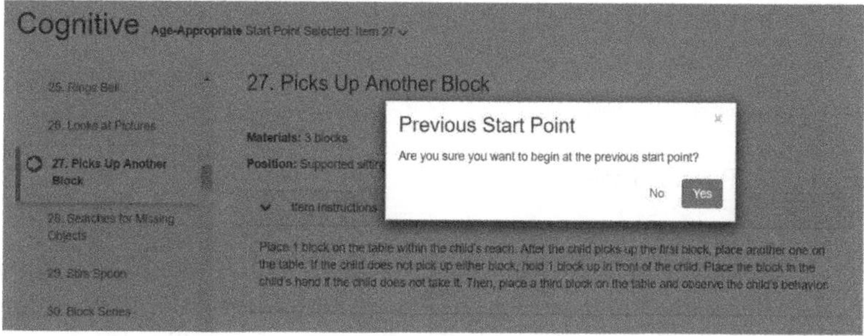

Figure 8.8 Previous Start Point Pop.

start point. Once the *Previous Start Point* or *Age-Appropriate Start Point* is selected and at least one score for that subtest is saved, the unselected start point button is disabled (E in Figure 8.7).

If the *Previous Start Point* is selected after at least one score for that subtest is saved, the Previous Start Point pop up is displayed (see Figure 8.8). If *Yes* is selected, the *Age-Appropriate Start Point* button is disabled (E in Figure 8.7). All previously saved data will be preserved, but the basal will need to be established at the previous start point.

Reverse Rule

To establish the basal, a score of 2 on the start point item and the two items immediately following need to be obtained. This is the same for all five subtests. If the child is assigned a score of 0 or 1 on either the start point item or the two items after the start point item, the Reverse pop up will be displayed (see Figure 8.9).

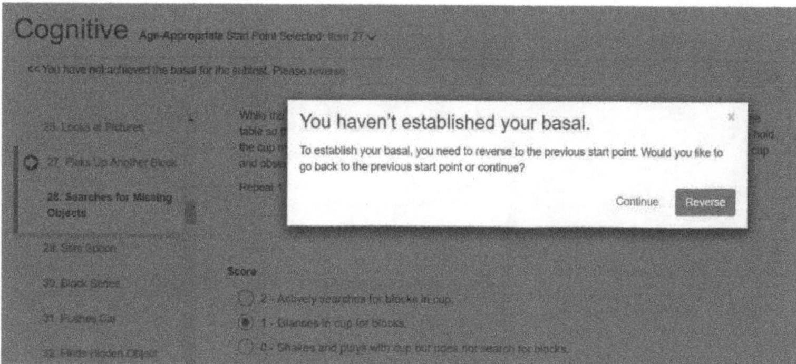

Figure 8.9 Reverse Pop Up.

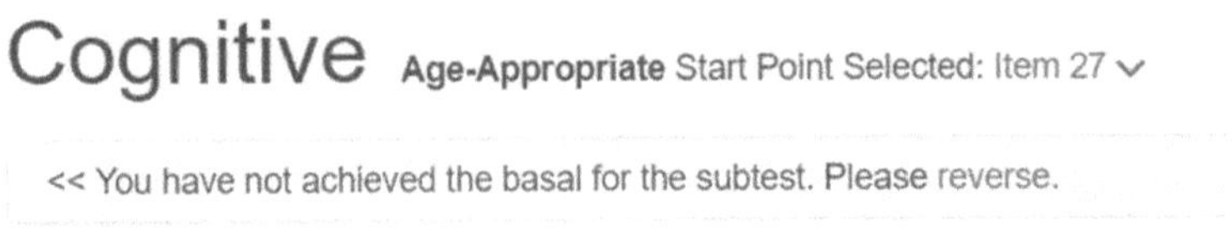

Cognitive Age-Appropriate Start Point Selected: Item 27 ⌄

<< You have not achieved the basal for the subtest. Please reverse.

Figure 8.10   Reverse Panel.

The pop up contains two buttons, *Continue* and *Reverse*. If *Continue* is selected, the next unadministered item appears; with *Reverse*, the assessment navigates to the previous start point item. The Reverse pop up will only appear once per subtest. After reversing to the previous start point, if the child still does not obtain a score of 2 on the start point item or either of the two subsequent items, the Reverse panel is activated and remains at the top of the screen under the subtest name until the basal has been established (see Figure 8.10). The Reverse panel link is helpful when scoring other items prior to establishing the basal (e.g., scoring Observations items).

Discontinue Rule

The Discontinue pop up and panel function much like the Reverse pop up and panel. Once five consecutive scores of 0 are obtained on a subtest, the Discontinue pop up will appear (see Figure 8.11).

If the *Next Item* button is selected, the next unadministered item appears. If the *Discontinue* button is selected, the assessment will navigate to the start point item for the next subtest or to the *Review* tab. The Discontinue pop up will only appear once per subtest, but the Discontinue panel will remain at the top of the screen under the subtest name (see Figure 8.12) to allow navigation to the next appropriate item. Even when the subtest discontinue rule has been met and the

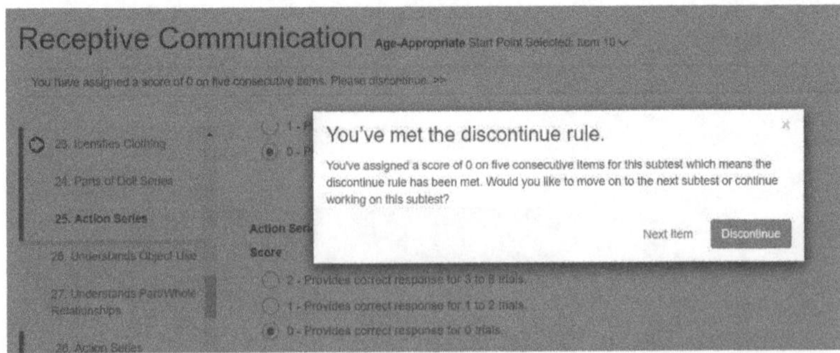

Figure 8.11   Discontinue Pop Up.

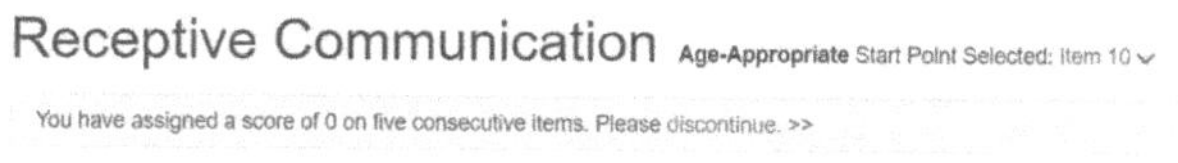

Figure 8.12   Discontinue Panel.

Discontinue button or the link in the Discontinue panel has been selected, navigation to complete subtests using the subtest and *Review* tabs is possible. This can be helpful when testing the limits.

THE BAYLEY–4 ON Q-GLOBAL ITEM INTERFACE

Materials and Position

Materials needed for an item and the recommended position of the child appear under the *Materials* and *Position* section at the top of each item (A in Figure 8.13).

Timer and Stopwatch

The timer or stopwatch is located to the right of the *Materials* and *Position* section when needed (B in Figure 8.13). The timer and stopwatch have slightly different functionality. The timer is used to score the item and a stopwatch is provided when stimuli are presented for a specific amount of time or an item has a time element.

Timer

Use the *Start and Stop* buttons (A and B in Figure 8.14) to start and stop the timer. For those items with a time limit, the numerals turn red once the time limit has been reached.

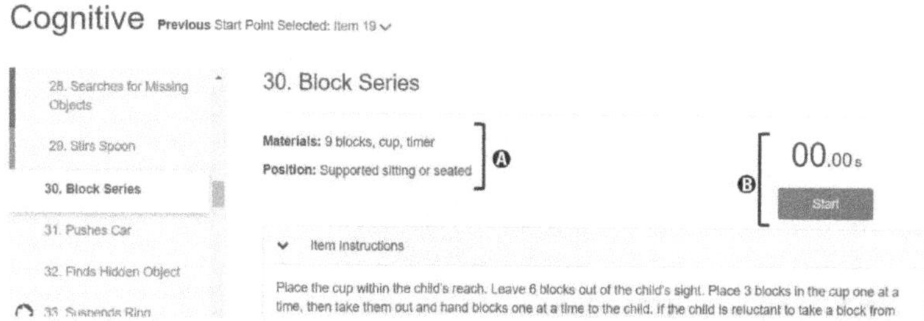

Figure 8.13   Materials, Position, and Timer or Stopwatch.

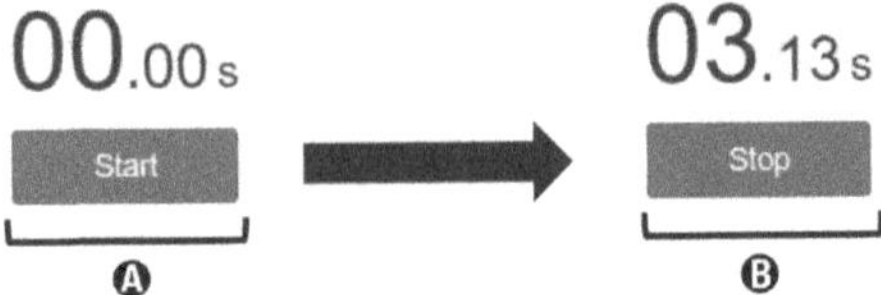

Figure 8.14   Start and Stop Buttons.

Once the timer or stopwatch is stopped, minus and plus buttons appear (see Figure 8.15). When one of these buttons is selected, the numbers in the timer will increment in 1-second intervals until the button is selected again.

For items that have both a response that can be selected and a timer, the response radio buttons are disabled as a reminder to stop the timer. Nonetheless, the item score radio buttons can be selected even while the timer is running.

Stopwatch

The stopwatch includes many of the same features as the timer and offers a *Reset* button (A in Figure 8.16). When the *Reset* button is selected, the time displayed is reset to zero seconds. This is particularly helpful when an item has more than one trial.

Item Instructions

The *Item Instructions* panel contains item administration and scoring directions and other instructions. This panel can be opened and closed by selecting the arrow (A in Figure 8.17).

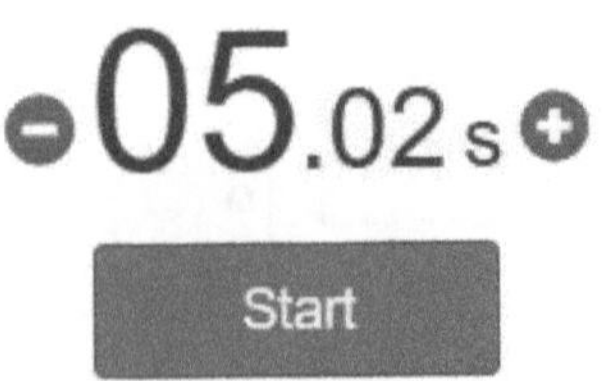

Figure 8.15   Minus and Plus Buttons.

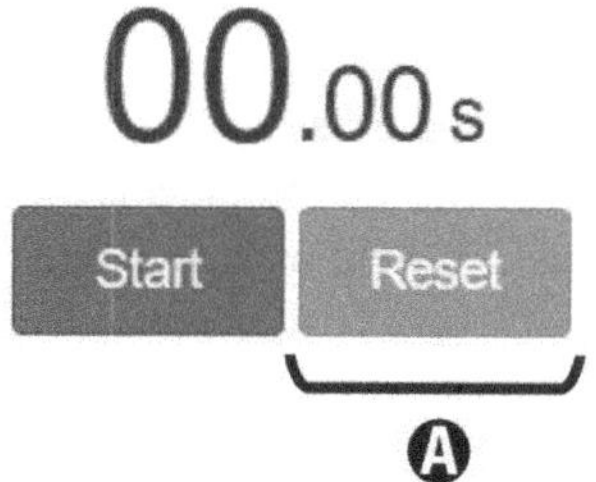

Figure 8.16   Reset Button.

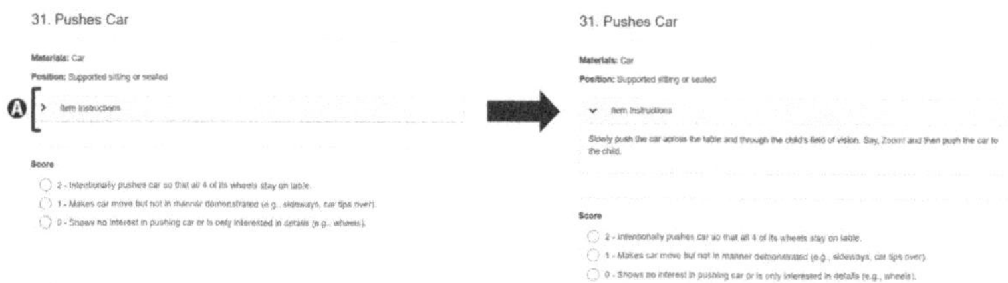

Figure 8.17   Example of Item Instructions.

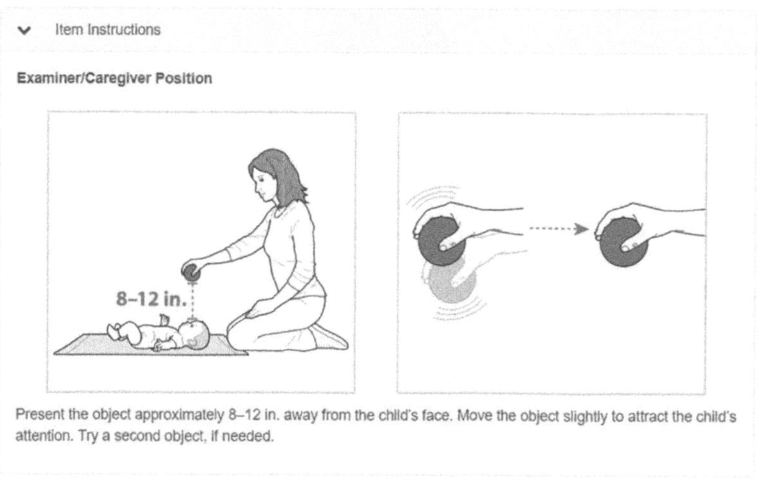

Figure 8.18   Example of Art in the Item Instructions Panel.

Art

For some items, art is included in the *Item Instructions* panel (see Figure 8.18). An image of the Stimulus Book or Response Booklet is shown when either is required. For other items, art is included to help with scoring.

Item Text

For each item, instructions are in black color (A in Figure 8.19), while text spoken to the child is in blue (B and C in Figure 8.19).

Score Section

The radio button or the text is selected in the *Score* section to assign a score (see Figure 8.20).

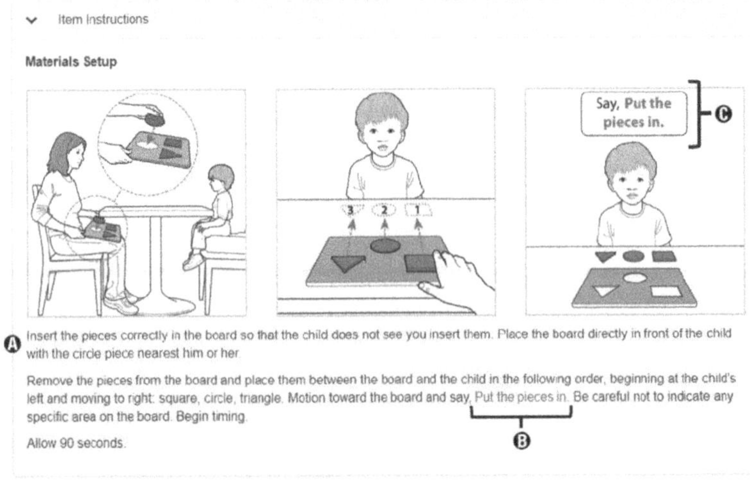

Figure 8.19   Example of Item Text.

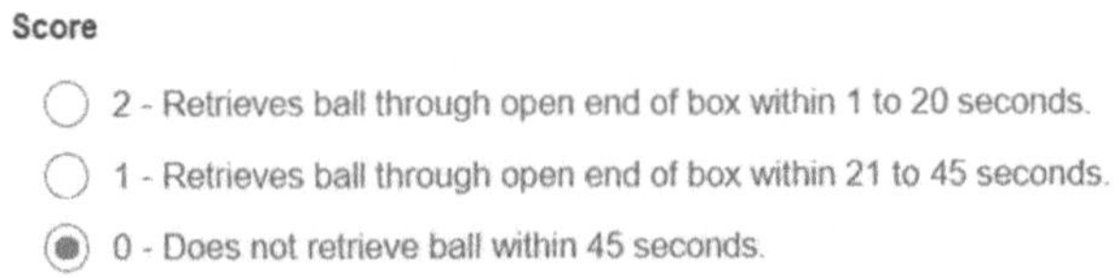

Score

- ○ 2 - Retrieves ball through open end of box within 1 to 20 seconds.
- ○ 1 - Retrieves ball through open end of box within 21 to 45 seconds.
- ◉ 0 - Does not retrieve ball within 45 seconds.

Figure 8.20   Example of Score Section.

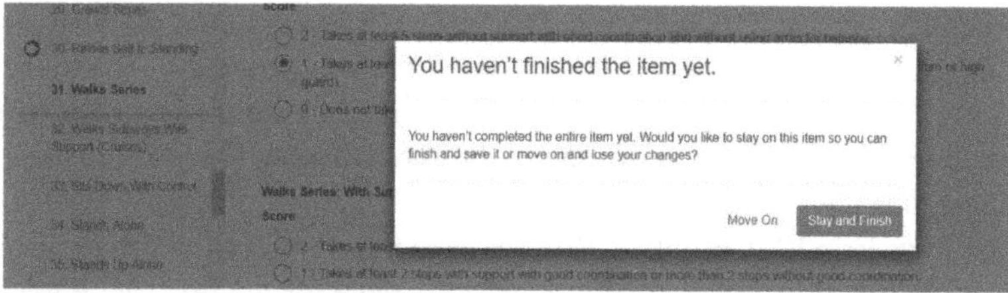

Figure 8.21 Stay and Finish Pop Up.

If the item is not complete, a Stay and Finish pop up appears (see Figure 8.21). If the *Move On* button is selected, the next unadministered item appears. If the *Stay and Finish* button is selected, the assessment returns to the current item.

Comments Section

A section is provided for notes or verbatim responses to be recorded for each item. The maximum number of characters that can be entered is 100.

THE BAYLEY–4 ON Q-GLOBAL ITEM TYPES

Item with Multiple Trials

For some items, there is a section for recording the child's trial responses. Each trial has a label (A in Figure 8.22) and two buttons. When the check mark button

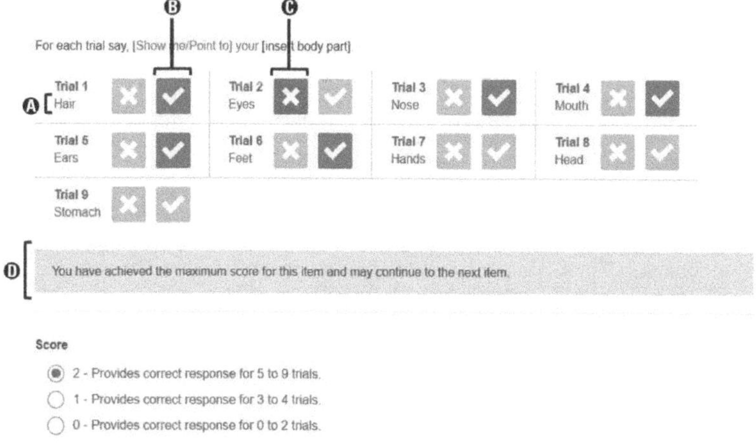

Figure 8.22 Example of Item with Multiple Trials.

(i.e., correct) is selected, the button turns green (B in Figure 8.22); when the X button (i.e., incorrect) is selected, it turns red (C in Figure 8.22). If a button is accidentally selected, it can be changed. Once the minimum number of correct trial responses needed for a maximum score is obtained, an alert is provided (D in Figure 8.22).

Cognitive Item 81. Completes Patterns has a feature that guides recording and scoring the trials in different manner: once the score for the first trial is selected (i.e., correct/incorrect), the next trial is brought to the center of the screen. A score suggestion is made after the last trial is scored.

Series Items

The series items differ in that they are administered just once, but scored in multiple places. A number of different series item types are used in the B4QG.

Response-based Series Items

A basic feature of the series item design is the ability to score all items in the series with the selection of a single response. For example, the Block Stacking Series

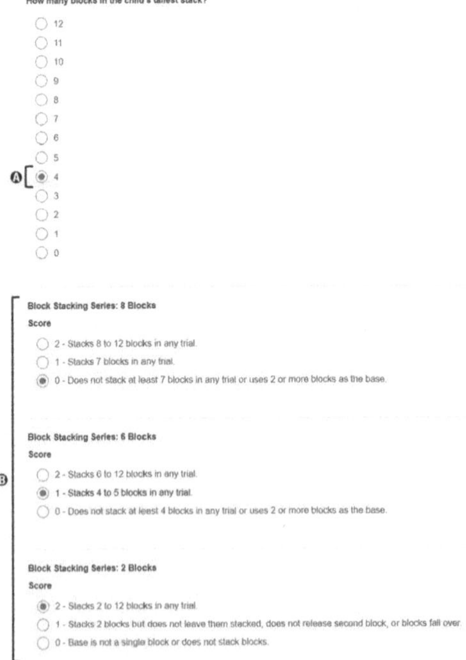

Figure 8.23   Example of Response-based Series Item.

requires the child to stack blocks and the number of blocks is recorded (A in Figure 8.23). When the response is selected, an item score suggestion is made for all three items in the series (B in Figure 8.23). If a selection is made inadvertently, another response can be selected, and the score suggestions for all items will adjust automatically. In this example, the scores are saved in three locations in the items panel (A–C in Figure 8.24).

Timer-based Series Items

In Figure 8.25, the timer was stopped at 17 seconds (A in Figure 8.25). Therefore, one point was assigned for the Supported Sitting Series: 30 Seconds item (B in Figure 8.25), and two points were assigned for the Supported Sitting Series: 10 Seconds item (C in Figure 8.25).

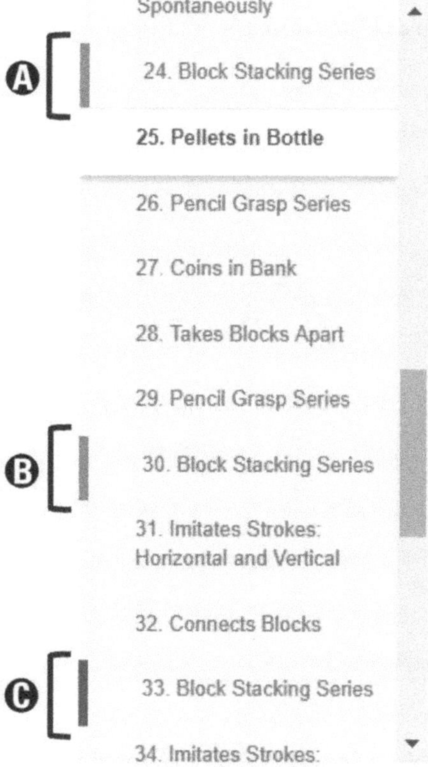

Figure 8.24   Example of Series Items in the Items Panel.

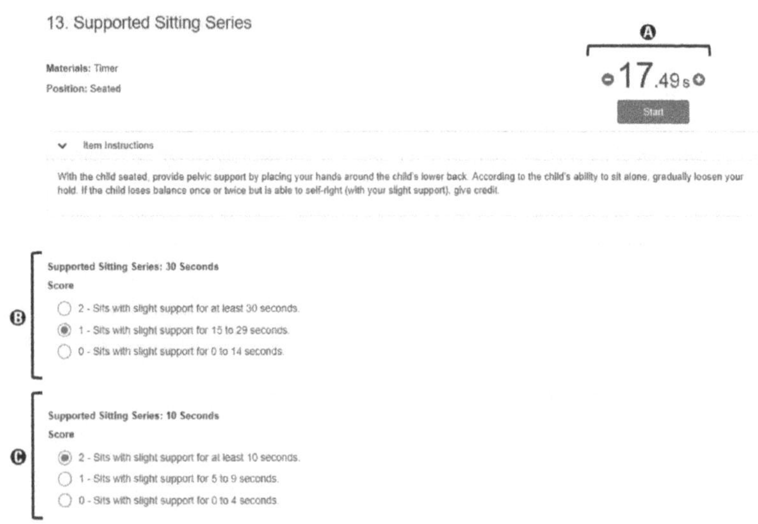

Figure 8.25   Example of Timer-based Series Item.

Figure 8.26   Example of Response- and Timer-based Series Item.

Response- and Timer-based Series Items

In Figure 8.26, the timer was stopped at 41 seconds (A in Figure 8.26). Three pieces were placed in the board (B in Figure 8.26), so two points were assigned for the Pink Board Series: 3 Pieces item (C in Figure 8.26), and two points were assigned for the Pink Board Series: 2 Pieces item (D in Figure 8.26).

Multitrial Series Items

A subset of series items has multiple trials (see Figure 8.27). As trials are scored, item score suggestions are made simultaneously. An alert appears when the minimum number of correct trial responses needed is obtained.

Image-based Series Items

In Figure 8.28, the partial thumb opposition grasp was selected and scores were assigned accordingly.

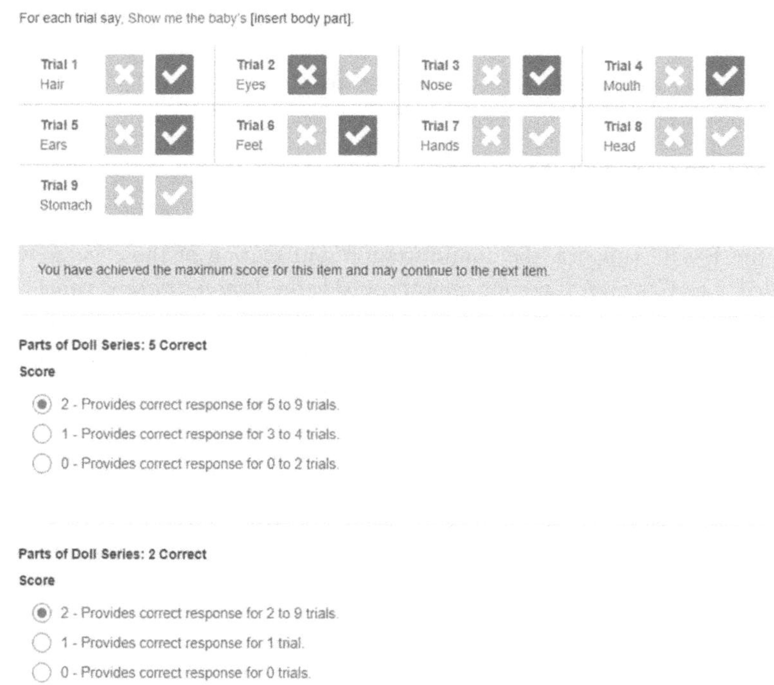

Figure 8.27   Example of Multitrial Series Item.

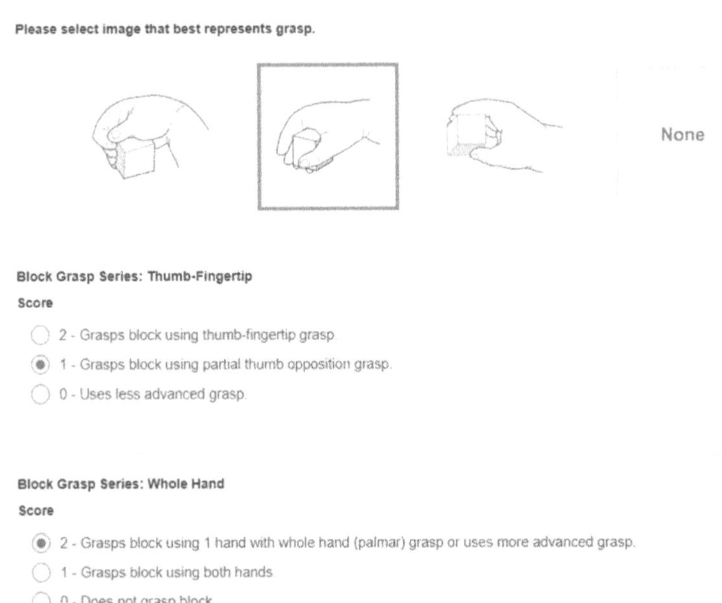

Figure 8.28   Example of Image-based Series Item.

Items with Caregiver Questions

The Caregiver Questions do not have to be asked every time they are presented, but the B4QG supports the administration and scoring of those items when needed. The Caregiver Question appears outside the *Item Instructions* panel (A in Figure 8.29). Radio buttons in the *Score* section are used to score either the structured item or the caregiver question and the scoring criteria is separated by the pipe character (B in Figure 8.29). Place a checkmark to indicate that the caregiver question was asked and used to score the item (C in Figure 8.29).

Shared Items

Six items are shared between the Cognitive and Receptive Communication subtests. The assessment automatically saves the assigned score in both subtests once the item is complete.

Paired Items

There are several items that can be scored after a prerequisite item has been scored. If the prerequisite item has not been scored, an alert will display (see

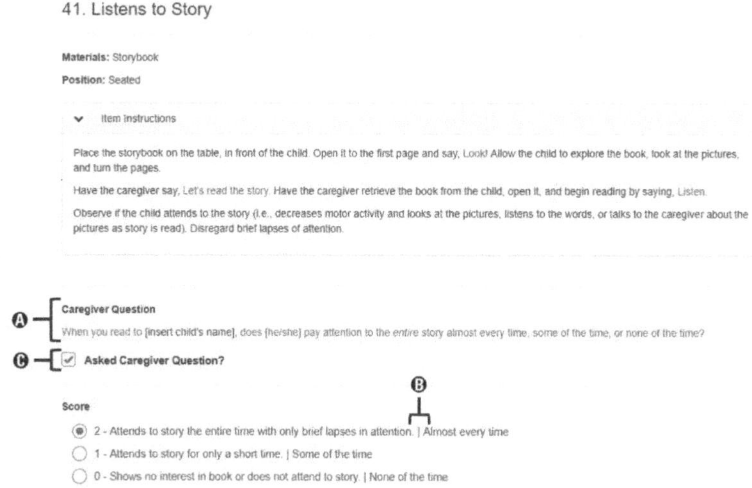

Figure 8.29   Example of Caregiver Question.

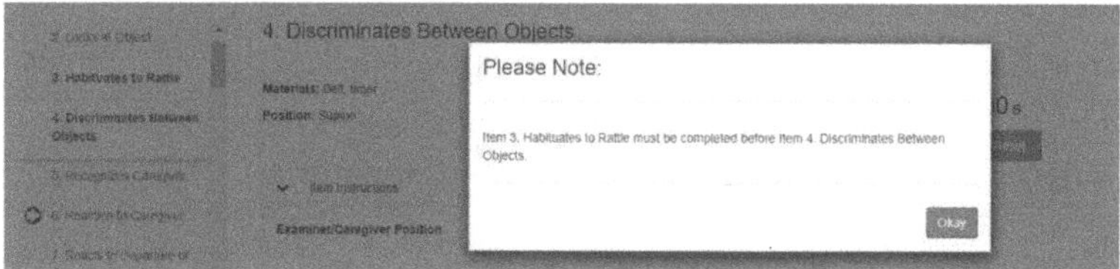

Figure 8.30   Example of Paired Items Message.

Figure 8.30). When the *Okay* button is selected, the assessment navigates to the appropriate item.

SUMMARY

This chapter provides a brief overview of the B4QG. Additional information can be found in the Bayley–4 Digital Administration User's Guide and the Bayley–4 Administration and Technical Manuals. Readers are encouraged to review these material as well.

Index

NB Illustrations are indicated by page locators in *italic*.

Adaptive Behavior (ADBE) Scale, *24*,
    27, 107, 199, 236
  age equivalents, 154, 169–170, 171
  digital administration, 100–101
  domains *see* ADBE domains
  evaluation of, 29, 208, 209, 210,
    214, 215
  link with Vineland–3 Scales, 25,
    27, 107, 199, 206, 208
  normative sample, 208, 209
  retention from Bayley-III, 199
  tests *see* Social-Emotional and
      Adaptive Behavior
      Questionnaire
  underlying skills, 167
ADBE domains, *24*, 107, 236
  Communication, *24*, 107, 110, 236
  Daily Living Skills, *24*, 107, 237
  Socialization, *24*, 107, 237
  subdomains, *24*, 27, 107
    tests *see* Social-Emotional and
      Adaptive Questionnaire
administering Bayley–4, 91–133, 166
  accommodations, 124–127,
      177–178
  basals *see* basals, Bayley–4
  breaks during testing, 96, 101, 128

  for children with disabilities, 125
  caregiver involvement *see under*
      caregivers
  challenges, 91, 114, 129
  checklists, 105–106, 177
    see also Observation Checklist,
      Bayley–4
  child age considerations, 101, 102
  with colleagues, 105
  determining start/discontinue
      points *see* start/discontinue
      points, Bayley–4
  and developmental delay, 115, 192
  digital *see under* Bayley–4
      administration formats
  directions for *see under* Bayley–4
      Administration Manual
  with disabilities, 122–127
  efficiency, 102
  ethical considerations, 92–93
  flexibility, 114, 116
  formats *see* administration formats,
      Bayley–4
  interpreting results *see* interpreting
      the Bayley–4
  linear, 248
  and litigation, 93

Essentials of Bayley™–4 Assessment, First Edition. Vincent C. Alfonso,
Joseph R. Engler and Andrea D. Turner.
© 2022 John Wiley & Sons, Inc. Published 2022 by John Wiley & Sons, Inc.

managing unusual behaviors, 127–129p

manuals, 104

    see also Bayley–4 Administration Manual; Bayley–4 Technical Manual

nonlinear, 248

observation *see* observation, during assessment

practitioner preparation, 91–99, 128

procedures *see* administration procedures, Bayley–4

qualifications for, 92

rapport with child, 96, 97

Record Form *see* Record Forms, Bayley–4

scoring *see* scoring the Bayley–4

Social-Emotional and Adaptive Behavior Questionnaire *see* Social-Emotional and Adaptive Behavior Questionnaire

starting positions *see* start/ discontinue points, Bayley–4

structured items *see* structured items, Bayley–4

subtests, 100, 113–115

    see also specific subtests

supervision of, 92

test content, 124, 206, 210–211, 215

    see also test materials, Bayley–4

testing environment, 94–96

timings, 101–102, 116, 206, 247–248, 253

training for, 92

validity evidence, 210–213

administration formats, Bayley–4, 99

    digital, 99–100, 104, 143, 217, 218

        see also B4QG administration

    paper, 99–100, 105, 119, 144–149, 158, 219

    questionnaires *see under* test materials, Bayley–4

    reports *see* diagnostic reports, Bayley–4

    subtests *see* Bayley–4 subtests

administration procedures, Bayley–4, 111–122

    age calculation, 112–113, *112*

    basal and ceiling rules, 114—115

    digital *see* B4QG administration

    guidelines, 118–122

    recording information, 111–112

    reverse rule *see* reverse rule, Bayley–4

    starting points *see* start/discontinue points, Bayley–4

    subtests, 113

age equivalents, developmental, 126, 139–140, 147, 169–171

    Adaptive Behavior Scale, 154, 169–170, 171

    availability, 150

    calculating, 139, 169–170

    Cognitive Scale, 169, 197

    controversy over, 170

    examples, 171, 240–241

    Language Scale, 169

    limitations, 139, 170–171

    Motor Scale, 169, 197

    and percent delay, 144

    and special groups, 192–198

    uses, 126

Alfonso, Vincent C., 28, 169, 214

American Educational Research Association, 208, 210

American Psychological Association (APA), xix

ASD *see* Autism Spectrum Disorders
ASD Checklist, 177, 186, 189–190, 237
  items, 189, 190
  limitations, 190
Autism Spectrum Disorders (ASD), 102, 193–194
  characteristics, 193
  prevalence rates, 189
  screening for, 177, 186, 231–233
    see also ASD Checklist
  study data, 193–194, 212
Aylward, Glen P., 22
  authorship of Bayley–4, 22, 26

basals, Bayley–4, 114–115, 116
  and developmental delay, 115
  digital administration, 116, 248, 255
  establishing, 115, 248, 255
  multiple, 115
  reverse rules, 115
Bayley–4, xix, 22–40, 91, 178, 200
  administration *see* administering Bayley–4
  age range categories, 114
  Bayley-III retentions *see* Bayley—III retentions, in Bayley–4
  case studies, 225–246
  clinical applications *see* clinical applications of Bayley–4
  comparison with other measures, 212
  development *see* development of Bayley–4
  diagnostic use, 192–194
    see also screening test, Bayley–4
  evaluation of, 7, 29–34, 35–39, 187, 192–200, 208–216
  inventories *see* Behavior Observation Inventory (BOI)

manuals, 104
  see also Bayley–4 Administration Manual; *Bayley–4 Technical Manual*
modifications, 177–178
publication, 22
qualitative characteristics *see* qualitative characteristics of Bayley–4
quantitative characteristics *see* quantitative characteristics of Bayley–4
Record Forms *see* Record Forms, Bayley–4
reports *see* diagnostic reports, Bayley–4
revision goals, 22–23, 104, 176, 205–207
scales, 23–28, *24*
  see also Adaptive Behavior (ADBE) Scale; Cognitive (COG) Scale; Language (LANG) Scale; Motor (MOT) Scale; Social-Emotional (SOEM) Scale
screening *see* screening test, Bayley–4
special groups, 102, 177–178, 188, 192–199
  see also Autism Spectrum Disorder (ASD); Bayley–4 special group studies Developmental Delay (DD); Down Syndrome (DS); Language Delay (LD); Motor Impairment; premature birth, deficit legacy of; Prenatal Drug/Alcohol Exposure (PDAE); Specific Language Impairment (SLI)
structure, 23–24, 206–207

technical review, 205–221

telepractice, 129–131

test materials *see* test materials, Bayley–4

underlying skills assessed, 166, 167

validity of evidence, 210–213

Bayley–4 Administration Manual, 91, 92, 93, 104

  Appendix A, 123, 127, 148, 150, 153, 169, 178

    tables, 146, 148, 150, 153, 155, 169

  Appendix B, 147, 150, 154, 156, 157, 158, 172, 174

    tables, 156, 157, 158, 171, 172, 174, 175

  Appendix C, 124, 126

  Appendix D, 104

  digital version, 100

  instructions, 96, 106, 216, 217

  item descriptions, 109, 117

  limitations, 219

  print version, 99, 100

  scoring, 110–111, 114, 217–218

Bayley–4 special group studies, 192–199, 212

  Autism Spectrum Disorders, 192–193, 212

  Developmental Delay, 193–194, 212

  Down Syndrome, 194–195, 212

  inclusion of secondary classification children, 193, 194–195, 198

  Language Delay, 195, 212

  limitations, 198–199, 212

  Motor Impairment, 196–197, 212

  multiple disabling conditions, 212

  Premature Birth, 196, 212

  Prenatal Drug/Alcohol Exposure, 196–197, 212

  reliability data, 209

  Specific Language Impairment, 195, 212

  Technical Manual data, 193, 209, 212

Bayley–4 Technical Manual, 104, 127

  appendices, 104, 127

  evaluation data, 207–212

  limitations, 194, 219

  special group data, 193, 196–197, 212

Bayley, Nancy, 7, 163

  biography, 7–10

  publications, 8, 163

Bayley Scales for Infant and Toddler Development (BSID)

  development, 7, 10–22, 206

  Fourth Edition *see* Bayley–4

  purposes, 6, 185

  Second Edition (BSID-II), 11, 20

  Social-Emotional Scale *see* Social-Emotional (SOEM) Scale

  sources, 19–20

  theoretical underpinning, 166

  Third Edition *see* Bayley–III

  see also Adaptive Behavior (ADBE) Scale; Cognitive (COG) Scale; Language (LANG) Scale; Motor (MOT) Scale; Social-Emotional (SOEM) Scale

Bayley–III, 12–18, 20–21, 111, 185

  administration time, 206

  Behavior Observation Inventory, 20

  Caregiver Report, 21

  changes from BSID–II, 21, 22

  compared with other scales, 67, 68

factor analysis, 17, 211
progress monitoring, 191,
retentions in Bayley–4 *see* Bayley–
    III retentions, in Bayley–4
standardization sample, 21
structure, 211, 216
test content, 206, 210
Bayley-III retentions, in Bayley–4,
    23–24, 206, 211, 221
  factor analysis, 17, 211, 216
  format, 205, 221
  scales, 23—25, 27—28, 166, 199,
    221
  structure, 211, 216, 221
  test content, 206
Behavior Observation Inventory
    (BOI), 21, 28, 105, 176
  caregiver ratings, 105, 176
  digital format, 105
B4QG administration, 247–267
  age calculation, 113
  discontinue rule, 256–257, *256,
    257*
  item interface, 257–261
  item types, 261–267
  objectives, 247
  recording data, 106, 116, 143
  reverse rule, 255–256, *255*
  scoring, 143, 158–159, 260–261,
    260, 261
  start points, 247–248, 254–255,
    254
  timer/stopwatch, 248, 257–258,
    257
B4QG navigation, 249–254
  drop-down menus, 254
  filters, 252–253, *252*
  icons, 250

Item Instructions panel, 258–260,
    259, 260, 266
Items panel, 251–252, *251*
  next item button, 253–254, *253*
  score section, 260–261, *260, 261,*
    266
  start screen, 249–250, *249*
  stopwatch, 258
  tabs, 250–251, *250*
  timer, 257, *257*
Binet, Alfred, 2
Binet–Simon Intelligence Scale, 2
Black, Maureen M., *Essentials of
    BSID-II assessment* (with
    Matula), 2–3, 6, 11–12
Bracken, Bruce, xix
  Observation of Preschool Children's
    Assessment-Related Behaviors
    (with Theodore), 35

Caregiver Questions, 110–111,
    177, 221
  and B4QG, 266, *267*
  scoring, 143–144
Caregiver Report, 28, 107,
    168, 217
  automatic digital generation, 107
  Bailey–III, 21
  examples, *103*, 246
  instructions for completion, 104
caregivers, involvement in testing,
    177, 217, 221
  assistance to practitioner, 108, 217
  digital, 100–101
  preparation for testing, 96
  presence at testing, 95
  ratings, 105
  and telepractice, 130

see also caregivers, practitioner
  engagement with; Caregiver
  Questions; Caregiver
  Report
caregivers, practitioner engagement
  with, 97, 98
  building rapport, 98
  communicating information, 165,
    168, 171
    see also Caregiver Report
  gaining information, 175, 177
    see also Caregiver Questions
Case-Smith, Jane, The Bayley–III
    Motor Scale (with Alexander),
    26–27
cerebral palsy (CP), 196–197
child age calculation, 112–113, *112*
  on Q-global, 113
  and prematurity, 113, *113*
    see also Premature Birth (PB)
child assessments, 163–165
  infant and toddler *see* infant and
    toddler assessment
  school-aged, 163–164
clinical applications of Bayley–4,
    185–200
  as screening tool, 186–190,
    199–200
cognitive assessment, xx
  course instruction, xx
  infant *see under* infant and toddler
    assessment
  publication trends, xx *see also*
    Cognitive subtest
Cognitive (COG) Scale, *24,*
    26, 100
  age equivalents, 169, 171
  assessment, 113–114
  correlation with Wechsler–IV, 212

evaluation of, 28, 35–39, 209, 214,
    215
  Record Form, 219
  reliability, 209
  standardization characteristics, 208
  tests *see* Cognitive subtest
  underlying skills, 167
Cognitive subtest, 24, 108, 115
  critical value, 172
  digital administration, 100
  examples, 228, 235
  and language impairment, 235
  scoring, 137–139, 140–141,
    144–145, 158
  timing, 116
Cooke, Robert, 3
COVID-19, 129, 130

developmental age equivalents *see* age
    equivalents, developmental
developmental coordination disorders,
    197
Developmental Delay (DD), 102, 194
  characteristics, 194
  screening for, 188, 192–193
  study data, 193, 194
development of Bayley–4, 205–207
  Bayley-III retentions, 23–24, 166,
    199, 205, 211, 216
  changes from Bayley-III, 205–206,
    216, 217–218
  normative samples, 207–209
  pilot phase, 206–207
  scoring procedures, 217–218
  standardization phase, 207–208
  test-retest samples, 208–209
  see also Bayley Scales for Infant
    Development
diagnostic reports, Bayley–4, 92

examples, 225–246

paper format, xx, 99

see also Caregiver Reports; Record Forms, Bayley–4

dichotomous scoring, 141, 208

digital assessments *see* Q-global platform

disabilities, children with, 3–4, 122–127

test accommodations, 124–127, 177–178

types of disability, 122, 124–126

see also Bayley–4 special groups

domains, developmental, 4, 6, 21, 107, 193

and ASD, 212

Bayley–4 assessment *see* Bayley–4

and developmental delay, 194

and multiple disablement, 198, 212

and premature birth, 196

see also Adaptive Behavior (ADBE) Scale; Cognitive (COG) Scale; Language (LANG) Scale; Motor (MOT) Scale; Social-Emotional (SOEM) Scale

Down Syndrome (DS), 102, 193–194

characteristics, 194

study data, 194–195

early intervention, 3–5, 185

effectiveness, 3

eligibility for, 3, 4, 140

and infant and toddler assessment, 140, 185

services, 4

Education of the Handicapped Act (EHA, 1975), 3–4

amendments (1986), 4

Engler, Joseph R., Cognitive Assessment of Preschool Children (with Alfonso), 35

Every Student Succeeds Act (2015), 5

Expressive Communication subtest, *24*, 26, 108, 110, 235

administering, 110, 115

and ASD, 189, 193

calculating standard scores, 148

Caregiver Questions, 110

classification accuracy, 188

and Cognitive subtest, 108

correlation coefficients, 209

critical values, 172

digital administration, 100

example, 228

GSVs, 172

item violations, 215

and Language Delay, 195

and Motor Impairment, 197

reliability coefficients, 209

and Screening Test, 186, 188

special group participants, 195

supplemental analysis, 156

test ceiling, 214

test floor, 213

test items, 127

Fine Motor subtest, *24*, 26, 195

basals, 115

changes from Bayley–III, 26

classification accuracy, 172

digital administration, 100

evaluation, 172, 187, 209

examples, 228, 236

GSVs, 172

reliability coefficients, 187

and Response Booklet, 105

skills, 236

special groups, 193, 197, 209
test ceilings, 214
test floors, 26
Flanagan, Dawn P., 28, 169, 214

Galton, Sir Francis, 2
Gesell, Arnold, 2
Goddard, Henry, 2
Gross Motor subtest, *24*, 26, 114, 148
age equivalents, 140
classification accuracy, 188
digital administration, 100
evaluation, 187, 214
examples, 229, 236
GSVs, 158, 172
and Screening Test, 186
skills, 236
special groups, 197
growth scale values (GSVs), 135, 140, 171–172, 185
analysis, 158–159, 172–175
calculating, 140, 147–148, 154, 172
examples, 172

Hall, G. Stanley, 2
Handicapped Infants and Toddlers Program, 4
Head Start programs, 3

Improving Head Start for the School Readiness Act (2007), 3
Individual Family Service Plans, 3, 231, 238
Individualized Education Programs (IEPs), 3
Individuals with Disabilities Education Act (IDEA, 1990), 4

Individuals with Disabilities Education Improvement Act (IDEIA, 2004), 4, 177
requirements, 4
Infant Behavior Record, 10infant and toddler assessment, 1–6, 163–164, 221
age calculation *see* child age calculation
Bayley Scales *see* Bayley Scales for Infant and Toddler Development
disabilities, 122–127, 177
see also special groups, Bayley–4
domains *see* domains, developmental, 6, 21, 107, 193, 194
and early intervention *see under* early intervention
evaluation criteria, 7, 28, 35
history, 1–5
importance, 3, 5–6
intelligence tests, 2
legislation, 4–5
McCarthy Scales, 163
multiple sources/settings, 165
preparation for, 91–99
psychometric elements, 22, 187
remote, 128
screening instruments, 65–88
infant and toddler development, 2, 27
assessment *see* infant and toddler assessment
and disabilities *see* disabilities, children with
domains *see* domains, developmental
Institute of Human Development, California, 8

integrated neuro-environmental synthesis model, 166

intelligence tests, 2

internal consistency, 31, 36, 209
  screening test, 187
  standard scores, 168
  see also reliability coefficients

interpreting the Bayley–4, 163–180
  comparisons, 172–175
  examples, 228–230, 234–238, 244–246
  integrated model, 164, 165–166
  methods, 164–165
  qualitative, 175–177
  quantitative, 168–175
  statistical significance *see* statistical significance

item gradients, 214
  Alfonso and Flanagan's recommendations, 214–215
  Bayley–4, 214–216
  violation, 214–215

Language Delay (LD), 102, 193
  and ear infections, 232, 238
  study data, 195

Language (LANG) Scale, *24*, 26, 100
  age equivalents, 169, 171
  assessment, 113–114
  changes from Bayley–III, 206
  correlation with Wechsler–IV, 212
  evaluation of, 29, 35–39, 208, 209, 214, 215
  Record Form, 219
  reliability, 209
  scoring, 137–139, 140–141, 144–145

standardization characteristics, 208
subscales, 23, *24*, 235
underlying skills, 167
see also Expressive Communication subtest; Receptive Communication subtest

linear assessments, 248

manipulatives, 103–104, *103*, 218–219
  changes from Bayley-III, 111
  and direct observation, 116, 176
  number of, 218
  and quantitative observation, 142
  as Related Items, 217
  safety risk, 94, 218

Matula, Kathleen, 2–3

McCarthy, Dorothea, 163

McCarthy Scales of Children's Abilities, 163

Mental Development Index (MDI), 10, 166

Motor Impairment (MI), 102, 193
  cerebral palsy, 196–197

Motor (MOT) Scale, *24*, 26, 100
  age equivalents, 169, 171
  assessment, 113–114
  changes from Bayley–III, 206
  correlation with Peabody–2, 212
  evaluation of, 29, 35–39, 198, 209, 214, 215
  Record Form, 219
  reliability, 209
  scoring, 137–139, 140–141, 144–145
  standardization characteristics, 208
  subscales, 23, *24*, 235–236
  underlying skills, 167

see also Fine Motor subtest; Gross Motor subtest

Nagle, Richard J., 5
National Association of School Psychologists, xix
National Institute of Mental Health, Maryland, 8
NCS Pearson, Inc., 93
  Q-global *see* Q-global platform
  web-based age calculator, 112
No Child Left Behind Act (2001), 5
nonlinear assessments, 248

observation, during assessment, 108, 116, 176
  Bayley–4 checklist *see* Observation Checklist, Bayley–4
  example, 239–240
  see also Behavior Observation Inventory (BOI)
Observation Checklist, Bayley–4, 105–106, *106*, 142–143
  and Q-global administration, 252

Pearson *see* NCS Pearson, Inc.
percentile ranks, 137–138, 155, 169
Pestalozzi, Johann Heinrich, 2
polytomous scoring, 140–142, 176
  advantages over dichotomous, 141, 221
  new to Bayley–4, 140–141, 205, 207, 217, 221
practitioner evaluation tests
  administering the Bayley–4, 131–132
  Bayley–4 overview, 39–40
  Bayley–4 technical review, 222–223

clinical applications of Bayley–4, 200–201
  interpreting the Bayley–4, 179–180
  scoring the Bayley–4, 159–160
premature birth, developmental legacy of, 102, 193, 196
  example, 226–230
  Moderate/Late Premature, 102, 196
  Very/Extremely Premature, 102, 196
Prenatal Drug/Alcohol Exposure (PDAE), 102, 193, 198
psychometric assessments, 6, 7, 164, 207
  Bayley–4 *see* quantitative characteristics of Bayley–4
  Bayley–III, 20, 22
  characteristics, 30–34
  and clinical assessments, 10
  Engler and Alfonso's evaluation criteria, 28
Psychomotor Development Index (PDI), 10–11, 166

Q-global platform, 99–100, 247–267
  advantages, 100, 101, 116, 159
  Bayley–4 administration *see* B4QG administration
  flexibility, 248
  integrated timer/stopwatch, 248, 257
  navigation *see* B4QG navigation
qualitative characteristics of Bayley–4, 35, 175–177
  evaluation, 216–220, 218–221
quantitative characteristics of Bayley–4, 28, 172–175

evaluation, 28–35, 206–216, 221
quantitative observation, 142

raw scores, 11, 139
    calculating, 144–145
    conversion to scaled scores,
        153–154
    and GSVs, 147–148
    screening test, 187
    Sensory Processing, 149, 150–151
    Social-Emotional, 149
Receptive Communication subtest,
    24, 26, 235
    age equivalents, 171
    and ASD, 193
    calculating standard scores, 148
    classification accuracy, 188
    and Cognitive subtest, 26, 105,
        110, 189, 266
    critical values, 172
    digital administration, 100
    examples, 172, 228
    GSVs, 158, 172
    reliability coefficients, 187
    and Screening Test, 186, 188
    test ceilings, 214
    test floors, 213
Record Forms, Bayley—4, 104–105,
    111–112, 113, 117
    color coding, 219
    digital, 247
    related items, 109
    scoring, 104–105, 144–157,
        158–159
    series items, 109
    tables, 113, 114
    timer information, 116
reliability, 187, 209, 210

Bayley–4 technical data, 36, 168,
    187, 208–210
criteria, 31
internal consistency *see* internal
    consistency
reliability coefficients, 187, 209
reverse rule, Bayley–4, 114–115,
    116
    on B4QG, 248, 255—256, *255*

scaled scores, 137, 146–147, 148,
    153–155
    conversion from raw scores,
        153–154
    conversion to standard scores, 154
    descriptive classification, 170
    presenting, 168–169
    profile plotting, 155
scoring the Bayley–4, 116, 135–160,
    166
    calculations, 137, 139, 140, 146
    Can't Tell items, 149–150
    Caregiver Questions, 110–111
    Caregiver Report, 107
    common errors, 145, 147
    criteria, 110—111, 117, 142, 219,
        266
    directions for, 216
    discrepancy comparisons, 156–157
    Estimated items, 122, 152, 153
    examples, 145–147, 149, 151, 153,
        171, 234
    percent delay, 140
    procedures, 140
    profile plotting, 155–156
    qualitative, 142, 175
    quantitative, 142, 172–175
    screening test, 187

and start points, 114, 115
statistical elements *see* statistical
    elements, Bayley–4
supplemental analysis, 156–157
test floors/ceilings, 213–214
types of scores, 135–137
see also basals, Bayley–4;
        dichotomous scoring;
        Observation Checklist,
        Bayley–4; polytomous scoring;
        raw scores; Record Forms;
        scaled scores; standard scores
screening, 177, 186–190
    for ASD, 177, 186, 189–190
    Bayley–4 test *see* screening test,
        Bayley–4
screening test, Bayley–4, 186–190
    evaluation of, 187–188
    manual, 187
    reliability coefficients, 187
    risk categories, 187, 188–189
    scoring, 187
    sensitivity, 188
Social-Emotional and Adaptive
        Behavior Questionnaire,
        106–107, 108, 118, 219
    Adaptive Behavior subtest, 120,
        122, *122*
    administration, 118–122
    analysis, 149–151
    caregiver involvement, 108, 110,
        120–121
    demographic information,
        111
    determining start/discontinue
        points, 119–120
    digital completion, 159
    profile analysis, 155

rating systems, 120
scoring, 137–139, 141–142,
        152, 154
as screening test, 190
Social-Emotional subtest *see*
        Social-Emotional
        Questionnaire
structured items, 110
supplemental analysis, 157
Social-Emotional Growth Chart,
        151–152
    example, 151
Social-Emotional Questionnaire,
        119–120, 121, 150, 236
Social-Emotional (SOEM) Scale, *24*,
        27, 28, 100, 106–107
    and ASD, 177, 190
    assessment *see* Social-Emotional and
        Adaptive Behavior
        Questionnaire
    development, 208
    limitation, 208
    quantitative weakness, 29, 35
    ratings, 121, *121*
    reliability, 209
    retention from Bayley-III, 199
    scoring, 137–139, 141–142,
        213–214
    standardization characteristics, 208
    test materials *see under* test
        materials, Bayley–4
    underlying skills, 167
Society of Pediatric Psychology, xix
Specific Language Impairment (SLI),
        102, 193
    study data, 195
standard error of measurements
        (SEMs), 209

standard scores, 137
  calculating, 148
  descriptive classification, 169, 170
  internal consistency, 168, 209
  profile plotting, 155
  reliability, 168
Standards for Educational and
    Psychological Testing, 34
start/discontinue points, Bayley–4,
    114–115, 116, 117–118
  Social-Emotional and Adaptive
    Behavior Questionnaire,
    119–120
  using Q-global, 247–248, 254–255,
    254
statistical elements, Bayley–4, 137,
    139, 140, 146
  confidence intervals, 139, 155, 169
  item gradient violations, 214–216
  reliability coefficients, 187, 209
  significance *see* statistical
    significance
  standard error of measurements
    (SEMs), 209
  see also raw scores; scaled scores;
    standard scores
statistical significance, 172–175
  examples, 174–175
  and GSVs, 140, 172
  Type I errors, 173, 188
  Type II errors, 173, 188
Stimulus Book, Bayley–4, *103*, 104
  pictures, 219, 260
  responses, 143
structured items, Bayley–4, 108–110,
    116–117, 176
  with Caregiver Questions, 266–267

multiple trial, 261–262, *261*, 265,
    265
paired, 266–267, *267*
performance-based, 117
on Q-global, 261–267
series, 263–264
  image-based, 265, *265*
  response-based, 263–264, *263*,
    264, 265
  time-based, 264, *264*, 265
shared, 105, 266

test ceilings, 214
test floors, 213
test materials, Bayley–4, 98–99,
    102–107, 219
  administration time,
    101–102
  artwork, 260
  Caregiver Report *see* Caregiver
    Report
  copyright, 93
  manipulatives *see* manipulatives
  preparation, 94–95, 98–99
  printed, 219
  questionnaires, 99, 106–107
    see also Social-Emotional and
    Adaptive Behavior
    Questionnaire
  Response Booklet, 105, 260
  security, 92
  Stimulus Book, 104, 219, 260

University of California,
    Berkeley, 8

validity evidence, 210, 213
  Bayley–4, 210–213

*Vineland Adaptive Behavior Scales,
     Third Edition* (Vineland–3)
   Caregiver Form, 206
   content in Bayley–4, 206
   content in Bayley–III, 25, 27,
     107, 199

Wechsler Preschool and Primary Scale
     of Intelligence, Fourth Edition
     (WPPSI–V), 163, 212

Zigler, Edward, 3